IMAGING IN
UROLOGY

TUBLIN · NELSON
BORHANI | FURLAN | HELLER | SQUIRES

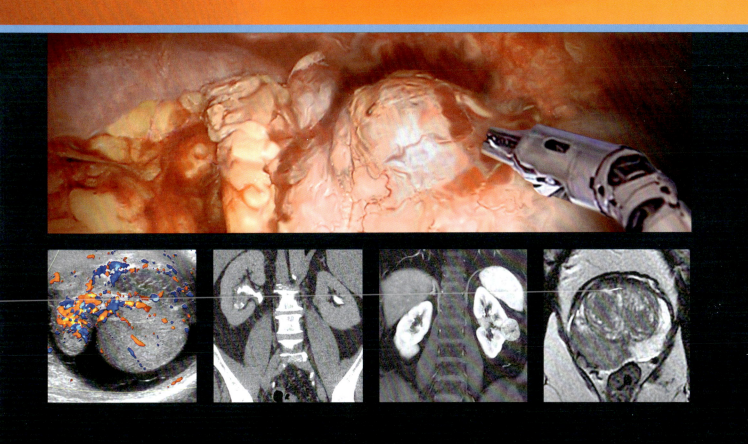

ELSEVIER

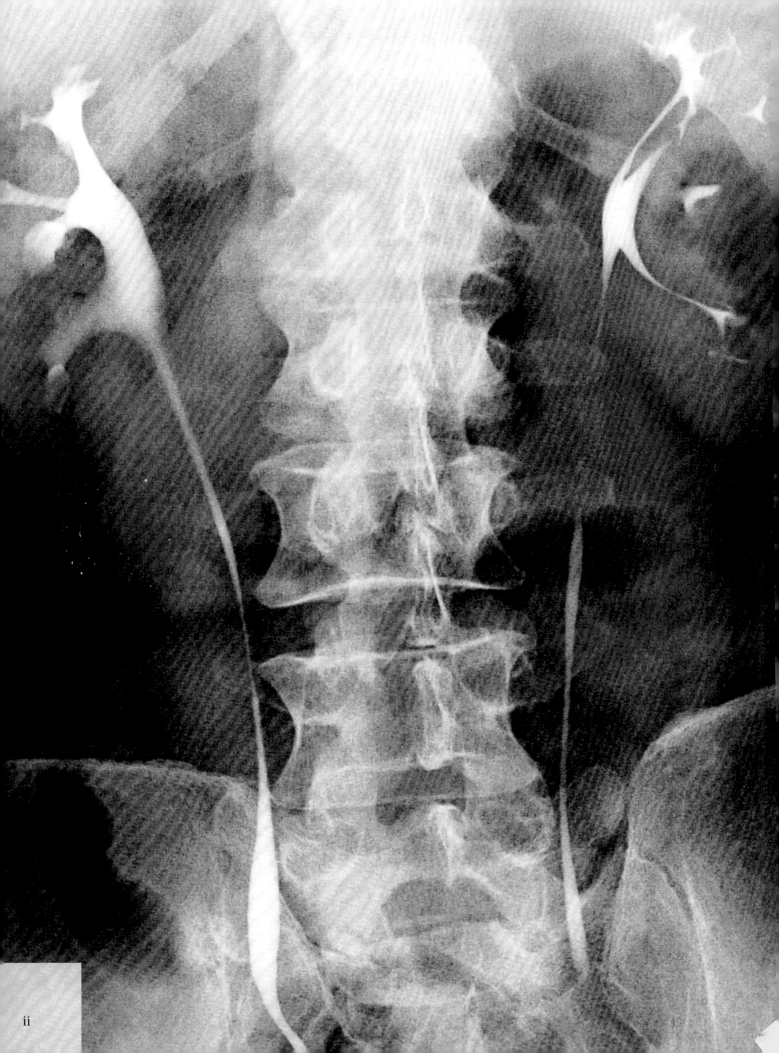

IMAGING IN
UROLOGY

Mitchell Tublin, MD

Professor and Vice Chair of Radiology
Chief, Abdominal Imaging Section
University of Pittsburgh School of Medicine
Pittsburgh, Pennsylvania

Joel B. Nelson, MD

Frederic N. Schwentker Professor and Chairman
Department of Urology
University of Pittsburgh School of Medicine
Chief Clinical Officer, Health Services Division, UPMC
Pittsburgh, Pennsylvania

Amir A. Borhani, MD

Assistant Professor of Radiology
Abdominal Imaging Section
University of Pittsburgh School of Medicine
Pittsburgh, Pennsylvania

Alessandro Furlan, MD

Assistant Professor of Radiology
Abdominal Imaging Section
University of Pittsburgh School of Medicine
Pittsburgh, Pennsylvania

Matthew T. Heller, MD, FSAR

Associate Professor of Radiology
Abdominal Imaging Section
Director, Radiology Residency Program
University of Pittsburgh School of Medicine
Pittsburgh, Pennsylvania

Judy Squires, MD

Assistant Professor of Radiology
Director, Pediatric Ultrasound
Children's Hospital of Pittsburgh
University of Pittsburgh School of Medicine
Pittsburgh, Pennsylvania

WITHDRAWN FROM LIBRARY — BMA LIBRARY, BRITISH MEDICAL ASSOCIATION

ELSEVIER

1600 John F. Kennedy Blvd.
Ste 1800
Philadelphia, PA 19103-2899

IMAGING IN UROLOGY

ISBN: 978-0-323-54809-0

Publisher Cataloging-in-Publication Data

Names: Tublin, Mitchell E. | Nelson, Joel B.
Title: Imaging in urology / [edited by] Mitchell Tublin and Joel B. Nelson.
Description: First edition. | Salt Lake City, UT : Elsevier, Inc., [2018] | Includes
   bibliographical references and index.
Identifiers: ISBN 978-0-323-54809-0
Subjects: LCSH: Urinary organs--Radiography--Handbooks, manuals, etc. | Urology--Handbooks,
   manuals, etc. | MESH: Urologic Diseases--diagnostic imaging--Atlases. | Urology--methods--
   Atlases. | Radiography--Atlases.
Classification: LCC RC874.I43 2018 | NLM WJ 141 | DDC 616.607572--dc23

International Standard Book Number: 978-0-323-54809-0

Cover Designer: Tom M. Olson, BA

Printed in Canada by Friesens, Altona, Manitoba, Canada

Last digit is the print number: 9 8 7 6 5 4 3 2 1

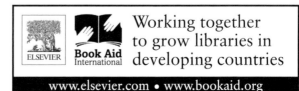

Dedications

*To the home front: My wife, Mary,
and our sons, Daniel, Josh, and Andrew. Your support and love
make everything possible and meaningful.*

MT

To Liz, my wonderful wife.

JBN

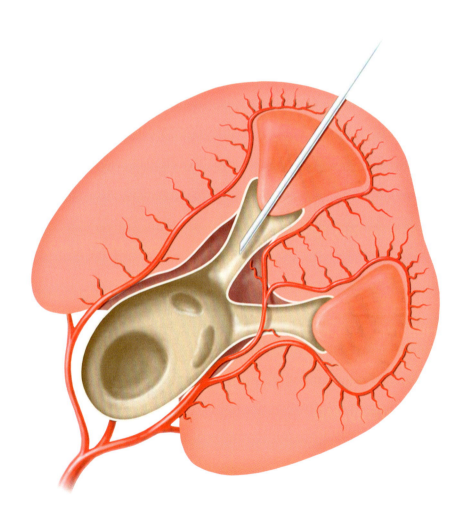

Contributing Authors

Hank Baskin, MD
Pediatric Imaging Section Chief
Primary Children's Hospital
Intermountain Healthcare
Adjunct Associate Professor of Radiology
University of Utah School of Medicine
Salt Lake City, Utah

David Bauer, MD
Missoula Radiology
Missoula, Montana

Shweta Bhatt, MD
Associate Professor
Department of Imaging Sciences
University of Rochester Medical Center
Rochester, New York

Todd M. Blodgett, MD
Foundation Radiology Group
Pittsburgh, Pennsylvania

Amit B. Desai, MD
Radiology Resident
Department of Imaging Sciences
University of Rochester Medical Center
Rochester, New York

Michael P. Federle, MD, FACR
Professor and Associate Chair for Education
Department of Radiology
Stanford University School of Medicine
Stanford, California

Marta Heilbrun, MD, MS
Associate Professor of Radiology and Body Imaging
University of Utah School of Medicine
Salt Lake City, Utah

R. Brooke Jeffrey, MD
Professor and Vice Chairman
Department of Radiology
Stanford University School of Medicine
Stanford, California

Vineet Krishan Khanna, MD
Radiology Resident
Department of Radiology
University of Pittsburgh Medical Center
Pittsburgh, Pennsylvania

Steven J. Kraus, MD
Division Chief of Fluoroscopy
Cincinnati Children's Hospital Medical Center
Associate Professor
Clinical Radiology and Pediatrics
University of Cincinnati College of Medicine
Cincinnati, Ohio

Katherine E. Maturen, MD, MS
Associate Professor
Abdominal Radiology Fellowship Director
University of Michigan Hospitals
Ann Arbor, Michigan

Christine O. Menias, MD
Professor of Radiology
Mayo Clinic School of Medicine
Scottsdale, Arizona
Adjunct Professor of Radiology
Washington University School of Medicine
St. Louis, Missouri

A. Carlson Merrow, Jr., MD, FAAP
Corning Benton Chair for Radiology Education
Cincinnati Children's Hospital Medical Center
Associate Professor of Clinical Radiology
University of Cincinnati College of Medicine
Cincinnati, Ohio

Sara M. O'Hara, MD, FAAP
Division Chief of Ultrasound
Cincinnati Children's Hospital Medical Center
Professor of Clinical Radiology and Pediatrics
University of Cincinnati College of Medicine
Cincinnati, Ohio

Gloria M. Salazar, MD
Assistant Radiologist
Division of Vascular Imaging and Intervention
Massachusetts General Hospital
Instructor in Radiology
Harvard Medical School
Boston, Massachusetts

Akram M. Shaaban, MBBCh
Professor of Radiology
Department of Radiology and Imaging Sciences
University of Utah School of Medicine
Salt Lake City, Utah

Ethan A. Smith, MD
Clinical Assistant Professor of Radiology
C.S. Mott Children's Hospital
University of Michigan Health System
Ann Arbor, Michigan

Ashraf Thabet, MD
Instructor in Radiology
Harvard Medical School
Division of Interventional Radiology
Massachusetts General Hospital
Boston, Massachusetts

Alexander J. Towbin, MD
Associate Chief of Radiology
Clinical Operations and Informatics
Neil D. Johnson Chair of Radiology Informatics
Cincinnati Children's Hospital Medical Center
Associate Professor
Clinical Radiology and Pediatrics
University of Cincinnati College of Medicine
Cincinnati, Ohio

T. Gregory Walker, MD, FSIR
Interventional Radiology Integrated Residency
Program Director
Interventional Radiology Fellowship Program Director
Massachusetts General Hospital
Division of Interventional Radiology
Assistant Professor of Radiology
Harvard Medical School
Boston, Massachusetts

Paula J. Woodward, MD
Professor of Radiology
David G. Bragg, MD and Marcia R. Bragg Presidential
Endowed Chair in Oncologic Imaging
Adjunct Professor of Obstetrics and Gynecology
University of Utah School of Medicine
Salt Lake City, Utah

Karl Yaeger, MD
Women's Imaging Fellow
Department of Radiology
Magee Women's Hospital of UPMC
Pittsburgh, Pennsylvania

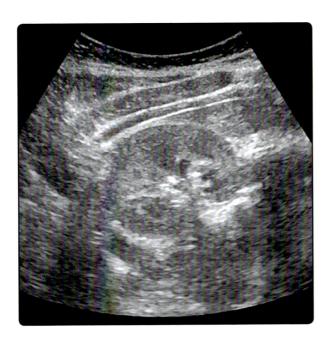

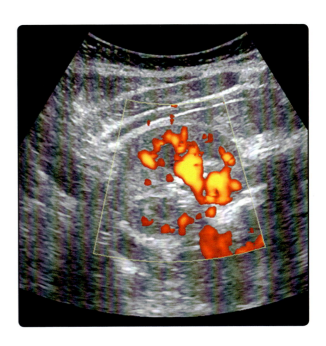

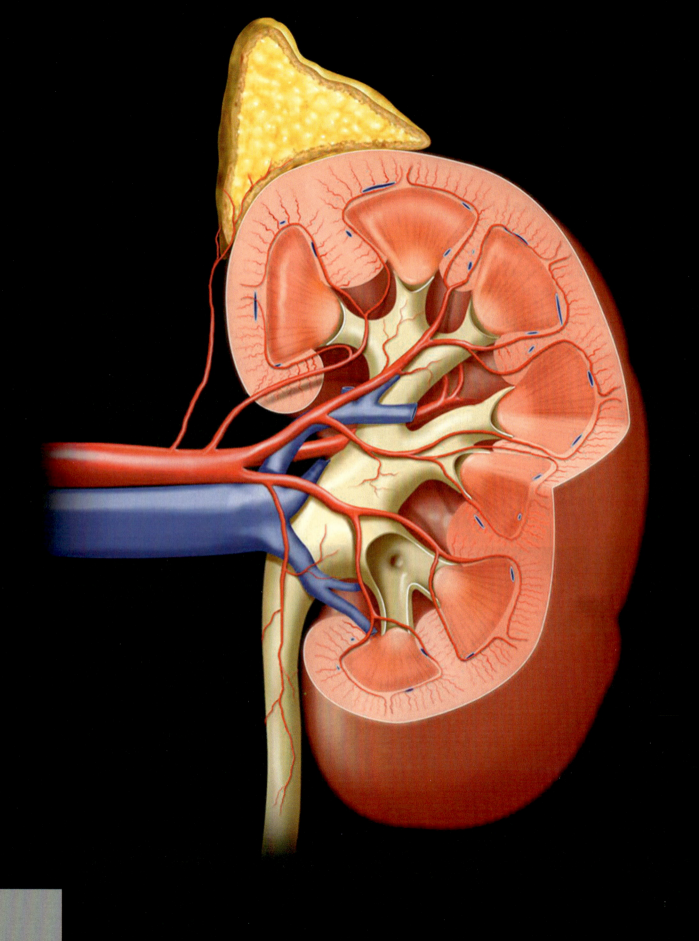

Preface

My colleagues and I within the abdominal imaging section at the University of Pittsburgh take pride in our partnerships with referring clinical services. Imaging is an integral part of all clinical pathways, and a shared vision and leveraged expertise benefits physicians and, most importantly, patients. The partnership between radiology and urology is a great example of professional synergy.

I've known Joel Nelson, the Urology Chair and Chief Clinical Officer of the UPMC Health Service Division, for my entire career at UPMC. Joel is the quintessential academic urologist and US healthcare thought leader. He has the optimism of an academic, the skepticism of an administrator, and the vision of an enterprise leader. Joel immediately embraced the opportunity to partner with our group to compile a state-of-the-art imaging compendium for urologists. He loved the idea of an imaging text friendly to urologists, written in conjunction with (and for) urologists. We were both struck by how important excellent imaging is for state-of-the-art urological care, how a background in imaging has become a critical component in urology training programs, and how, despite these prerequisites, there was no go-to, reader-friendly imaging resource for urologists. We believe that this textbook fills that void.

Introduction chapters set the framework: Genitourinary anatomy and basic imaging precepts relevant for urologists are described. The entire spectrum of urological conditions is then covered in bulleted, image-rich chapters. Key facts of each diagnosis are listed, but the real take-home points are driven home in hundreds of classic illustrative annotated images/figures and corresponding legends. Radiology trainees learn best by picking up pearls and experience while looking at images at the "view box"; we think that present-day urologists interested in imaging will do the same with this textbook.

We have many people to thank for helping to produce this book. The abdominal imaging faculty at the University of Pittsburgh are the best of the best, and we learn from them always. Our coauthors, Drs. Borhani, Furlan, Heller, and Squires, are the heart and soul of the Elsevier GU team, and they make it all possible. Dr. Jathin Bandari, our urology taskmaster, kept us in line and offered perspective on what was truly important for his colleagues. Finally, the entire staff at Elsevier deserves a shout-out for facilitating this project, and more importantly, for articulating a collaborative imaging vision relevant for all current practitioners.

Mitchell Tublin, MD
Professor and Vice Chair of Radiology
Chief, Abdominal Imaging Section
University of Pittsburgh School of Medicine
Pittsburgh, Pennsylvania

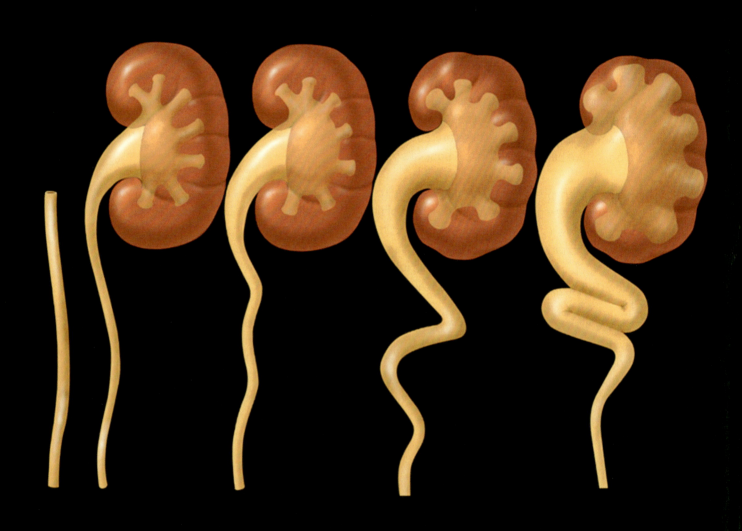

Acknowledgments

Lead Editor

Lisa A. Gervais, BS

Text Editors

Arthur G. Gelsinger, MA
Rebecca L. Bluth, BA
Nina I. Bennett, BA
Terry W. Ferrell, MS
Matt W. Hoecherl, BS
Megg Morin, BA

Image Editors

Jeffrey J. Marmorstone, BS
Lisa A. M. Steadman, BS

Medical Editor

Jathin Bandari, MD

Illustrations

Richard Coombs, MS
Lane R. Bennion, MS
Laura C. Wissler, MA

Art Direction and Design

Tom M. Olson, BA

Production Coordinators

Angela M. G. Terry, BA
Emily C. Fassett, BA

ELSEVIER

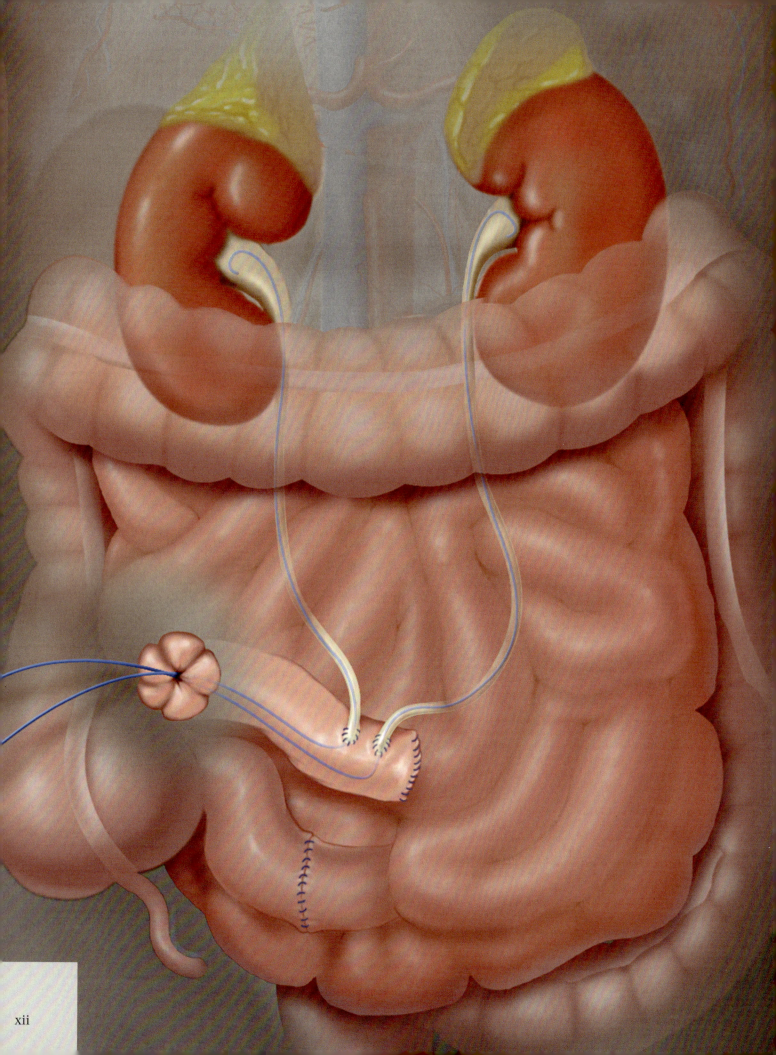

Sections

TABLE OF CONTENTS

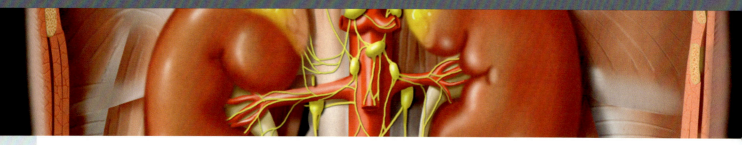

TABLE OF CONTENTS

TABLE OF CONTENTS

TABLE OF CONTENTS

TABLE OF CONTENTS

IMAGING IN
UROLOGY

TUBLIN · NELSON
BORHANI | FURLAN | HELLER | SQUIRES

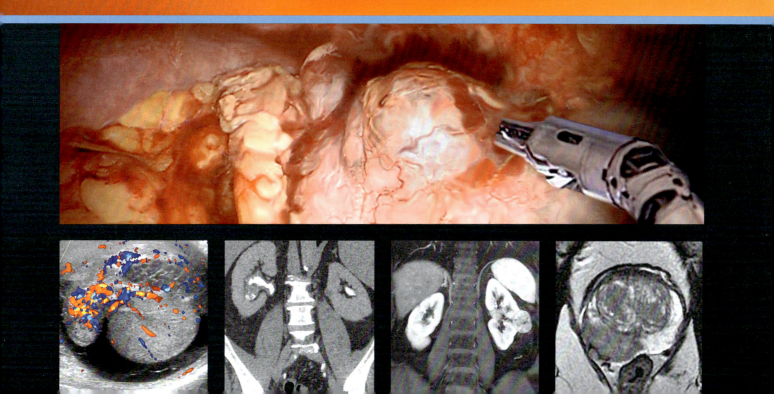

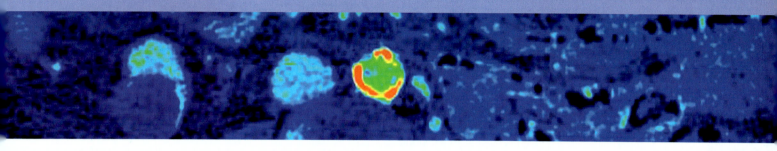

SECTION 1
Overview and Introduction

Renal Mass Evaluation

CT: Although rapid improvements in scanner technology have resulted in dramatic increases in spatial and temporal resolution, the imaging marker for potential neoplasia (enhancement of soft tissue components of renal masses after contrast administration) has not changed over several generations of CT scanners. Typical renal mass protocols consist of NECT of the kidneys followed by contrast-enhanced images obtained during nephrographic and excretory phases (roughly defined as 85-120 seconds and 3-5 minutes, respectively, postcontrast injection). Corticomedullary-phase images (25-70 seconds post contrast) may also be obtained, though small, central, endophytic tumors may not be perceived given the lack of medullary enhancement during this phase. An increase in soft tissue attenuation of soft tissue components postcontrast administration of > 10-20 Hounsfield units (HU) is classically considered to be indicative of true enhancement, though "pseudoenhancement" of small lesions may result in false-positive examinations, and slowly enhancing lesions (e.g., papillary carcinomas) may be missed if delayed images are not acquired. Despite these caveats, if such a protocol is employed, most renal masses can be accurately characterized as potential surgical lesions (i.e., enhancing: Benign/malignant neoplasia) or leave-alone entities (either fat-containing angiomyolipomas or simple-/high-attenuation cysts). Assessment of cyst complexity at CT, utilizing features described by Bosniak a generation ago, also aids in the triage of this particularly problematic category of renal masses. Suffice to say that increasing levels of complexity (septa thickness, wall/nodularity enhancement, and calcification) increase the likelihood of malignancy.

Optimized protocols should utilize the advantages of multidetector technology. Thin (.625- to 1.250-mm) source images are acquired and thicker (e.g., 2.5-mm) axial coronal images are reconstructed. Such protocols allow for diagnostic coronal reconstructed image sets with isotropic or near isotropic resolution; these are particularly helpful for staging of renal cell carcinoma. The potential utility of dual energy for the characterization of renal masses is a topic of current intense investigation. These platforms may permit assessment of enhancement by calculating iodine concentration in the mass, though criteria for meaningful changes have not been universally accepted. The reproducibility of postprocessed HU calculations will also need to be validated.

MR: Lesion enhancement is the feature that is also primarily assessed with tailored renal MR protocols. MR offers several unique advantages: Numerous fat-saturation T1-weighted dynamic enhanced phases can be obtained directly in a coronal plane, and dedicated Gadolinium (Gd)-enhanced delayed coronal imaging is the standard of care for identification and characterization of renal vein-caval thrombus. Chemical shift imaging and frequency selective fat-saturation technique may be utilized to identify the fat that is characteristic of angiomyelolipomas. Assessment of T2 and T1 signal intensity improves diagnostic accuracy: Enhancing T2-hyperintense lesions are likely renal cell carcinomas, whereas enhancing T2-hypointense lesions are typically either nonfat-containing acute myeloid leukemias or papillary renal cell carcinoma. Diffusion-weighted imaging assessment may also be employed, though the apparent diffusion coefficient value overlap between benign and malignant renal lesions has limited the utility of this technique. A final caveat regarding MR assessment of renal masses is that Gd enhancement of renal masses on MR remains a largely qualitative biomarker of neoplasia (though one that is better assessed by evaluating subtracted images).

Ultrasound: Despite marked improvements in ultrasound platforms over the past 40 years, the role of ultrasound in the renal mass imaging algorithm has not changed: Ultrasound is typically performed to determine if a lesion is cystic or solid. Technique should be optimized: Compound and harmonic imaging should be routinely employed to reduce artifacts and to obtain sufficient penetration. Color Doppler may be utilized to help identify pseudolesions (e.g., column of Bertin, renal scars) and, rarely, to identify flow within solid or complex cystic masses. Microbubble contrast agents have been employed in several centers to increase the accuracy of ultrasound assessment of renal masses: Unlike CT and MR, enhancement of masses may be observed at continuous real-time examination using low mechanical index protocols, although standards for enhancement are not uniform, and FDA approval for this indication is still forthcoming.

Hematuria (and Potential Urothelial Malignancy) Evaluation

CT urography (CTU): CTU has supplanted conventional intravenous urography as the noninvasive imaging gold standard for the evaluation of patients with hematuria when nephrologic causes (e.g., urinary tract infection, glomerulonephritis) have been excluded. Nonetheless, societies differ on age cutoffs for its use and whether ultrasound may be employed as a primary screening in selected, typically younger, populations. Guidelines for optimizing CTU also widely differ. The basic CTU study includes an initial NECT (to assess for calculi and as a baseline for assessing lesion enhancement if ultimately present), a nephrographic phase for identification of potential renal lesions, and an excretory phase for depicting upper and lower tracts. Coverage and imaging technique may vary, though 64-slice multidetector CT (MDCT) should be employed to obtain thin-slice source images for multiplanar and maximum-intensity projection reconstructions. Approaches to minimize radiation dosing include multiple new iterative reconstruction algorithms, selective coverage, and split-bolus protocols. CTU performed with dual-energy scanners may be a theoretically attractive option to decrease dosing because a virtual NECT may be obtained, though punctate calculi are sometimes obscured. Finally, several options to optimize ureteral opacification (oral hydration, saline administration, low-dose diuretics, prone positioning, and compression) have been employed, but comparison of efficacy between studies is difficult, results have varied, and the logistics of several of these techniques can be daunting. Many centers continue to use simple oral hydration with 1 liter of water 30-60 minutes prior to imaging and a 3-phase protocol with satisfactory results.

MR urography (MRU): MRU is employed in some centers for evaluation of upper tract malignancy and for identification of urinary tract anomalies. A typical MR urogram includes heavily T2-weighted sequences and excretory T1-weighted images after Gd administration. Like with CTU, saline &/or diuretic administration may improve contrast distribution throughout upper tracts. The renal parenchyma is screened with T1- and T2-weighted images and nephrographic-phase Gd-enhanced MR. An abbreviated static T2 MRU protocol may be performed in patients with renal insufficiency to avoid the potential risk of nephrogenic systemic sclerosis. Such an approach may also be a viable alternative for pregnant patients with potential renal colic. Use of dedicated phase array coils improves resolution, though it should be noted that both static T2-weighted MR and excretory T1-weighted MR are prone to motion artifact and lack the spatial resolution of CTU; identification of small calculi may be particularly problematic.

Intravenous urography, retrograde urography: Intravenous urography is rarely performed; it includes tomographic images obtained ~ 1 minute postcontrast administration and delayed views of the kidneys, ureters, and bladder. Problematic areas may be evaluated at fluoroscopy, and compression improves upper tract distention. Retrograde urography is invasive, though it provides a necessary road map for cystoscopic procedures and may be helpful for confirmation of equivocal lesions suggested at either CTU or MRU.

Renal Dysfunction Evaluation

Ultrasound: Ultrasound is the modality typically employed during the initial assessment of the patient with renal insufficiency. Collecting system dilatation, renal size, symmetry, and echogenicity are easily assessed. The utility of ultrasound in nonselected patients in the acute setting has been called into question, however; the likelihood of bilateral ureteral obstruction (manifested by hydronephrosis at ultrasound) in patients without a prior history of hydronephrosis, abdominal/pelvic malignancy, or pelvic surgery is extremely low. An additional limitation of the modality is that it is an anatomic test; it is impossible to differentiate between obstructive and nonobstructive pelvicaliectasis based upon ultrasound alone.

Preliminary work in the radiology literature, subsequently built upon by other disciplines, has suggested a role for Doppler in assessing the changes in renal hemodynamics that occur with varying causes of renal dysfunction. Most papers have employed the resistive index (RI) (peak systolic velocity - end diastolic velocity / peak systolic velocity) as a surrogate for renal vascular resistance. Recent work has shown, however, how changes in segmental renal arterial RIs are due to tissue compliance (not vascular resistance) and that the RI is neither a specific nor sensitive parameter for the many causes of renal failure. Advocates for contrast-enhanced ultrasound have recently proposed a more elegant ultrasound approach for assessing renal physiology: Tissue perfusion (not flow velocities assessed by Doppler) may be calculated by analyzing replenishment kinetics after bubbles are transiently destroyed by a high mechanical index pulse. However, these techniques have not been adopted by practices outside of select research centers given the lack of FDA approval of microbubble agents and the logistics involved with bubble studies. Despite these limitations, the low cost, portability, and lack of radiation associated with ultrasound have solidified its central longstanding role in the evaluation of the patient with renal dysfunction. Ultrasound is also used for renal biopsy guidance in those patients in whom renal dysfunction is unexplained and persistent.

CT: Like with ultrasound, traditional CT largely evaluates gross anatomic causes for renal failure. It may be helpful for depicting obstructing pelvic malignancies or infiltrating renal neoplastic or inflammatory processes. Several centers have assessed the potential role of MDCT for extracting functional parameters (renal perfusion, renal blood flow, and glomerular filtration) from renal time-density curves obtained during intravenous contrast administration. Quantification of renal contrast kinetics has shown promise in evaluating the pathophysiology of a variety of renal diseases, but the need for central venous line placement, radiation exposure, and (most importantly) large IV contrast doses for renal contrast kinetic studies has prevented its use in patients with preexisting renal dysfunction.

MR: Gd-based contrast kinetics may also be analyzed to assess split renal function and global glomerular filtration rate (GFR), although like with CT function studies, these approaches have not been validated in large-scale studies. The length of the examination, reproducibility issues, motion artifact, and the potential of Gd agents to induce nephrogenic systemic fibrosis in patients with renal disease have limited the utility of Gd-enhanced renal function studies. Nonenhanced functional MR approaches may ultimately be incorporated into clinical practice; however, diffusion-weighted MR has been proposed as a noninvasive exam for identifying renal fibrosis, and blood oxygen level-dependent MR techniques may assess changes in renal and cortical oxygen tension (and, by extension, renal blood flow).

Nuclear medicine: Various nuclear medicine techniques are still employed to assess renal function. Tc-99m MAG3 is the agent of choice for dynamic radionuclide renal imaging at most centers. Clearance of this agent is primarily via tubular secretion. Renograms can be evaluated to assess urinary uptake, transit, excretion, and split renal function. Lasix renography may be employed to help differentiate between obstructive and nonobstructive pelvicaliectasis. Changes in renogram curves after administration of captopril (an angiotensin-converting enzyme inhibitor) may be helpful for detecting renovascular hypertension and assessing the impact of surgical or angiographic intervention. Tc-99m DMSA is still the preferred radiopharmaceutical for static parenchymal imaging. This agent concentrates within the renal cortex and best shows functioning tubular mass. As such, it is useful for assessing renal scarring (due to urinary tract infections or reflux nephropathy) and calculating relative renal function. Finally, a variety of radionuclide techniques for GFR estimation may be employed, although in routine clinical practice, estimates of GFR are typically made using equations that incorporate serum creatinine, weight, and multiple additional readily measured parameters. It should be noted that, despite their widespread use, all of these equations (including the most commonly employed Modification of Diet in Renal Disease formula) are limited in patients with unstable renal function. Estimates in certain populations (e.g., cirrhotic or pregnant patients) may be particularly prone to error.

Adrenal Mass Evaluation

CT: The high incidence of incidental adrenal masses has prompted a variety of imaging approaches for their characterization. The work-up of these often asymptomatic lesions (or adrenal "incidentalomas") remains imaging intensive, despite large-scale retrospective studies that have shown that the vast majority of small (< 4 cm), incidental adrenal lesions identified at cross-sectional imaging are benign (i.e., adrenal adenomas, cysts, myelolipomas).

Two basic approaches for characterizing adrenal masses at CT are utilized. The attenuation of the adrenal lesion at NECT is assessed. An attenuation of < 10 HU is highly specific for an adenoma (due to the high lipid content of most adenomas).

Attenuation of < 10 HU might also suggest a true endothelial or posttraumatic pseudocyst (another typically benign lesion). Although differentiation between simple cysts and adenomas is usually not clinically relevant, thin-wall calcification is a common feature of cysts.

The small percentage of adenomas that do not contain much intracellular lipid may be identified by evaluating contrast kinetics. The washout of contrast from so-called lipid-poor adenomas is typically brisk, as opposed to metastases. Delayed absolute or relative washout of iodinated contrast may be calculated using readily available web-based calculators. Brisk washout may also be seen in a small percentage of pheochromocytomas and vascular metastases (e.g., renal cell carcinoma, hepatocellular carcinoma), although in these cases, an appropriate endocrine evaluation and clinical history may help avoid an errant diagnosis of an adenoma. Finally, the incidental large (> 4 cm), but imaging benign, adrenal mass remains a management dilemma. Current dogma continues to suggest that in appropriate surgical candidates, these lesions should be resected given the concern for adrenal cortical carcinoma.

MR: Like NECT, chemical shift MR is employed to identify the lipid content of adrenal adenomas. Relative percent signal suppression at out-phase imaging may be used to increase diagnostic confidence, but qualitative assessment often suffices. Early MR studies suggested a role of MR for identifying pheochromocytomas, but the classic "light bulb" T2-bright appearance is neither a sensitive nor specific feature of these lesions.

Bladder Mass Evaluation

CT: The sensitivity and specificity of CTU for the diagnosis of bladder cancer in patients with hematuria is > 90%. MDCT is readily available, and the recommendations of multiple societies have highlighted its effectiveness in assessing visceral and nodal metastases pre- and post therapy. Even well-performed, state-of-the-art MDCT often fails with local T staging, however. The depth of muscle invasion is frequently under- or overestimated, though CT performs better with higher T score tumors. Thus, cystoscopy remains in every algorithm of the investigation of hematuria. Imaging-suspected or occult bladder lesions are directly visualized, and if present, biopsy for diagnosis and depth of invasion is performed. Similarly, size and shape remain the only imaging criteria for nodal metastases, and like with other GU malignancies, low-volume nodal disease will not be identified. Recent work has also unfortunately suggested that PET/CT adds little beyond conventional MDCT to local N staging.

MR: The role of MR for the local staging of bladder cancer continues to evolve. The superior soft tissue contrast resolution of MR using standard T1- and T2-weighted imaging sequences allows for better differentiation between bladder wall layers. Multiple studies have shown that compared to CT, MR performs better for identifying intramural tumor invasion and perivesical spread. Nonetheless, MR often fails, and muscle invasion may be under or over called. Multiparametric imaging (combining multiplanar T1/T2 image sets, diffusion-weighted MR, and dynamic contrast-enhanced MR) may improve staging accuracy, though this approach is currently employed at select centers. Preliminary work has also suggested the utility of ultra small super paramagnetic iron oxide particles and diffusion MR for node characterization, though for the meantime, radical cystectomy and extended template node dissection remain the standard of care for the staging and therapy of confirmed muscle invasive tumor.

Selected References

1. Ioachimescu AG et al: Adrenal Incidentalomas: a disease of modern technology offering opportunities for improved patient care. Endocrinol Metab Clin North Am. 44(2):335-354, 2015

2. Davarpanah AH et al: MR imaging of the kidneys and adrenal glands. Radiol Clin North Am. 52(4):779-98, 2014

3. Heller MT et al: In search of a consensus: evaluation of the patient with hematuria in an era of cost containment. AJR Am J Roentgenol. 202(6):1179-86, 2014

4. McClennan BL: Imaging the renal mass: a historical review. Radiology. 273(2 Suppl):S126-41, 2014

5. Kaza RK et al: Dual-energy CT of the urinary tract. Abdom Imaging. 38(1):167-79, 2013

6. Lawrentschuk N et al: Current role of PET, CT, MR for invasive bladder cancer. Curr Urol Rep. 14(2):84-9, 2013

7. Raman SP et al: MDCT evaluation of ureteral tumors: advantages of 3D reconstruction and volume visualization. AJR Am J Roentgenol. 201(6):1239-47, 2013

8. Wolin EA et al: Nephrographic and pyelographic analysis of CT urography: differential diagnosis. AJR Am J Roentgenol. 200(6):1197-203, 2013

9. Wolin EA et al: Nephrographic and pyelographic analysis of CT urography: principles, patterns, and pathophysiology. AJR Am J Roentgenol. 200(6):1210-4, 2013

10. Verma S et al: Urinary bladder cancer: role of MR imaging. Radiographics. 32(2):371-87, 2012

11. Siegelman ES: Adrenal MRI: techniques and clinical applications. J Magn Reson Imaging. 36(2):272-85, 2012

12. Taffel M et al: Adrenal imaging: a comprehensive review. Radiol Clin North Am. 50(2):219-43, v, 2012

13. Chandarana H et al: Iodine quantification with dual-energy CT: phantom study and preliminary experience with renal masses. AJR Am J Roentgenol. 196(6):W693-700, 2011

14. Durand E et al: Functional renal imaging: new trends in radiology and nuclear medicine. Semin Nucl Med. 41(1):61-72, 2011

15. Grenier N et al: Radiology imaging of renal structure and function by computed tomography, magnetic resonance imaging, and ultrasound. Semin Nucl Med. 41(1):45-60, 2011

16. Kaza RK et al: Distinguishing enhancing from nonenhancing renal lesions with fast kilovoltage-switching dual-energy CT. AJR Am J Roentgenol. 197(6):1375-81, 2011

17. Notohamiprodjo M et al: Diffusion and perfusion of the kidney. Eur J Radiol. 76(3):337-47, 2010

18. Israel GM et al: Pitfalls in renal mass evaluation and how to avoid them. Radiographics 28: 1325-1338; 2008

19. Quaia E et al: Comparison of contrast-enhanced sonography with unenhanced sonography and contrast-enhanced CT in the diagnosis of malignancy in complex cystic renal masses. AJR Am J Roentgenol. 191(4):1239-49, 2008

20. Setty BN et al: State-of-the-art cross-sectional imaging in bladder cancer. Curr Probl Diagn Radiol. 36(2):83-96, 2007

21. O'Connor OJ et al: MR Urography. AJR Am J Roentgenol. 195(3):W201-6, 2010

22. Silverman SG et al: Hyperattenuating renal masses: etiologies, pathogenesis, and imaging evaluation. Radiographics. 27(4):1131-43, 2007

23. Tublin ME et al: Review. The resistive index in renal Doppler sonography: where do we stand? AJR Am J Roentgenol. 180(4):885-92, 2003

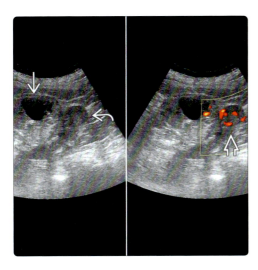 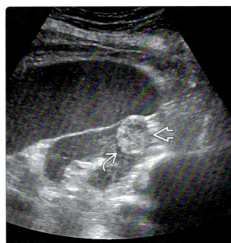

(Left) Grayscale and power Doppler renal US performed on a patient with renal insufficiency shows a cyst ➡ and an incidental isoechoic lower pole renal cell carcinoma (RCC) ➡. US is typically performed to differentiate solid from cystic lesions. Intralesional Doppler flow ➡ helps confirm malignancy. (Right) US shows an echogenic RCC ➡. Differentiating between an echogenic RCC and acute myeloid leukemia may be difficult on ultrasound, but a thin halo ➡ and the lack of weak shadowing favor RCC.

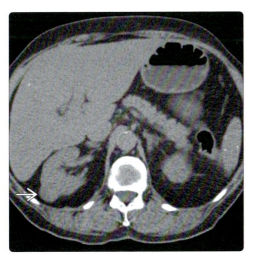 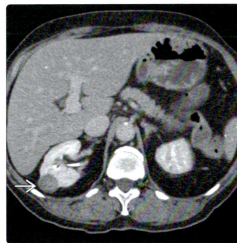

(Left) NECT shows an exophytic solid attenuation right renal lesion ➡. Either US or CECT is needed to differentiate between a high-attenuation cyst and solid neoplasia. (Right) CECT of the same patient performed during the nephrographic phase shows that the lesion ➡ enhances by 40 Hounsfield units (HU). Enhancement is the hallmark imaging marker of neoplasia. Papillary RCC was confirmed at laparoscopic partial nephrectomy.

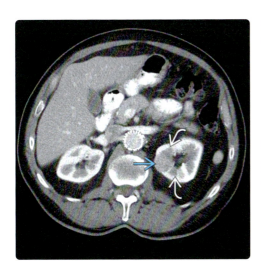 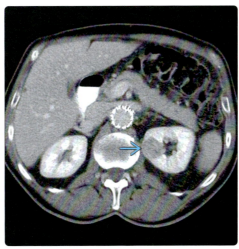

(Left) CECT performed during corticomedullary phase shows a subtle, largely nonborder-deforming left upper pole renal lesion ➡. Its attenuation is similar to minimally enhanced surrounding medulla ➡. (Right) CECT of the same patient during nephrographic phase shows an obvious, now relatively low-attenuation left upper pole mass ➡ (confirmed clear cell RCC). Endophytic renal masses are often imperceptible on corticomedullary phase. Deenhancement of masses over time is an additional imaging marker of neoplasia.

(Left) *Gadolinium (Gd)-enhanced T1WI MR shows an exophytic right lower pole RCC ➡. Assessment of contrast enhancement at MR is largely qualitative; subtraction images may be helpful in problematic cases.* (Right) *DECT spectral data is used to generate an iodine-specific overlay map. Qualitative assessment confirms no iodine uptake in a high-attenuation right renal cyst ➡. Early work has suggested that direct quantification of iodine concentration may compete with HU assessment of neoplasia enhancement.*

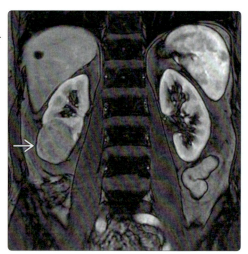
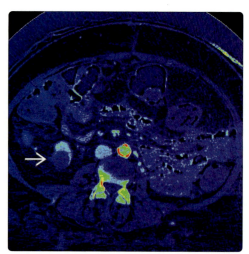

(Left) *Gd-enhanced T1WI MR shows expansile, enhancing tumor thrombus ➡ within the left renal vein in a patient with an adjacent RCC (not shown). Coronal imaging is particularly helpful for the preoperative evaluation of T3 RCC.* (Right) *CT urogram in an elderly man with hematuria shows an infiltrating right renal urothelial cell carcinoma ➡. Recent consensus statements advocate CTU for the evaluation of nonnephrologic causes of hematuria, though age guidelines and the utility of US are still debated.*

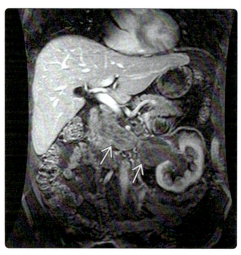
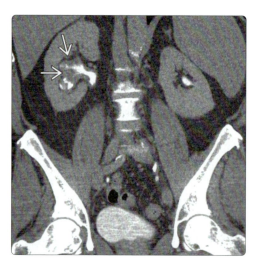

(Left) *Gd-enhanced T1-weighted urogram shows normal upper tracts. Both Gd-enhanced and heavily T2-weighted sequences are part of typical MRU protocols, though image resolution is less than that obtained by CT urography, and calculi may not be identified.* (Right) *US of a patient with acute renal failure shows a normal-sized echogenic kidney (a nonspecific finding of medical renal disease) and perirenal edema ➡. The primary role of US in this setting is to assess renal size and collecting system dilatation.*

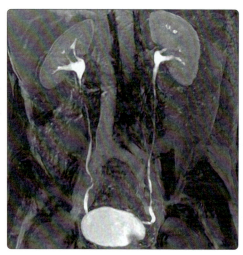
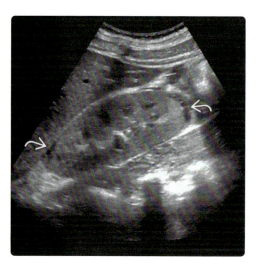

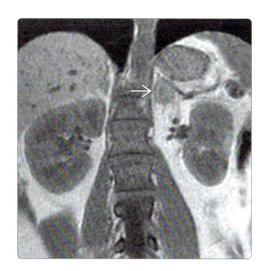
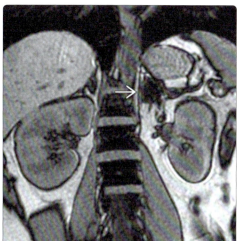

(Left) In-phase T1WI MR in a 37-year-old woman with Cushing syndrome shows an intermediate signal intensity left adrenal lesion ➡. (Right) Out-of-phase T1WI MR of the same patient shows uniform signal loss of a lipid-rich adenoma ➡. Chemical shift imaging exploits resonance differences between lipid and water to detect the intracytoplasmic fat characteristic of lipid-rich adenomas. Adrenal:spleen suppression ratios may be calculated for problematic cases, but visual assessment typically suffices.

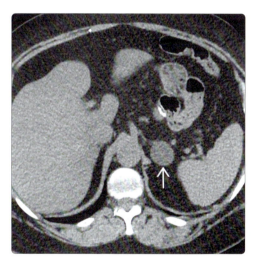
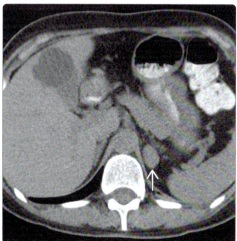

(Left) NECT of a patient with Cushing syndrome shows a left adrenal lesion ➡ measuring -2 HU. NECT is an effective screening modality for characterizing lipid-rich adenomas, but the utility of intensive imaging for incidental adrenal lesions has been questioned. (Right) Baseline NECT shows an incidental, indeterminate, left adrenal mass ➡. Relative and absolute washout percentages on a dedicated adrenal CT (not shown) confirmed a lipid-poor adenoma. Web-based programs are readily available for calculations.

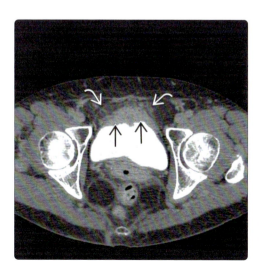
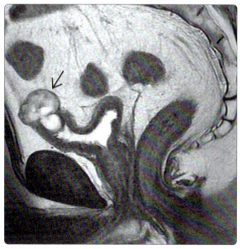

(Left) Delayed CECT shows a large, sessile, anterior bladder urothelial carcinoma ➡. Prevesical fat infiltration ➡ suggests T3 tumor (i.e., tumor extending beyond detrusor). CT is utilized for preoperative evaluation of nodal and visceral metastases, but it is typically not helpful for assessing tumor depth (T stage). (Right) Sagittal T2WI MR shows a likely muscle-confined (T2) bladder dome urachal adenocarcinoma ➡. MR performs better than CT for assessing tumor depth, but cystoscopic biopsy remains the standard of care for T staging.

SECTION 2
Retroperitoneum

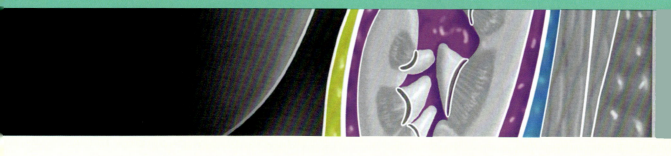

Relevant Anatomy and Embryology

The parietal peritoneum separates the peritoneal cavity from the retroperitoneum. The retroperitoneum contains all the abdominal contents located between the parietal peritoneum and the transversalis fascia. It is divided into 3 compartments by 2 well-defined fascial planes: The renal and lateroconal fasciae.

The **perirenal space** contains the kidney, adrenal, proximal ureter, and abundant fat, and it is enclosed by the renal fascia, which is also referred to as Gerota fascia. The perirenal spaces can communicate across the abdominal midline as shown through in vivo and cadaveric injection studies.

The **anterior pararenal space** contains the pancreas, duodenum, colon (ascending and descending), and a variable amount of fat.

The **posterior pararenal space** contains fat but no organs; it is contiguous with the properitoneal fat along the flanks.

The anterior renal fascia separates the perirenal space from the anterior pararenal space, and the posterior renal fascia separates the perirenal space from the posterior pararenal space.

The lateroconal fascia separates the anterior from the posterior pararenal space and marks the lateral extent of the anterior pararenal space.

The renal fascia joins and closes the perirenal space resembling an inverted cone with its tip in the iliac fossa. Caudal to the perirenal space, in the pelvis, the anterior and posterior pararenal spaces merge to form a single infrarenal retroperitoneal space, which communicates directly with the pelvic prevesical space (of Retzius). Due to an opening in the cone of the renal fascia caudally, the perirenal space communicates with the infrarenal retroperitoneal space. Thus, all 3 retroperitoneal compartments communicate with each other within the lower abdomen and pelvis. All of the pelvic retroperitoneal compartments, such as the perivesical and perirectal spaces, communicate with each other, which is evident and clinically relevant in cases of pelvic hemorrhage or tumor as well as with extraperitoneal rupture of the urinary bladder.

The renal and lateroconal fascia are laminated planes, which can split to form potential spaces as pathways of spread for rapidly expanding fluid collections or inflammatory processes, such as hemorrhage or acute pancreatitis. Splitting of the anterior renal fascia creates a "retromesenteric plane" that communicates across the midline; splitting of the posterior renal fascia creates a "retrorenal plane," which also communicates across the midline and anteriorly. Knowing this principle is crucial to understanding how diseases originating in the anterior pararenal space, such as acute pancreatitis, can extend posterior to the back of the kidney or how fluid collections within the posterior pararenal space or retrorenal plane can extend around the lateral or even anterior abdominal wall.

Imaging Techniques and Indications

Multiplanar CT and MR are ideally suited to display the anatomy and pathology of retroperitoneal disease processes. Use of intravenous contrast material allows easier recognition of fascial plane landmarks and pathology and should be used unless contraindicated.

Approach to Retroperitoneal Abnormalities

Perirenal Space

Disease within the perirenal space is usually the result of diseases of the kidney. Common disease states include hemorrhage, infection, inflammation, and neoplasia.

The renal fascia is very strong and is usually effective in containing most primary renal pathology within the perirenal space. Similarly, it usually excludes most other processes from invading or involving the perirenal space.

The perirenal space is divided irregularly and inconsistently by perirenal bridging septa that often result in loculation of perirenal fluid, which may be misinterpreted as subcapsular in location. The perirenal septa also act as conduits for fluid or infiltrative disease, including tumor, to enter or leave the perirenal space.

Perirenal fluid may represent blood, urine, or pus or may be simulated by inflammation of the perirenal fat. Hemorrhage is often due to trauma but may occur due to anticoagulation, rupture of a renal tumor, or vasculitis. Pus or inflammation usually originates from acute pyelonephritis, which may be associated with an abscess. Perirenal urine ("urinoma") may result from trauma with laceration through the renal collecting system, but it usually resolves rapidly unless there is an obstruction to the flow of urine to the bladder. Acute urine extravasation may also accompany ureteral obstruction by a calculus due to forniceal rupture.

Renal cell carcinoma is common, and the renal fascia usually confines the tumor, preventing invasion of contiguous structures. Spread to lymph nodes or hematogenous spread through the renal vein and inferior vena cava (IVC) may occur and constitute important elements of the imaging and staging of this tumor.

Anterior Pararenal Space

Disease within the anterior pararenal space is common. For example, acute pancreatitis results in peripancreatic infiltration ± fluid collections that spread throughout the anterior pararenal space, often affecting the duodenum and ascending and descending colon segments that share this anatomic compartment. The spread of inflammation is usually limited posteriorly by the anterior renal fascia and laterally by the lateroconal fascia. Thickening of these planes is a reliable clue as to the presence of pancreatitis, which might otherwise be occult on imaging. The perirenal space is usually not involved in acute pancreatitis, sometimes resulting in a striking appearance of a perirenal "halo" of fat density, while other retroperitoneal spaces and planes are infiltrated. Ventral (anterior) spread of inflammation or tumor from the anterior pararenal space is not limited by any fascial boundary but only by the posterior parietal peritoneum. The root of the mesentery and transverse mesocolon originate from just ventral to the 3rd portion of duodenum and pancreas, and disease originating in these organs may easily dissect into the mesentery without crossing any anatomic boundaries. Some refer to the spaces enclosed by the mesenteric layers as the subperitoneal space, emphasizing that there is no inviolate separation between the intraperitoneal and retroperitoneal spaces.

A duodenal ulcer may perforate and result in extraluminal gas and fluid that occupy 1 or more spaces, including the anterior pararenal, intraperitoneal (as the duodenal bulb is an intraperitoneal structure), and even the perirenal space since the latter is open at the renal hilum and communicates with the anterior pararenal space.

Posterior Pararenal Space

Disease originating within the posterior pararenal space is uncommon, essentially limited to hemorrhage and tumor.

"Retroperitoneal hemorrhage" is a misnomer since most spontaneous, coagulopathic hemorrhage originates within the abdominal wall, the iliopsoas compartment, or the rectus sheath. Only when hemorrhage extends beyond these fascial boundaries does it enter the retroperitoneum. Rectus sheath hematomas enter the extraperitoneal pelvic spaces through a defect in the caudal (infraumbilical) portion of the sheath. Iliopsoas hemorrhage often extends into any or all of the retroperitoneal compartments, predominantly along the main fascial planes. The hallmarks of coagulopathic hemorrhage are: Bleeding out of proportion to trauma, multiple sites of bleeding, and the presence of the hematocrit sign, a fluid-cellular debris level within the hematoma.

Retroperitoneal sarcomas, most commonly liposarcoma, often originate within 1 of the retroperitoneal compartments, and the site of origin can be determined by the relative mass effect on various organs and structures, such as the kidneys, colon, and great vessels. Most liposarcomas have some identifiable fat within them and seem to be encapsulated, allowing for excision, although recurrent disease is common.

If retroperitoneal nodes are included in the discussion, the most common retroperitoneal tumor is non-Hodgkin lymphoma (NHL). NHL often results in massive lymphadenopathy. This characteristically involves the mesenteric and retroperitoneal nodes that are confluent and anteriorly displace the aorta and IVC from the spine. Retroperitoneal nodes are also frequently involved by malignancies originating in pelvic organs, such as the prostate, rectum, and cervix.

The other large, though uncommon, group of primary retroperitoneal tumors are of neurogenic origin, including nerve sheath tumors, ganglioneuroma, neuroblastoma, and others. These often share the characteristics of appearing as well-defined, moderately enhancing masses that do not appear to arise from nodes nor abdominal viscera. Many, in fact, arise along the sympathetic nerve trunks, while others are part of a syndrome, such as neurofibromatosis, that may involve multiple nerves in a paraspinal or presacral distribution.

The great vessels, the aorta and IVC, are located in the retroperitoneum and are usually depicted as lying within the retromesenteric plane. Although primary disease of the IVC is rare, it may be the site of primary tumor (sarcoma) or the site of spread from a renal or adrenal carcinoma. More common are anomalies of the embryologic development of the IVC. Some 10% of the population have some anomaly of the embryologic sub- and supracardinal veins, usually at or below the level of the renal veins, resulting in variations such as duplicated IVC and retro- and circumaortic renal vein. While these are uncommonly of clinical significance (limited to affecting surgical and interventional procedures), they may be mistaken for pathologic conditions, most commonly enlarged retroperitoneal lymph nodes.

Abdominal aortic aneurysm is a major health concern, and rupture is usually fatal. Accurate diagnosis and precise mapping of the size and shape of an aneurysm allows effective, minimally invasive prophylactic treatment with endovascular stenting.

Retroperitoneal fibrosis is an inflammatory disorder that may be misinterpreted as a malignant process, as it envelops the aorta and IVC, often causing displacement and encasement of the ureters. It may occur as an isolated process or as part of a multisystem autoimmune disorder.

Selected References

1. Osman S et al: A comprehensive review of the retroperitoneal anatomy, neoplasms, and pattern of disease spread. Curr Probl Diagn Radiol. 42(5):191-208, 2013
2. Goenka AH et al: Imaging of the retroperitoneum. Radiol Clin North Am. 50(2):333-55, vii, 2012
3. Tirkes T et al: Peritoneal and retroperitoneal anatomy and its relevance for cross-sectional imaging. Radiographics. 32(2):437-51, 2012
4. Lee SL et al: Comprehensive reviews of the interfascial plane of the retroperitoneum: normal anatomy and pathologic entities. Emerg Radiol. 17(1):3-11, 2010
5. Sanyal R et al: Radiology of the retroperitoneum: case-based review. AJR Am J Roentgenol. 192(6 Suppl):S112-7 (Quiz S118-21), 2009

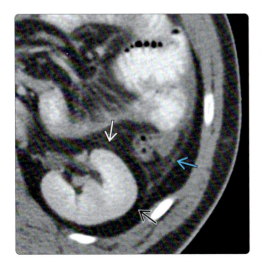
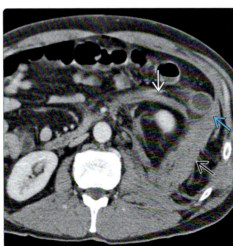

(Left) Axial CECT shows the normal anterior ➡ and posterior ➡ renal fascia, which fuse to form the lateroconal fascia ➡. Note that the normal fascia are extremely thin. (Right) Axial CECT demonstrates fluid from pancreatitis dissecting along the retromesenteric plane ➡, formed by the layers of the anterior renal fascia and the retrorenal plane ➡, formed by layers of the posterior pararenal space. Fluid also extends along the lateral conal fascia ➡.

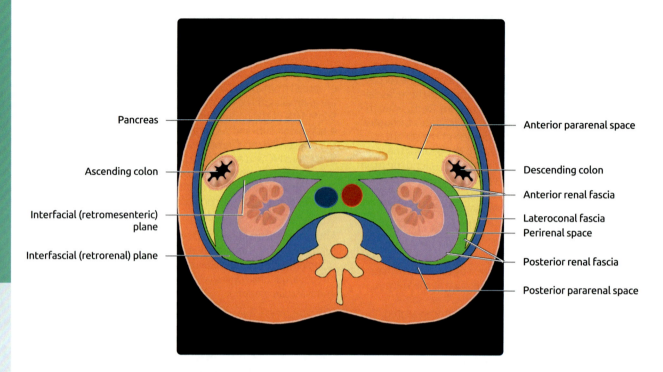

Pancreas

Ascending colon

Interfacial (retromesenteric) plane

Interfascial (retrorenal) plane

Anterior pararenal space

Descending colon

Anterior renal fascia

Lateroconal fascia

Perirenal space

Posterior renal fascia

Posterior pararenal space

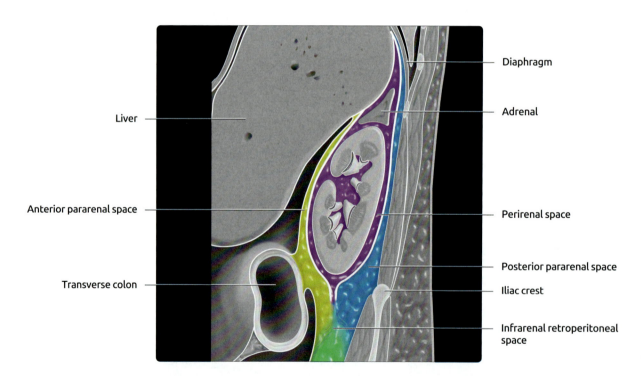

Liver

Anterior pararenal space

Transverse colon

Diaphragm

Adrenal

Perirenal space

Posterior pararenal space

Iliac crest

Infrarenal retroperitoneal space

(Top) The 3 main compartments of the retroperitoneum are the anterior pararenal space (yellow), perirenal space (purple), and posterior pararenal space (blue). The interfascial planes (green) are potential spaces created by inflammatory processes that separate the double laminated layers of the renal and lateroconal fasciae. The posterior pararenal space is synonymous with the properitoneal fat that extends along the lateral and anterior abdominal wall. (Bottom) Sagittal graphic through the right kidney shows the 3 retroperitoneal compartments. Note the confluence of the anterior and posterior renal fasciae at ~ the level of the iliac crest. Caudal to this, there is only a single infrarenal retroperitoneal space.

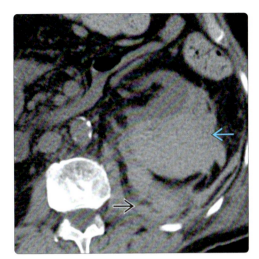
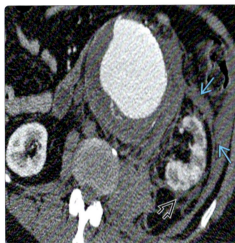

(Left) *Axial NECT in a patient following flank trauma shows that the left kidney is compressed and displaced due to a large subcapsular renal hematoma ➡. There is also hematoma in the posterior pararenal space ➡. Note the lack of a fluid-hematocrit level, a finding that is associated with anticoagulation hemorrhage.* (Right) *Axial CECT during the arterial phase reveals hemorrhage dissecting along the left interfascial planes ➡ and into the perirenal space ➡ due to contained rupture of an abdominal aortic aneurysm.*

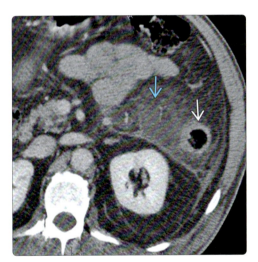
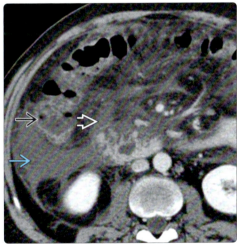

(Left) *Axial CECT demonstrates fluid ➡ from subacute pancreatitis tracking into the left anterior pararenal space. Note that the descending colon ➡ also resides in the anterior pararenal space and is partially surrounded by fluid.* (Right) *Axial CECT demonstrates fluid from acute pancreatitis dissecting through the right aspect of the anterior pararenal space ➡. Fluid abuts the ascending colon ➡ (also in the anterior pararenal space) and dissects along the proximal aspect of the transverse mesocolon ➡.*

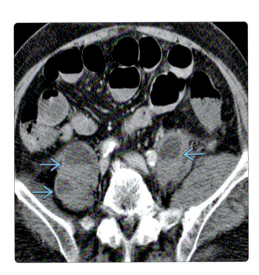
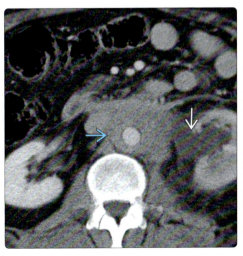

(Left) *Axial CECT in a patient with decreased hematocrit reveals hematomas ➡ within both psoas muscles. Note the fluid-hematocrit levels within the hematomas due to anticoagulant hemorrhage.* (Right) *Axial CECT shows left hydronephrosis ➡ and delayed nephrogram due to obstruction of the proximal ureter. The obstruction results from retroperitoneal fibrosis (RPF) and is shown as a periaortic soft tissue mantle ➡; unlike lymphoma, RPF does not displace the aorta from the spine.*

TERMINOLOGY

- Congenital anomalies of inferior vena cava (IVC)

IMAGING

- Duplication of IVC (prevalence: ~ 1-3%)
  - Left- and right-sided IVCs are present inferior to renal veins
  - Left IVC typically drains into left renal vein, which crosses anterior to aorta to join right IVC
  - Recognition important prior to IVC filter placement
- Left IVC (prevalence: ~ 0.2-0.5%)
  - Typically drains into left renal vein, which crosses anterior to aorta to join normal right suprarenal IVC
  - Important variant in repair of abdominal aortic aneurysm and transjugular placement of IVC filter
- Azygos continuation of IVC (prevalence: ~ 2-9%)
  - Absence of suprarenal IVC
  - Blood flow enters azygous vein and enters thorax posterior to diaphragmatic crus

- Enlarged azygos vein empties into superior vena cava normally in right peribronchial location
- Hepatic veins drain directly into right atrium
- Important variant in planning cardiopulmonary bypass
- Circumaortic left renal vein (prevalence: ~ 2.0-3.5%)
  - Important variant in nephrectomy planning
  - Rare occurrences of hematuria and hypertension
- Retrocaval ureter (prevalence: ~ 0.7%)
  - Right ureter courses posterior and medial to IVC
  - Variable degrees of right hydroureteronephrosis

TOP DIFFERENTIAL DIAGNOSES

- Retroperitoneal lymphadenopathy
- Varices/collaterals
- Gonadal vein

DIAGNOSTIC CHECKLIST

- Check for IVC anomalies prior to abdominal surgery, kidney/liver transplant, and IVC filter placement

(Left) *Graphic shows transposition of the inferior vena cava (IVC) ➡ and its more common duplications ⤴. The duplicated IVC originates at the left iliac vein caudally and empties into the left renal vein. The boxes labeled A through D refer to the respective levels of the axial sections.* (Right) *Graphic shows a circumaortic left renal vein with a smaller ventral vein ➡ crossing cephalad to the dorsal vein ⤴. The dorsal vein is typically located 1-2 cm caudal to superior renal vein and is joined by the left gonadal vein.*

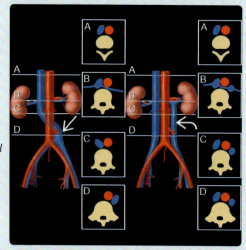
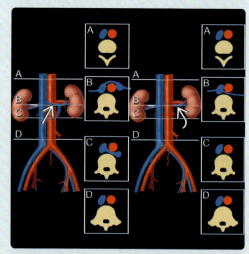

(Left) *Postcontrast axial T1 FS MR shows a normal IVC ➡ and an incidental additional cylindrical structure to the left of the aorta, consistent with a duplicated IVC ⤵. The left-sided IVC typically drains into the left renal vein, which empties to the right-sided IVC.* (Right) *AP view during retrograde pyelography shows medial deviation of the right ureter due to its retrocaval course; note mild ureteral dilatation ⤵ upstream coursing posterior ➡ to the IVC. The left ureter (not shown) had a normal course.*

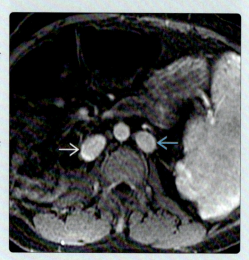
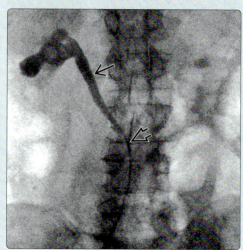

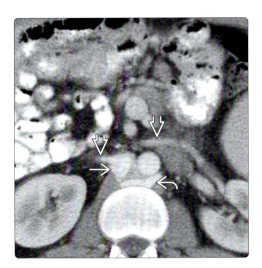

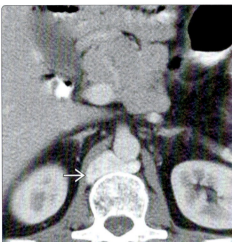

(Left) Axial CECT shows azygos continuation of the IVC. Note that the renal veins ➡ drain into the infrahepatic IVC ➡, which also receives tributaries from the hemiazygos vein ➡ coursing posterior to the aorta. (Right) Axial CECT of a more cephalad section in the same patient shows absence of the intrahepatic portion of the IVC. Instead, the azygous vein ➡ returns all the venous blood from the lower body to the heart via its thoracic connections. The hepatic veins drain directly into the right atrium.

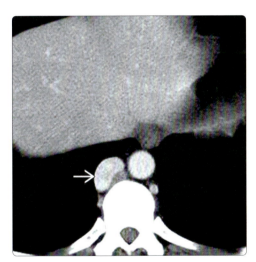

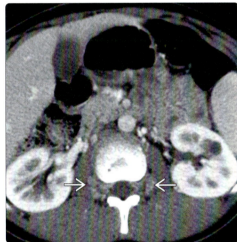

(Left) Axial CECT more superiorly in the same patient shows absence of the intrahepatic portion of the IVC. Instead, blood flow from the lower body returns to the heart via the enlarged azygous vein ➡, which eventually drains into the superior vena cava. The hepatic veins (not shown) drain directly into the right atrium. (Right) Axial CECT shows complete absence of the IVC and numerous paraspinal collaterals ➡. The external and internal iliac veins join to form enlarged ascending lumbar veins, which give rise to collaterals.

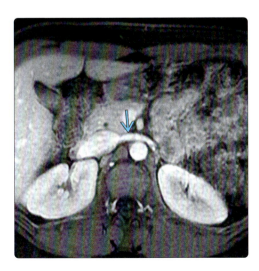

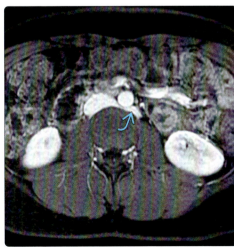

(Left) Postcontrast axial T1 C+ FS MR with fat suppression shows that the anterior component ➡ of a circumaortic left renal vein is located cephalad to the posterior component. The cephalad left renal vein is joined by the left adrenal vein prior to emptying into the IVC. (Right) Postcontrast axial T1 C+ FS MR with fat suppression in the same patient demonstrates that the posterior component (retroaortic) ➡ of the circumaortic left renal vein is located more caudally.

Retroperitoneal Fibrosis

IMAGING

- Irregular, periaortic soft tissue mass extending from renal vessels to iliac bifurcation
  - Aorta not typically displaced from spine in primary retroperitoneal fibrosis
  - Soft tissue can surround inferior vena cava and medially displace ureters
  - Soft tissue may extend to renal hila and into pelvis
- NECT: Isoattenuating to muscle
- CECT or MR: Enhancement varies with stage of disease
  - Early/active disease: Avid enhancement
  - Late/chronic disease: Minimal to no enhancement
- T1WI: Low signal intensity
- T2WI: Signal intensity varies with stage of disease
  - Early/active disease: High signal intensity
  - Late/chronic disease: Low signal intensity
- Prognosis: Decrease in T2 signal intensity, enhancement or size reflects favorable response to treatment

TOP DIFFERENTIAL DIAGNOSES

- Chronic periaortitis
- Retroperitoneal metastases and lymphoma
- Coagulopathic ("retroperitoneal") hemorrhage
- Inflammatory abdominal aortic aneurysms

PATHOLOGY

- Primary (idiopathic): 2/3 of cases
  - Manifestation of systemic autoimmune or inflammatory diseases
- Secondary: 1/3 of cases
  - Most commonly due to medications, neoplasms

CLINICAL ISSUES

- Difficult diagnosis: Insidious, nonspecific symptoms

DIAGNOSTIC CHECKLIST

- Surgical biopsy may be required for definitive diagnosis and exclusion of malignancy

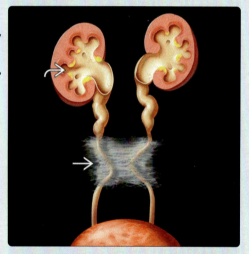
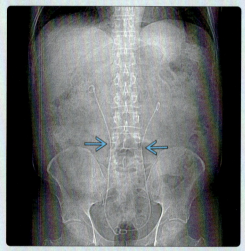

(Left) Graphic shows encasement and medial displacement of mid ureters by a band of fibrous tissue ➡. Note the bilateral hydroureteronephrosis ➡. The fibrous tissue is usually limited to the inferior lumbar region. (Right) AP radiograph shows bilateral ureteral stents that are medialized in their mid portion ➡ due to retroperitoneal fibrosis (RPF). The medialization of the ureters typically occurs at the L4-L5 level.

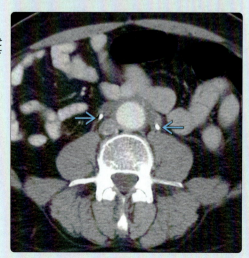
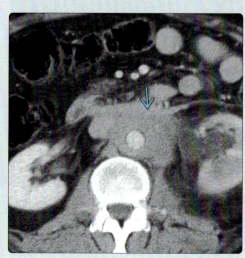

(Left) Axial CECT in the same patient shows stents within the medialized ureters ➡ that are surrounded by a mantle of soft tissue due to RPF. Note that the aorta is also encased by the soft tissue but is not displaced from the lumbar spine. (Right) Axial CECT shows an unusually massive RPF ➡ in this patient with an obstructed left kidney. In the rare, extensive variant of RPF, fibrosis can infiltrate the root of the small bowel mesentery and affect the abdominal viscera.

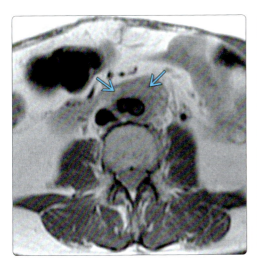
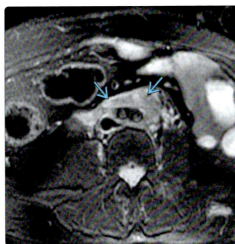

(Left) *Axial T1WI MR shows a mantle of soft tissue ➡ surrounding the anterior and lateral aspects of the iliac bifurcation. The soft tissue has low to intermediate signal intensity.* (Right) *Axial T2WI MR with fat suppression in the same patient demonstrates high signal intensity of the soft tissue mass ➡ that surrounds the iliac bifurcation, consistent with active fibrosis.*

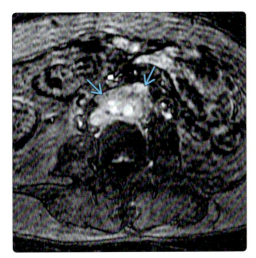
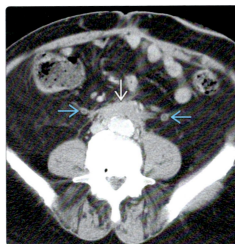

(Left) *Axial T1WI C+ MR with fat suppression in the same patient shows avid enhancement of the soft tissue mass ➡ surrounding the iliac bifurcation, consistent with active fibrosis.* (Right) *Axial CECT shows a mantle of soft tissue ➡ surrounding the anterolateral aspects of the aorta and inferior vena cava. The mantle caused medial displacement and mild dilatation of both ureters ➡.*

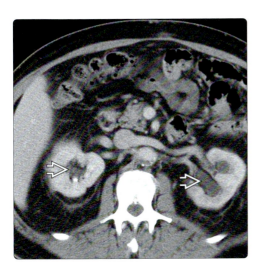
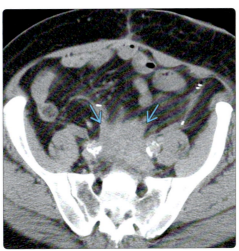

(Left) *Axial CECT in the same patient reveals bilateral hydronephrosis ➡ due to the fibrotic soft tissue mass shown in the previous image.* (Right) *Axial CECT in the same patient shows atypical, caudal extension of the fibrotic process ➡ into the pelvis along the iliac vessels.*

Pelvic Lipomatosis

KEY FACTS

TERMINOLOGY

- Uncommon, progressive, benign overgrowth of mature, unencapsulated fat in perirectal and perivesical spaces

IMAGING

- Symmetrically distributed, nonencapsulated fat surrounding pelvic organs
  - No soft tissue component or enhancement of fat
- Superior displacement of bladder, prostate, seminal vesicles, sigmoid colon
- Inverted pear- or teardrop-shaped bladder
  - Dilated, medially displaced ureters
- Elongated, narrowed rectum due to smooth, concentric extrinsic compression
  - Elongated, straight, narrowed rectosigmoid colon

TOP DIFFERENTIAL DIAGNOSES

- Normal variant (large pelvic muscles, narrow bony pelvis)
- Proctitis (e.g., radiation, lymphogranuloma venereum)

- Ulcerative colitis (Rectosigmoid: ↑ narrowing, thickness, symptoms)
- Postoperative colon (e.g., proctosigmoid resection)

CLINICAL ISSUES

- Compressed bladder (e.g., ↑ frequency, dysuria, nocturia, and hematuria)
- Compressed rectum (e.g., constipation, rectal bleeding, tenesmus, ribbon-like stools, nausea)
- Compressed veins (e.g., leg edema, thrombosis)
- Complications: Hydronephrosis, urolithiasis, renal failure, colon obstruction, venous thrombosis, bladder adenocarcinoma
  - Frequent cystoscopy for those with proliferative cystitis
  - Radical cystoprostatectomy with urinary diversion to relieve obstruction
- Associated with cystitis glandularis
- Increased morbidity of pelvic surgery (e.g., ↑ incidence of bladder neck contractures post radical prostatectomy)

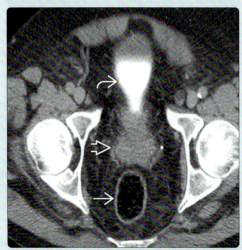
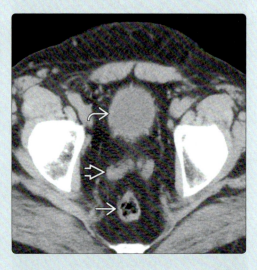

(Left) Axial CECT shows the inverted pear- or teardrop-shaped appearance of the bladder ➡. The prostate ➡ is displaced cephalad, and the rectum ➡ is surrounded and separated from other viscera by the lipomatosis. No soft tissue nodule or enhancement was identified within the fat. (Right) Axial NECT in a 72-year-old man with minimal symptoms of pelvic lipomatosis shows the rectum ➡, bladder ➡, and seminal vesicles ➡ to be compressed and displaced from each other by the proliferation of pelvic fat.

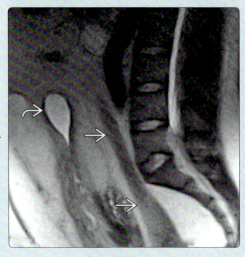
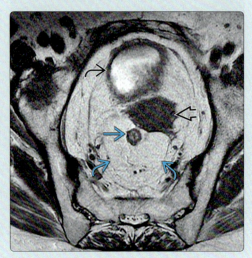

(Left) Sagittal T2 MR shows the inverted pear- or teardrop-shaped bladder that is displaced superoanteriorly ➡. The rectum ➡ is compressed and elongated due to the lipomatosis. (Right) Axial T2 MR in the same patient shows proliferation of the perirectal fat ➡, narrowing of the rectum ➡, and superoanterior displacement of the prostate ➡ and bladder ➡. Note that the proliferated fat has homogeneous signal intensity. As a corollary, there would be no abnormality on postcontrast or diffusion imaging.

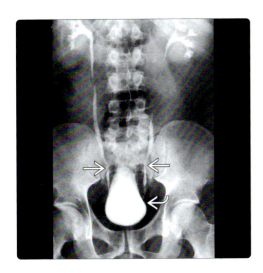

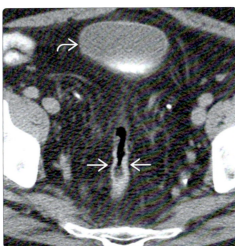

(Left) AP excretory urography shows medial deviation of both ureters ➡ and the bladder ➡ due to pelvic lipomatosis. (Right) Axial CECT in a patient with dysuria and constipation shows abundant fibrofatty tissue in the pelvis that compresses, straightens, and elongates the sigmoid colon ➡. The bladder ➡ is displaced superoanteriorly by the lipomatosis.

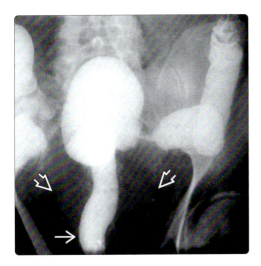

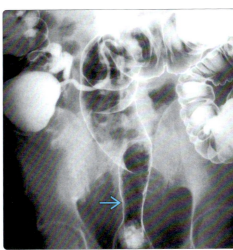

(Left) AP view during contrast enema is shown. This is the typical appearance of pelvic lipomatosis on barium enema. There is elongation and symmetric extrinsic compression of the rectum ➡ and radiolucency in the pelvis ➡. (Right) AP view during an air-contrast barium enema shows smooth rectal narrowing ➡ from extrinsic compression due to pelvic lipomatosis.

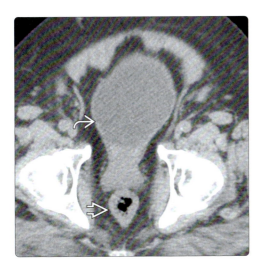

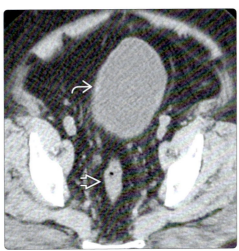

(Left) Axial NECT in an symptomatic patient shows a pear-shaped bladder ➡ and narrowing of the sigmoid colon ➡. The inverted pear shape of the bladder is usually more evident on coronal views, but can been also appreciated on axial images. (Right) Axial NECT shows mild compression and deformity of the urinary bladder ➡ that is anteriorly displaced from the narrowed and straightened sigmoid colon ➡.

Coagulopathic (Retroperitoneal) Hemorrhage

TERMINOLOGY

- Can be misnomer: Retroperitoneal hemorrhage often only in posterior abdominal wall musculature

IMAGING

- Best imaging tool
  - CT ± IV contrast; contrast may identify active hemorrhage
- Major causes and CT findings
  - Coagulopathy or anticoagulation; high-density collection in retroperitoneum or body wall with cellular-fluid level (hematocrit sign)
  - Ruptured abdominal aortic aneurysm; large eccentric aneurysm with blood ± active extravasation contiguous with aorta
  - Renal tumors
  - Trauma
  - Vasculitis
- CT appearance of hemorrhage: Heterogeneous

- Active: Linear, flame-like shape, isodense to vessels
  - Extravasation of vascular contrast (~ 150-400 HU)
- Sentinel clot sign: High attenuation (60-80 HU)
  - Initially accumulates near site of bleeding
- MR: Variable signal intensity due to phase of blood products
- US: Variable echogenicity due to age of hematoma
  - Acute/subacute: Echogenic
  - Chronic: Hypo- to anechoic fluid collection

TOP DIFFERENTIAL DIAGNOSES

- Retroperitoneal abscess
- Retroperitoneal sarcoma
- Asymmetrical muscles

DIAGNOSTIC CHECKLIST

- Spontaneous perirenal hemorrhage: Consider underlying tumor, vasculitis, or coagulopathy

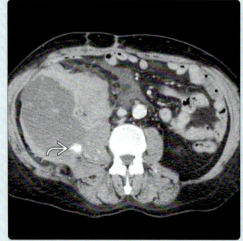
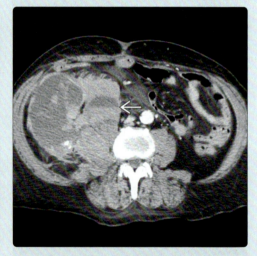

(Left) *Axial CECT shows a large, heterogeneous, "retroperitoneal" mass centered in the iliopsoas compartment in a patient with coagulopathic hemorrhage. Active extravasation of contrast ➡ is usually venous in this setting and does not typically require embolization.* (Right) *Axial CECT in the same patient shows the presence of the hematocrit sign ➡, which is consistent with an acute, coagulopathic hemorrhage. The hematocrit sign is due to a cellular-fluid level within the collection.*

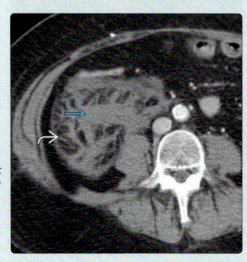
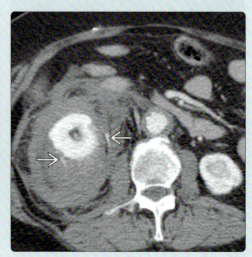

(Left) *Axial CECT shows a large perirenal hemorrhage that distends the perirenal space. The hematoma ➡ is nearly isoattenuating to adjacent skeletal muscle. The septa ➡ within the perirenal space are well depicted and prevent the blood from spreading evenly throughout the perirenal space.* (Right) *Axial CECT shows a large, spontaneous hemorrhage that distends the perirenal space in a patient with coagulopathic hemorrhage. Two foci of active bleeding are noted ➡.*

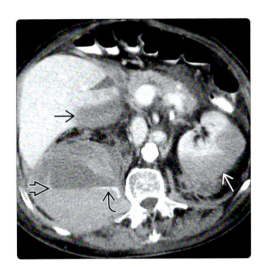

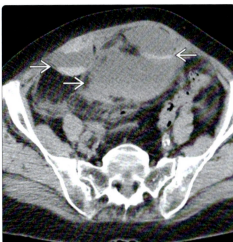

(Left) *Axial CECT shows classic findings of coagulopathic hemorrhage at multiple sites, including the left perirenal ➡, right iliopsoas, and intraperitoneal ➡ spaces. Note the hematocrit sign ➡ and active (venous) bleeding ➡ in the right iliopsoas muscle. Active extravasation from coagulopathy was due to venous bleeding and stopped with reversal of the anticoagulation. (Right) Axial NECT shows enlargement of both rectus sheaths and hematocrit signs ➡ indicating acute hemorrhage due coagulopathy.*

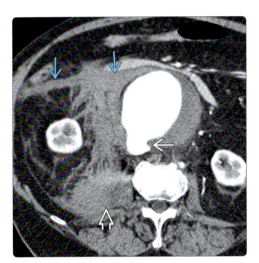

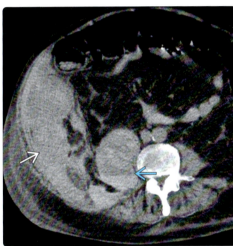

(Left) *Axial CECT shows a large aneurysm extending along the aorta and recent rupture into the right retroperitoneum ➡ and iliopsoas muscle ➡. The aorta is "draped" over the spine and there is a mural contour defect ➡ along the dorsal aspect of the aortic lumen at the site of extravasation. (Right) Axial NECT shows an acute hematoma in the right retroperitoneum ➡ and a hematocrit sign ➡ within the expanded psoas muscle due to coagulopathic hemorrhage.*

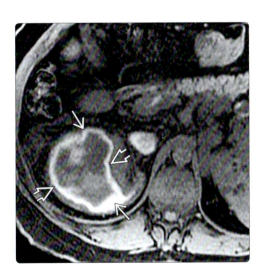

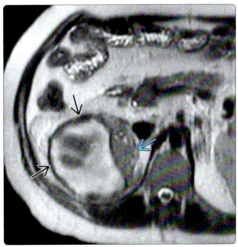

(Left) *Axial T1WI MR with fat saturation shows a heterogeneous mass in the right perinephric space. Note that there is a thin, low signal intensity outer rim ➡ surrounding a high signal intensity inner rim ➡, both of which surround an intermediate signal intensity center. Findings are consistent with a subacute hematoma. (Right) Axial T2WI MR in the same patient better demonstrates a low signal intensity outer rim ➡. Note that the right kidney ➡ is compressed and displaced medially.*

Postoperative Lymphocele

IMAGING

- Well-marginated, simple cystic lesion in extraperitoneal pelvis or retroperitoneum of postoperative patient
- Commonly located along iliac vessels, inguinal region, and paraaortic retroperitoneum
- CECT
  - Typically unilocular but may contain few, thin septa
  - Mild enhancement of wall and thin septa
  - No mural nodule
- MR
  - Homogeneous low signal intensity (SI) on T1WI and high SI on T2WI
  - Low SI on diffusion-weighted imaging
  - MR lymphangiography: Allows specific diagnosis of lymphocele
- US
  - Marginated, anechoic lesion with through transmission
  - May have internal echoes or layering debris if infected

- Occasional septa but no internal color flow

TOP DIFFERENTIAL DIAGNOSES

- Other pelvic cystic masses
  - Urinoma
  - Bladder diverticulum
  - Lymphangioma

PATHOLOGY

- Occurs in up to ~ 30% of patients undergoing radical pelvic surgery
- Cystic lesion with thin, tan to yellowish-brown fluid
- Lymphocytes, few red blood cells, variable protein/fat

CLINICAL ISSUES

- Most are small, asymptomatic, and resolve spontaneously
- Large lymphoceles may be symptomatic due to mass effect
- Lymphadenectomy is most significant risk factor
- Presentation varies weeks to months after surgery
- Treatment: Drainage, sclerotherapy, or surgery

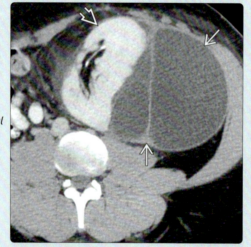
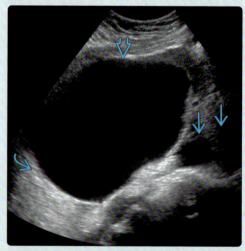

(Left) Axial CECT in a patient with a lymphocele following renal transplantation shows a multiseptate mass ➡ compressing the renal allograft ⇻. Note that there is mild enhancement of the thin wall and septa but no mural thickening or nodule. (Right) Transverse endovaginal US in a patient who has undergone hysterectomy and node dissection shows a large, anechoic cystic lesion ⇲ adjacent to the iliac vessels ⇲, representing a postoperative lymphocele. Note the thin wall and through transmission ⇲.

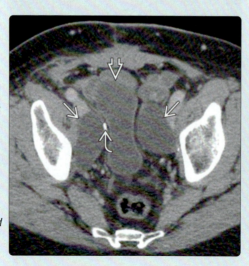
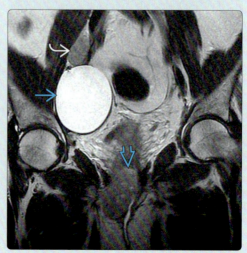

(Left) Axial CECT following prostatectomy shows compression of the urinary bladder ⇲ by bilateral lymphoceles ➡. Note the surgical clip ⇗ from node dissection. There is minimal enhancement of the thin walls of the lymphoceles. (Right) Coronal T2WI MR post hysterectomy and node dissection due to cervical cancer reveals that a sharply marginated lymphocele ⇲ has high T2 signal intensity. Note local tumor recurrence ⇲ adjacent to the urethra and a metastatic lymph node ➡.

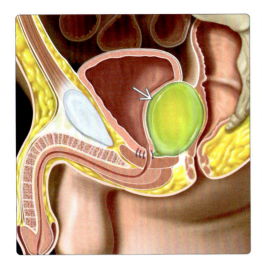

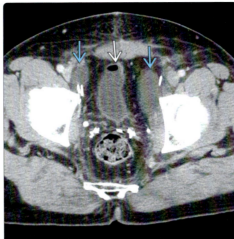

(Left) *Graphic shows a male patient who has had a radical prostatectomy, which includes extensive pelvic node dissection. A lymphocele ➡ has developed within the pelvis and exerts mass effect on the bladder and rectum.* (Right) *Axial CECT following radical prostatectomy shows bilateral, ovoid, water attenuation structures ➡ adjacent to surgical clips and lateral to the urinary bladder ➡; these structures lack rim enhancement and represent incidental lymphoceles.*

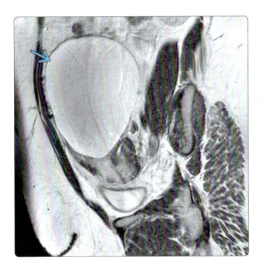

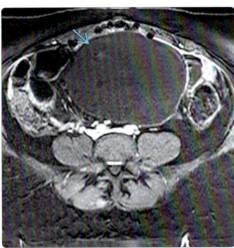

(Left) *Sagittal T2WI MR post hysterectomy shows a large, midline cystic lesion with high signal intensity representing a postoperative lymphocele ➡.* (Right) *Contrast-enhanced axial T1WI MR with fat suppression following hysterectomy shows lack of enhancement in the large, midline cystic structure representing a postoperative lymphocele ➡.*

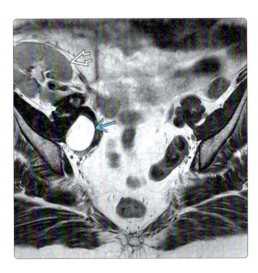

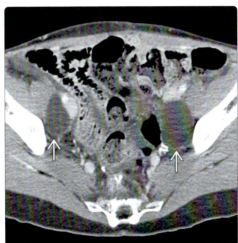

(Left) *Axial T2WI MR shows an ovoid cystic lesion ➡ with high signal intensity and an imperceptible wall, consistent with an incidental lymphocele. The lymphocele is adjacent to the iliac vessels at the level of the anastomosis with the renal transplant ➡.* (Right) *Axial CECT shows bilateral lymphoceles ➡ along the iliac vessels in a woman following bilateral salpingo-oophorectomy and pelvic lymph node dissection.*

TOP DIFFERENTIAL DIAGNOSES

- Ganglioneuroma
  - Rare, benign tumor of sympathetic ganglia or adrenal
  - Well circumscribed: Excellent prognosis
- Ganglioneuroblastoma
  - Malignant sympathetic tumor affecting 2-4 year olds
  - Heterogeneous mass: Ranges from solid to cystic
- Neuroblastoma
  - Malignant tumor of sympathetic nerves or adrenal
  - Unencapsulated, irregular, lobulated
  - Necrosis, hemorrhage, coarse calcifications
  - Invades adjacent structures + metastases
- Paraganglioma ("extraadrenal pheochromocytoma")
  - Benign or malignant; hormonally active in ~ 40%
  - Very avid enhancement due to hypervascularity
  - T2WI: "Light bulb bright" in ~ 80%
  - Usually syndromic (e.g., von Hippel-Lindau) and benign
- Schwannoma (neurilemmoma)
  - Usually benign tumor of peripheral nerve sheaths
  - Usually paravertebral but can arise in any nerve
  - Typically < 5 cm, round, homogeneous
    - ↑ size: ± cystic degeneration, calcifications
- Neurofibroma
  - Typically solitary, benign nerve sheath tumor: Well marginated, homogeneous
    - ~ 10% are multiple, often due to neurofibromatosis type 1 (NF1)
  - Malignant degeneration → neurofibrosarcoma
    - ~ 2-20% in those with NF1
    - Large, heterogeneous, infiltrative mass

DIAGNOSTIC CHECKLIST

- Review history for syndromes (NF1 and von Hippel-Lindau)
- Most common scenario for neurogenic tumor
  - Child to young adult
  - Solid, enhancing, retroperitoneal mass
  - Mass neither contains fat nor arises from viscera

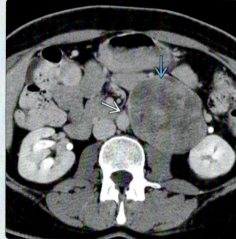
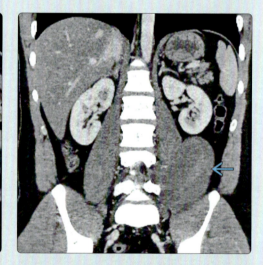

(Left) Axial CECT reveals a large, heterogeneously enhancing mass ⮕ in the left aspect of the retroperitoneum at the level of the origin of the inferior mesenteric artery ⮕, a landmark for the organ of Zuckerkandl. Note that the mass abuts and mildly displaces adjacent viscera but does not arise from them. Pathology was consistent with a paraganglioma. (Right) Coronal CECT reveals a large, heterogeneously enhancing ovoid mass ⮕ arising between the spine and left psoas muscle.

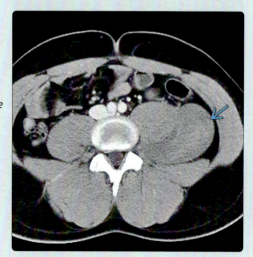
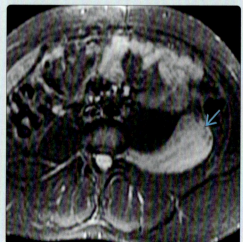

(Left) Axial CECT in the same patient demonstrates the heterogeneously enhancing mass ⮕ posterior to the left psoas muscle and contiguous with the adjacent neural foramen. (Right) Axial T2WI MR with fat suppression in the same patient reveals slightly heterogeneous, high signal intensity within the left retroperitoneal mass ⮕. Surgical pathology was consistent with benign schwannoma.

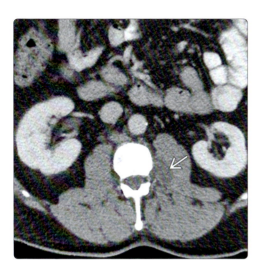

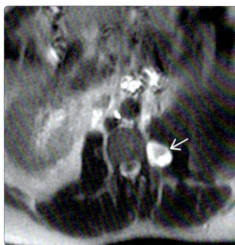

(Left) Axial CECT shows a well-marginated, hypoattenuating mass ⇨ medial to the left psoas muscle and adjacent to a neural foramen. (Right) Axial T2WI MR in the same patient reveals high signal intensity in the periphery of the left paravertebral lesion ⇨ due to myxoid matrix and central low signal intensity due to cellular neural tissue. Pathology was consistent with a solitary neurofibroma.

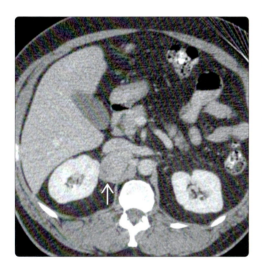

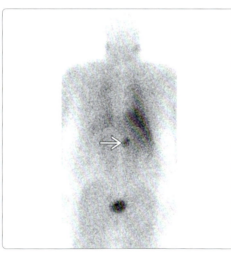

(Left) Axial CECT shows an enhancing retrocaval mass ⇨. A radionuclide MIBG scan confirmed uptake within this lesion. This is a paraganglioma, which is equivalent to an extraadrenal pheochromocytoma. (Right) Coronal MIBG (iodine-131-metaiodobenzylguanidine) scintigraphy shows focal uptake ⇨ within the retrocaval soft tissue mass shown on prior CT. Pathology revealed a paraganglioma.

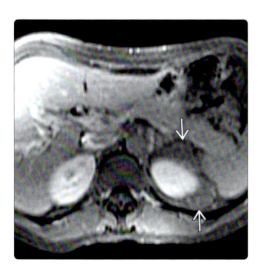

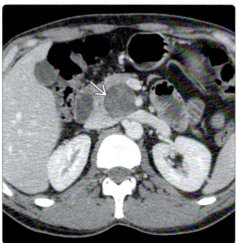

(Left) Axial postcontrast T1WI MR with fat suppression shows heterogenous enhancement of a left perirenal soft tissue mass ⇨. Pathology proved ganglioneuroma. (Right) Axial CECT shows a well-marginated, heterogeneous mass ⇨ arising from the posterior border of the pancreatic head. Surgical pathology was consistent with pancreatic schwannoma.

IMAGING

- 80% of retroperitoneal (RP) tumors are malignant
  - Typical appearance: Large heterogeneous mass of fat + soft tissue attenuation displacing RP structures or viscera
- Most malignant RP tumors are of mesodermal origin
- Liposarcoma and leiomyosarcoma account for > 90%
- Liposarcoma: 3 CT patterns based on amount and distribution of fat in tumor (often coexist)
  - Discrete fatty areas < -20 HU; other soft tissue foci > +20 HU
  - Solid pattern: Attenuation values > +20 HU (mostly myxoid tissue)
  - Pseudocystic pattern: Homogeneous density between +20 and -20 HU
  - Can be mistaken for fluid collection
- Leiomyosarcoma
  - Extravascular (62%)
  - Large RP mass ± necrotic or cystic degeneration

- Intravascular mass (6%)
- Solid mass within inferior vena cava and dilatation or obstruction of lumen

TOP DIFFERENTIAL DIAGNOSES

- Renal angiomyolipoma
  - Renal parenchymal defect ("notch" or "claw" sign) and enlarged vessels favor angiomyolipoma
- Adrenal myelolipoma
- RP hemorrhage

CLINICAL ISSUES

- Most RP sarcomas are asymptomatic until sufficiently large
- Signs/symptoms include: Pain (abdomen, back, flank), palpable abdominal mass, lower extremity edema
- Differentiate from renal and adrenal tumors

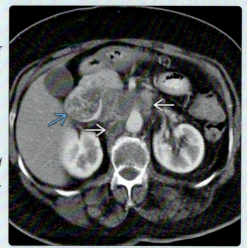
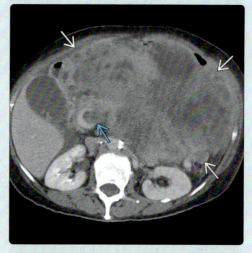

(Left) Axial CECT reveals a heterogeneously enhancing mass ➡ that expands the inferior vena cava (IVC). Tumor ➡ extends into paraaortic and prevertebral spaces of the retroperitoneum. Pathology revealed leiomyosarcoma that originated in the IVC. (Right) Axial CECT demonstrates a huge heterogeneous mass ➡ that arose in the retroperitoneum and displaced peritoneal structures anteriorly and laterally. Tumor thrombus ➡ is shown within the IVC. Pathology was consistent with a malignant fibrous histiocytoma (MFH).

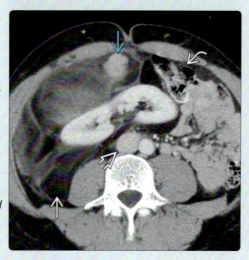
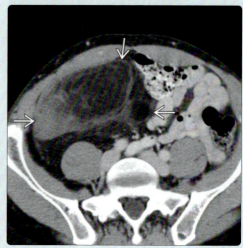

(Left) Axial CECT shows a large, right-sided retroperitoneal mass that displaces the kidney, IVC ➡, and ascending colon ➡. The mass has foci of fat ➡ and soft tissue attenuation ➡, the latter representing areas of myxoid degeneration within a liposarcoma. (Right) Axial CECT in the same patient shows that the more caudal aspect of this large mass ➡ displaces, but does not invade, retroperitoneal structures and viscera. The mass was resected but recurred within 1 year.

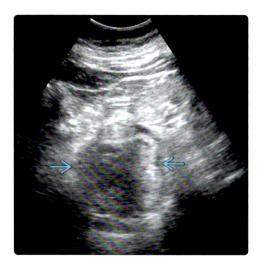

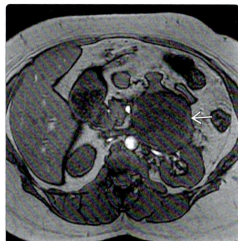

(Left) Transverse US reveals a lobulated soft tissue mass ➡ in the left upper quadrant of an asymptomatic patient. (Right) Axial T1WI out-phase MR in the same patient reveals a soft tissue mass ➡ of intermediate soft tissue signal intensity. Compared to the in-phase sequence (not shown), there was no loss of signal during the out-phase sequence. Surgical resection was consistent with an MFH.

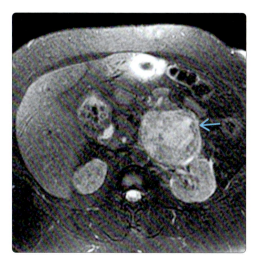

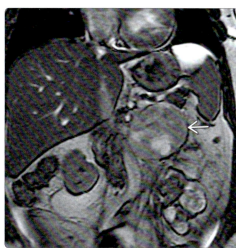

(Left) Axial T2WI MR with fat suppression in the same patient demonstrates heterogeneous signal intensity throughout the MFH ➡. Central high signal intensity was due to necrosis. (Right) Coronal T2WI MR in the same patient reveals heterogeneous signal intensity in the MFH ➡. There was no invasion of any adjacent structures. MFH is more commonly an extremity soft tissue tumor, but it can also arise in the retroperitoneum and peritoneum.

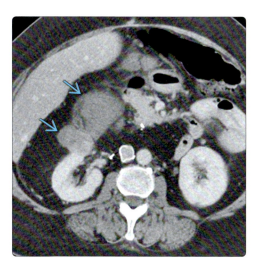

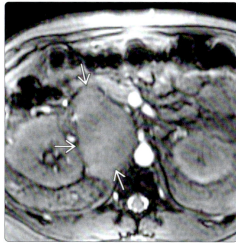

(Left) Axial CECT shows a heterogeneously enhancing mass ➡ spanning the anterior pararenal and perirenal spaces. The mass consists of regions of fat and soft tissue attenuation and was proven to be a liposarcoma. (Right) Axial T2 gradient MR in a patient with leiomyosarcoma of the IVC shows a large, oblong mass ➡ with intermediate soft tissue signal intensity that occupies the expected position of the IVC.

TERMINOLOGY

- Generally classified as non-Hodgkin lymphoma (NHL) vs. Hodgkin disease (HD)
  - However, WHO recognizes over 80 types of lymphoma

IMAGING

- Discrete or confluent soft tissue nodules in mesentery or paraaortic spaces
- Enlarged nodes (generally ≥ 1 cm in short axis) for mesenteric and retroperitoneum
  - Retrocrural nodes enlarged if ≥ 6 mm
- Confluent soft tissue mantle fills paraaortic spaces in advanced cases
  - Displacement of aorta from spine (unusual for benign etiologies)
- Nodes due to NHL typically larger than HD
  - Also more likely to be noncontiguous in distribution in NHL
- Mesenteric adenopathy more common in NHL (> 50%) than HD (< 5%)
- HD: Typically involves superior paraaortic nodes initially without skip areas of involvement
- Sensitivity of 90-95% for PET compared to 80-85% for CECT
  - Useful to determine early response to chemotherapy
  - Often helpful to distinguish residual lymphoma vs. fibrosis postradiation

TOP DIFFERENTIAL DIAGNOSES

- Retroperitoneal metastases
- Testicular metastases
- Retroperitoneal sarcoma
- Retroperitoneal neurogenic tumor
- Retroperitoneal fibrosis
- Abdominal manifestations of tuberculosis

DIAGNOSTIC CHECKLIST

- Tissue sampling: Several core biopsies for flow cytometry

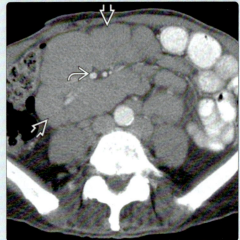
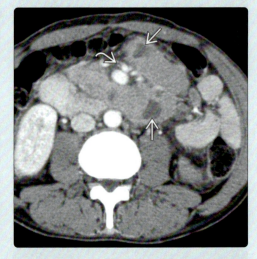

(Left) Axial CECT in a 34-year-old man with AIDS and non-Hodgkin lymphoma shows extensive mesenteric and paraaortic adenopathy. Note the "sandwich" sign created by the mesenteric nodes ⇒ surrounding the vessels ⇒. Mesenteric adenopathy is common in patients with non-Hodgkin lymphoma but rare in Hodgkin disease. (Right) Axial CECT shows multifocal soft tissue masses with foci of necrosis ⇒ "sandwiching" the mesenteric vessels ⇒ due to non-Hodgkin lymphoma.

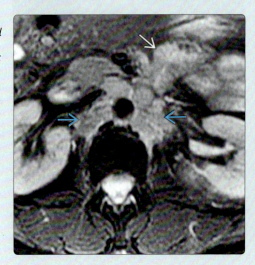
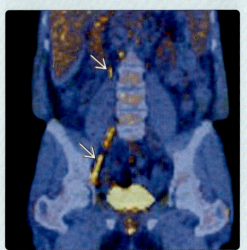

(Left) Axial T2WI MR with fat suppression shows high signal intensity in confluent paraaortic ⇒ and mesenteric ⇒ adenopathy due to non-Hodgkin lymphoma. (Right) Fused coronal PET/CT in a patient with Hodgkin disease shows a long contiguous line of FDG-avid right paraaortic and iliac nodes ⇒ that are normal in size and would be missed on CT as not involved by tumor.

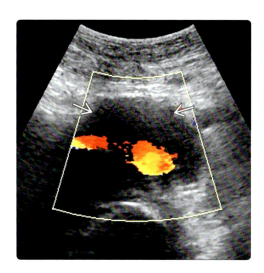

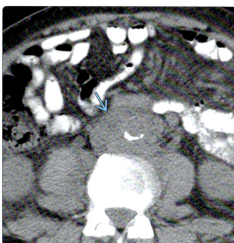

(Left) Transverse US shows a soft tissue mass ➡ surrounding the aorta and inferior vena cava due to non-Hodgkin lymphoma. (Right) Axial NECT in the same patient shows that the adenopathy ➡ from non-Hodgkin lymphoma fills the paraaortic spaces and displaces the aorta from the spine.

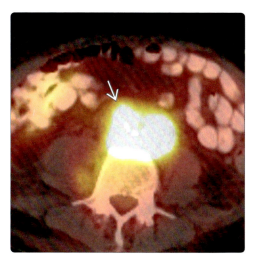

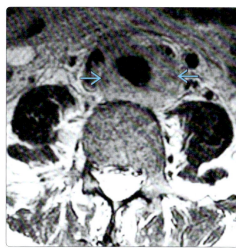

(Left) Axial PET/CT in the same patient demonstrates that the non-Hodgkin lymphoma adenopathy ➡ is FDG avid. (Right) Axial T2WI MR SS FSE in the same patient shows that the periaortic mass ➡ has intermediate to high signal intensity.

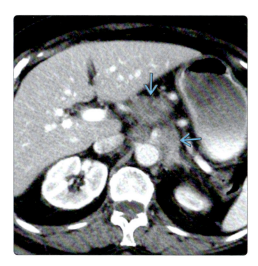

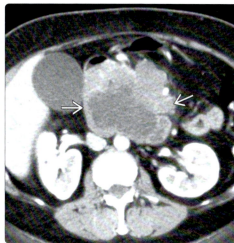

(Left) Axial CECT shows confluent paraceliac adenopathy ➡ due to non-Hodgkin lymphoma. (Right) Axial CECT shows pancreatic non-Hodgkin lymphoma as a bulky mass ➡ in the head of the pancreas region. The lymphoma occupies the peripancreatic nodal group, but the appearance may simulate a primary pancreatic tumor.

Retroperitoneal Metastases

IMAGING

- Soft tissue masses or abnormal nodes in retroperitoneum
  - Masses displace aorta + inferior vena cava from spine
- Size criteria
  - Paraaortic, pelvic adenopathy: ≥ 10-mm short axis
  - Retrocrural nodes: ≥ 6-mm short-axis diameter
  - Nodal size not reliable criterion alone (yet still most used)
- Morphology
  - Round, irregular margins
- Architecture
  - Distortion or loss of normal fatty hilum
- Enhancement
  - Variable due to type of primary tumor
  - Similar enhancement suggests same grade and aggressiveness
- Etiologies of metastases
  - Lymphoma and anaplastic tumors tend to cause confluent nodal masses
    - Other nodal metastases tend to be discrete masses
  - Testicular seminomas: Bulky retroperitoneal nodes
    - Nonseminomatous germ cell tumors: Small, clustered nodes
  - Extranodal retroperitoneal metastases: Melanoma, renal cell, anaplastic, breast, small cell lung cancers

TOP DIFFERENTIAL DIAGNOSES

- Lymphoma
- Infectious
- Primary retroperitoneal tumors
- Inflammatory
- Retroperitoneal fibrosis

PATHOLOGY

- Depending on primary tumor site: Nodal metastases may constitute N1 (regional), N2, or M1 (distant metastases) spread of disease

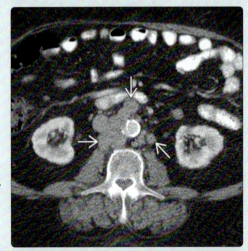
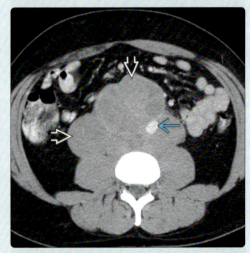

(Left) Axial CECT shows several discrete, enlarged nodes ➡ in the paraaortic spaces (measuring 1.0-1.5 cm) typical of malignant adenopathy. These lymph node metastases were due to prostate cancer. (Right) Axial CECT shows extensive, confluent paraaortic adenopathy ➡ due to metastatic testicular seminoma. Note that the aorta ➡ is displaced from the lumbar spine by the mantle of soft tissue, a finding that is not seen in typical retroperitoneal fibrosis.

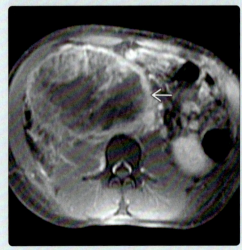
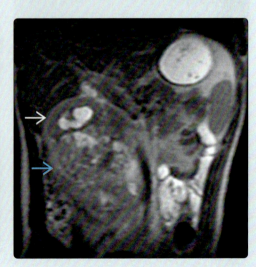

(Left) Axial postcontrast T1WI MR with fat saturation reveals a large, retroperitoneal mass ➡ that is partially necrotic. Nodal disease from right testis tumors occurs in the interaortocaval space, while nodal disease from left testis tumors occurs in the paraaortic space. (Right) Coronal T2WI MR in the same patient shows superolateral displacement and hydronephrosis of the right kidney ➡ due to mass effect from the right retroperitoneal mass ➡.

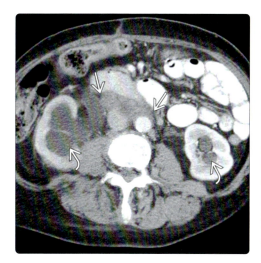
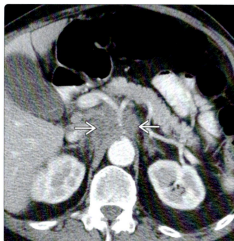

(Left) Axial CECT demonstrates bilateral hydronephrosis ➡ due to confluent retroperitoneal nodal metastases ➡ resulting in ureteral obstruction. (Right) Axial CECT shows confluent nodes ➡ encasing the celiac axis due to metastatic esophageal carcinoma. Cancer of the distal esophagus often metastasizes to upper abdominal nodes prior to liver or lungs.

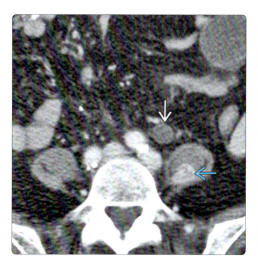
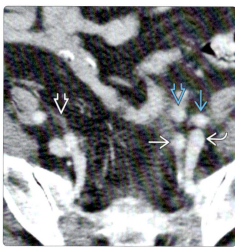

(Left) Axial CECT shows left hydroureter ➡ and an enhancing metastatic lesion in the left psoas muscle ➡. (Right) Axial CECT in the same patient shows an enhancing metastasis ➡ obstructing the left ureter. The left common iliac artery ➡ and vein ➡ and left gonadal vein ➡ are identified. The normal right ureter ➡ is shown for comparison.

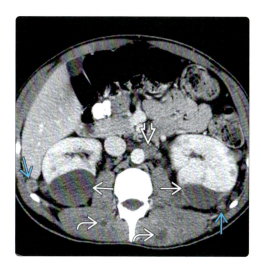
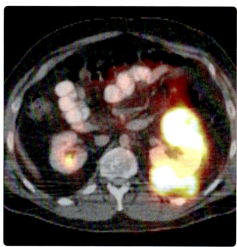

(Left) Axial CECT shows bilateral renal subcapsular hematomas ➡, perinephric soft tissue nodules ➡, retroperitoneal adenopathy ➡, and muscular lesions ➡ due to metastatic melanoma in a 21-year-old male patient. (Right) FDG-avid tumor is present within the left kidney and perirenal space, representing hematogenous metastases from melanoma to the retroperitoneum. For tumors that are FDG avid, PET/CT is the ideal imaging tool, because it often detects metastases in unexpected sites and normal-sized nodes.

Hemangiopericytoma

TERMINOLOGY

- Hemangiopericytomas are group of neoplasms that arise from pericytes in walls of capillaries and can occur in various tissues
  - Rare, vascular neoplasms of variable clinical behavior

IMAGING

- No specific imaging features allow diagnosis
- US
  - Solid renal mass of variable echogenicity
  - Flow may be detected in solid components
- CECT
  - Heterogeneously enhancing soft tissue mass
  - ± necrosis, calcification
- MR
  - T1WI: Typically low signal intensity
  - T2WI: Heterogeneous intermediate to high signal intensity

TOP DIFFERENTIAL DIAGNOSES

- Renal cell carcinoma
- Oncocytoma
- Renal angiosarcoma

PATHOLOGY

- Most renal hemangiopericytomas are benign
  - However, clinical behavior is variable
  - Therefore, long-term follow-up is recommended

CLINICAL ISSUES

- Most common symptoms
  - Painless mass > flank pain > hematuria > hypoglycemia > hypertension

DIAGNOSTIC CHECKLIST

- No specific imaging or clinical findings to facilitate diagnosis
- Diagnosis of renal hemangiopericytoma is one of exclusion, requiring immunohistochemistry and electron microscopy

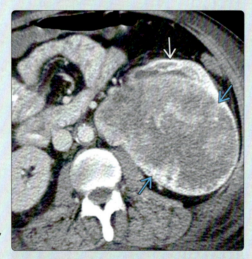
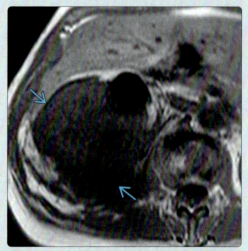

(Left) Axial CECT shows a large, ovoid, heterogeneously enhancing mass ➡ in the left kidney. A small amount of normal renal parenchyma ➡ is located anteriorly. The left renal vessels were displaced, but not invaded, and no adenopathy was present. Resection specimen was consistent with renal hemangiopericytoma (HPC). (Right) Axial T1WI MR reveals a large mass ➡ replacing the majority of the right kidney. The mass has homogeneously low signal intensity and displaces, but does not invade, the renal vessels.

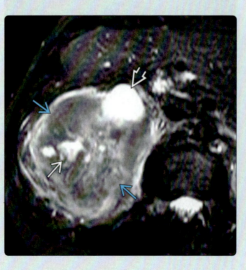
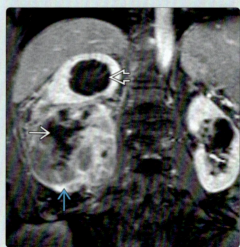

(Left) Axial T2WI MR with fat suppression in the same patient shows intermediate, heterogeneous signal intensity throughout the mass ➡ and a small area of necrosis ➡. An incidental cyst ➡ is shown anteriorly. (Right) Contrast-enhanced coronal T1WI MR with fat suppression in the same patient reveals an area of necrosis ➡ within the mass ➡. An incidental cyst is shown in the superior pole of the right kidney ➡. Differential considerations for the mass include various primary renal neoplasms. Pathology revealed renal HPC.

Perivascular Epithelioid Cell Tumor (PEComa)

TERMINOLOGY

- Rare group of mesenchymal neoplasms associated with blood vessel walls

IMAGING

- CECT
  - Variable enhancement
    - Hypovascular to avid enhancement
  - Necrosis in large tumors
  - Well circumscribed
  - Rare calcification
- MR
  - T1WI: Hypo- to isointense
  - T2WI: Heterogeneously hyperintense
- Ultrasound
  - Heterogeneous echotexture

TOP DIFFERENTIAL DIAGNOSES

- Renal origin
  - Renal cell carcinoma
  - Transitional cell carcinoma
  - Lymphoma
- Retroperitoneal origin
  - Various sarcomas

PATHOLOGY

- Typically express melanocytic and smooth muscle markers

CLINICAL ISSUES

- Usually present as incidentally discovered mass
- Most perivascular epithelioid cell tumors (PEComas) are benign
  - Minority are malignant and metastasize

DIAGNOSTIC CHECKLIST

- Consider PEComa for retroperitoneal masses that do not contain fat
- Consider PEComa for renal masses that lack adenopathy and vascular invasion

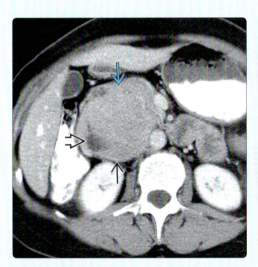
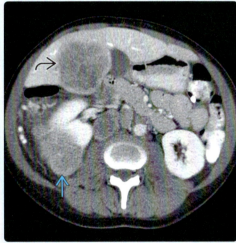

(Left) Axial CECT reveals a large, heterogeneously enhancing mass ⊟ arising in the right aspect of the retroperitoneum. The mass results in compression and posterior displacement of the inferior vena cava ⊟. A small area of necrosis ⊟ is shown along the lateral aspect of the mass. (Right) Axial CECT shows an enhancing mass ⊟ arising from the lateral cortex of the right kidney. A similar-appearing metastasis ⊟ is within hepatic segment 5. Only a minority of PEComas are malignant and metastasize.

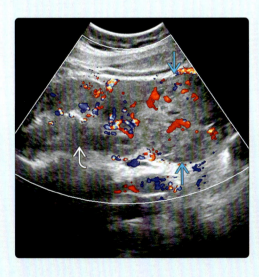
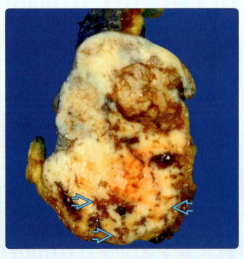

(Left) Longitudinal color Doppler US demonstrates a solid mass ⊟ extending from the inferior pole of the left kidney ⊟. There is extensive color flow within the exophytic mass. Although not shown on this image, there was no invasion of the renal vessels or adenopathy. (Right) Photograph of the resection specimen reveals innumerable small vessels ⊟ coursing through the mass, demonstrating the often vascular nature of PEComas. Pathology confirmed PEComa.

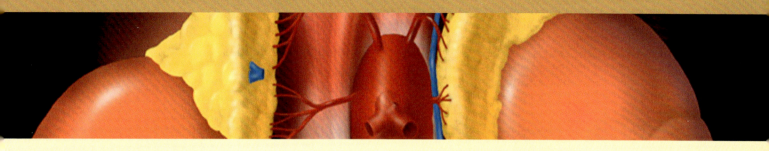

Anatomy, Embryology, and Physiology

The adrenal (suprarenal) glands lie in the perirenal space, usually cephalic to the kidneys. The right adrenal gland lies above the kidney, lateral to the crus of the diaphragm, medial to the liver, and touches the posterior aspect of the inferior vena cava. The left adrenal gland usually lies anterior to the upper pole of the left kidney, posterior to the splenic vein and pancreas. The splenic vein is a useful landmark in identifying the source of left upper quadrant masses that may be of uncertain origin. Adrenal masses generally displace the splenic vein forward, while pancreatic or gastric masses displace it posteriorly.

The adrenal cortex and medulla are essentially different organs that lie within the same structure. The cortex is an endocrine gland, secreting primarily cortisol, aldosterone, and androgenic steroids, all of which are derived from cholesterol esters. This contributes to the high lipid content that is characteristic of most adrenal cortical adenomas.

The medulla is derived from the neural crest and secretes epinephrine and norepinephrine.

Adrenal physiology is controlled by an elaborate interaction between the hypothalamus, pituitary, and adrenals. Stress results in the release of epinephrine and cytokines, which cause the pituitary to secrete adrenocorticotrophic hormone (ACTH), which in turn stimulates the adrenals to secrete cortisol. Cortisol and epinephrine are often regarded as the "stress hormones." Elevated serum cortisol has a suppressing effect on the hypothalamus and pituitary, reducing further release of ACTH.

Cushing syndrome, due to excess cortisol, is characterized by truncal obesity, hirsutism, amenorrhea, hypertension, weakness, and abdominal striae. It is usually caused by adrenal hyperplasia (75-80% of cases) but may also result from an adrenal adenoma (20-25%), adrenal carcinoma (< 5%), or exogenous corticosteroid medication.

Conn syndrome is the eponym sometimes used for excess aldosterone and is characterized by hypertension, hypokalemia, alkalosis, muscle weakness, and cardiac dysfunction. Unlike Cushing syndrome, Conn syndrome is usually caused by an adrenal adenoma (65-70%). Adrenal hyperplasia accounts for most of the remaining (25-30%) cases, while adrenal carcinoma is a rare cause.

Because patients with Cushing syndrome are symptomatic, the diagnosis of either pituitary or adrenal-induced cortisol excess is typically made biochemically, prior to imaging. Imaging (either MR or CT) performed after diagnosis usually easily localizes the pituitary or adrenal adenoma responsible for Cushing syndrome, thus obviating catheter angiography or other invasive tests. Conn adenomas, however, may be quite small, and traditional imaging may be problematic in the setting of elevated aldosterone.

Addison syndrome or disease refers to adrenal insufficiency and is characterized by hypotension, weight loss, and altered pigmentation. Among the causes of "slow-onset" adrenal insufficiency are autoimmune disease, which is the most common cause in developed countries. Tuberculosis and other infections remain common causes of Addison syndrome in the developing world, while metastatic disease and AIDS are encountered in all populations.

The most common cause of abrupt onset adrenal insufficiency is adrenal hemorrhage, which may result from sepsis, shock, anticoagulation, or vasculitis. Abrupt withdrawal of corticosteroid medication and postpartum pituitary necrosis, known as Sheehan syndrome, also result in acute adrenal insufficiency. Prompt recognition and treatment of these conditions is critical.

Imaging Techniques and Protocols

Adrenal Protocol, CT

NECT is often sufficient to diagnose an adrenal adenoma, seen as a homogeneously low-attenuation (< 10 HU) nodule. If the lesion is indeterminate or if only a contrast-enhanced scan was obtained, determine the attenuation of the mass on CECT, then repeat a series of thin sections through the adrenals after a delay of 15 minutes and measure the attenuation of the adrenal mass. Calculate the relative or absolute washout.

Adrenal Protocol, MR

Lipid-rich adrenal adenomas can be diagnosed with confidence on T1WI gradient-echo (GRE) sequences that include both in-phase and opposed-phase imaging. Loss of signal from an adrenal mass on opposed-phase imaging is essentially diagnostic of adenoma. Lipid-poor adenomas may remain indeterminate on MR and are best evaluated by adrenal protocol CT.

Approach to Adrenal Mass

Is it Adenoma?

Adrenal adenomas are extremely common, though most are "nonfunctional" or, more accurately, "not hyperfunctioning." It is estimated that some 2% of the general population has an adrenal adenoma, making this the most common cause of an adrenal mass, even in patients with a known extraadrenal malignancy. The high prevalence of adrenal adenomas in the general population, and large scale studies showing that the vast majority of adrenal "incidentalomas" are benign findings of no clinical significance, have prompted some authors to advocate a much more conservative approach to the small incidental adrenal lesion. Nonetheless, most professional societies continue to advocate an imaging and clinically intensive approach to incidental adrenal lesions depicted at CT. Most adenomas are rich in intra- and intercellular lipid, which creates a characteristic appearance as a homogeneous near-water-density (-5 to +10 HU) on a nonenhanced CT scan. The same lipid-rich adenomas have a characteristic appearance on MR as well. For the minority of adrenal adenomas that lack sufficient lipid, the best imaging test is an "adrenal protocol" CT scan. Adenomas are distinguished from metastases and most other adrenal masses by their characteristic "washout" of contrast, quickly returning to near baseline attenuation after the IV administration of contrast medium.

It's Not Adenoma, What Is It?

While other adrenal masses may share overlapping imaging characteristics, it is usually not problematic to make an accurate diagnosis when taking into account the imaging features and clinical and laboratory data in a particular patient. Both pheochromocytoma and metastases may result in a large, heterogeneous adrenal mass; however, correlation with the medical history, endocrine lab, and physical findings will usually obviate extensive or expensive additional imaging evaluation.

Are All Fat-Containing Adrenal Masses Adenomas?

Adenomas rarely contain macroscopic fat.

While the lipid in adrenal adenomas is microscopic fat, the presence of macroscopic deposits of fat characterizes a less common adrenal neoplasm, the myelolipoma (not to be confused with a renal angiomyolipoma, which is different in every regard). Myelolipoma is an uncommon benign adrenal neoplasm that can usually be diagnosed with confidence on CT or MR by the presence of mature, macroscopic fat deposits, ± calcification and soft tissue elements.

How Should We Image for Suspected Pheochromocytoma?

Before initiating an expensive imaging work-up, it is recommended to do the appropriate history, physical exam, and appropriate biochemical screening. In most patients, this will establish the presence or absence of this tumor.

Either CT or MR will easily detect most symptomatic pheochromocytomas, as these are typically 3-5 cm in diameter. While the IV administration of contrast media is often not necessary due to the large size of these lesions, it is safe to do so if needed as there have been no reported adverse effects of IV administration of nonionic contrast media in patients with pheochromocytoma.

How Should We Image for Suspected Adrenal Metastases?

While the adrenal glands are common sites of metastatic disease (and lymphoma), they are rarely the only site. Remember that an isolated small adrenal lesion in a cancer patient is still most likely to represent an adrenal adenoma, especially if it is of homogeneous low density.

PET/CT is being used more frequently in the staging of patients with cancer and lymphoma, and most adrenal metastases are FDG avid. The expense of PET/CT makes it more appropriate to use as part of an approved cancer staging evaluation rather than as a specific test to further evaluate an adrenal lesion that was detected by another imaging modality.

Selected References

1. Berland LL et al: Managing incidental findings on abdominal CT: white paper of the ACR incidental findings committee. J Am Coll Radiol. 7(10):754-73, 2010

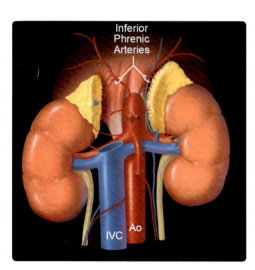
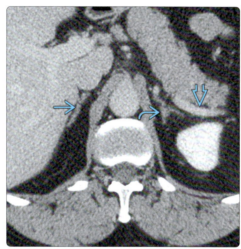

(Left) *Graphic shows typical adrenal anatomy. Note the multiple arterial sources. The right adrenal vein drains directly into the inferior vena cava (IVC), while the left enters the renal vein. Note that Ao = aorta.* (Right) *The right adrenal gland ➡ abuts the IVC and lies lateral to the right diaphragmatic crus and medial to the liver. The left adrenal gland ➡ usually lies ventral to the upper pole of the left kidney and behind the splenic vein ➡. The left adrenal appears as an inverted Y, while the right is more like an inverted V.*

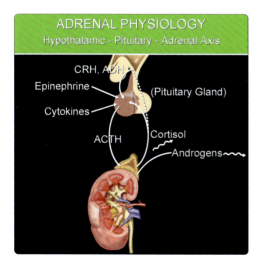
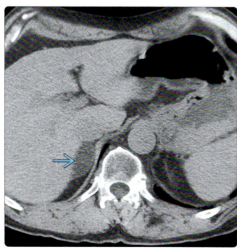

(Left) *Graphic shows stimulation of the anterior pituitary by epinephrine and cytokines or by hypothalamic release of corticotropin-releasing hormone (CRH) or antidiuretic hormone (ADH), resulting in the release of ACTH, causing the adrenal secretion of cortisol. Excess circulating cortisol inhibits further pituitary secretion.* (Right) *Axial NECT shows an incidental low-attenuation right adrenal mass ➡, which measures < 10 HU. This feature has > 90% specificity for the diagnosis of a lipid-rich adenoma.*

(Left) *Dedicated washout adrenal CT may be performed for indeterminate (> 10 HU) adrenal lesions at NECT to identify potential lipid-poor adenomas. The graph shows the formula for calculating adrenal washout on CT. Web-based calculators are readily available. Note that ROI = region of interest.* (Right) *Adrenal CT protocol is shown. NECT (A) shows an adrenal mass ➡ measuring 30 HU. The mass measures 60 HU on CECT (B) and 40 HU on delayed CT (C). The absolute washout of 67% is diagnostic of a lipid-poor adenoma.*

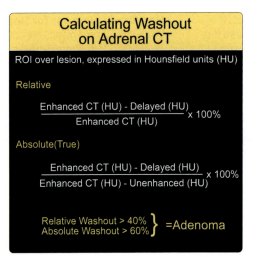

Calculating Washout on Adrenal CT

ROI over lesion, expressed in Hounsfield units (HU)

Relative

$$\frac{\text{Enhanced CT (HU) - Delayed (HU)}}{\text{Enhanced CT (HU)}} \times 100\%$$

Absolute (True)

$$\frac{\text{Enhanced CT (HU) - Delayed (HU)}}{\text{Enhanced CT (HU) - Unenhanced (HU)}} \times 100\%$$

Relative Washout > 40%
Absolute Washout > 60% } =Adenoma

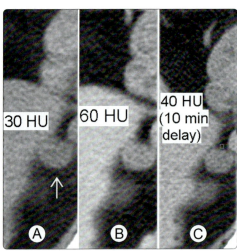

(Left) *Graph shows an imaging approach to the incidental adrenal mass. History and prior studies are crucial. Most adrenal lesions are benign, although characterization may be critical in the oncology population. Note that F/U = follow-up.* (Right) *Assessment of cortisol or epinephrine excess is also key for adrenal mass characterization. (Adapted with permission from L. Berland, MD, JACR.)*

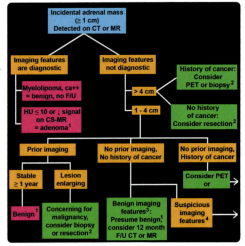

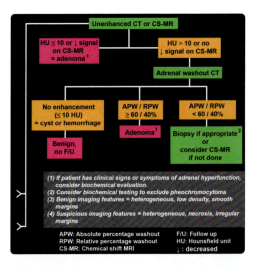

(Left) *On this in-phase T1WI GRE MR in a patient with bilateral adrenal nodules or small masses, only the left adrenal nodule is evident ➡.* (Right) *On opposed-phase T1WI GRE MR in the same patient, there is signal dropout from both adrenal nodules ➡, indicating a mixture of lipid and water protons. This is diagnostic of lipid-rich adenomas.*

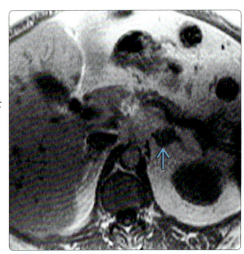

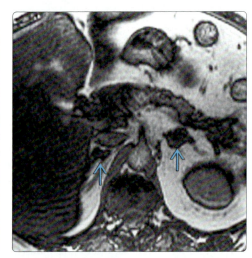

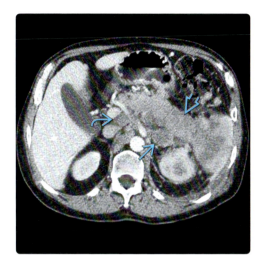
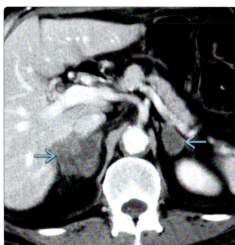

(Left) *Axial CECT in a patient with adrenal (and disseminated) lymphoma shows a left adrenal mass* ⮕ *as well as soft tissue-density masses that infiltrate the pancreas* ⮕*, spleen, and nodes* ⮕*.* (Right) *Axial CECT in a patient with adrenal metastases and esophageal carcinoma shows bilateral, heterogeneous, lobulated adrenal masses* ⮕*. PET/CT was performed prior to planned esophagectomy. These lesions were FDG avid, resulting in a cancellation of the planned curative esophagectomy.*

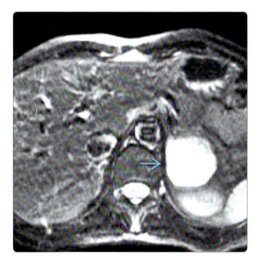
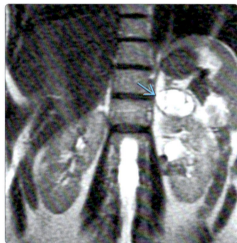

(Left) *Axial T2WI MR in a patient with pheochromocytoma shows a large left adrenal mass* ⮕ *that is heterogeneously hyperintense on T2WI and was hypointense on T1WI. The appearance is typical, although not pathognomonic, of a pheochromocytoma. The diagnosis was confirmed at resection.* (Right) *Coronal T2WI MR in the same patient shows the heterogeneously hyperintense mass* ⮕*, typical of a pheochromocytoma.*

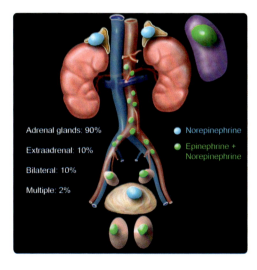
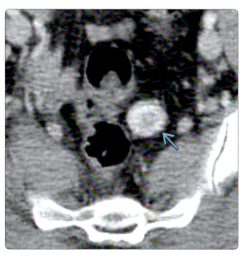

(Left) *Graphic indicates potential sites for pheochromocytoma (blue) and paraganglioma (green). Note the organ of Zuckerkandl at the aortic bifurcation.* (Right) *Axial CECT shows a hypervascular mass* ⮕ *in the pelvis. This was a paraganglioma with clinical symptoms identical to those of pheochromocytoma.*

Adrenal glands: 90%

Extraadrenal: 10%

Bilateral: 10%

Multiple: 2%

● Norepinephrine

● Epinephrine + Norepinephrine

Adrenal Hyperplasia

IMAGING

- Enlarged limbs of 1 or both adrenal glands > 10 mm width on CT
  - Glands may appear normal sized or multinodular
  - Adrenal gland shape is maintained
- Abdominal CT best for imaging adrenals
  - Contiguous < 3-mm axial images with multiplanar reformations
- Congenital adrenal hyperplasia
  - Causes most cases of adrenogenital syndrome (increased secretion of androgenic steroids)
  - Should be diagnosed in neonatal period; not imaging diagnosis
- Cushing syndrome (hypercortisolism)
  - Usually caused by pituitary adenoma
- Conn syndrome (primary hyperaldosteronism)
  - 80% of cases due to adrenal adenoma

TOP DIFFERENTIAL DIAGNOSES

- Adrenal adenoma
- Adrenal metastases and lymphoma
- Adrenal hemorrhage
- Pheochromocytoma

DIAGNOSTIC CHECKLIST

- Correlate clinical, biochemical, and imaging findings
- "Prominent" adrenals may be normal or temporary response to stress
- Multinodular hyperplasia is difficult to distinguish from adenoma by CT
- Most other causes of bilateral disease cause spherical masses in adrenals

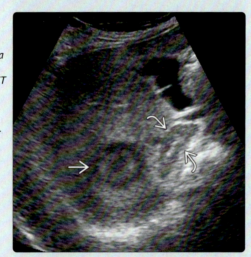
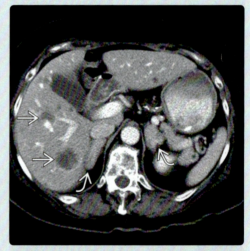

(Left) Right upper quadrant ultrasound performed on a cushingoid patient shows a right lobe metastasis ➡ and a diffusely enlarged right adrenal gland ⤵. (Right) CECT of the same patient shows diffusely enlarged adrenal glands ⤴ and multiple hepatic metastases ➡. Work-up for ectopic ACTH production revealed a small cell lung primary. Symmetric enlargement of the adrenal glands is the classic imaging manifestation of ACTH-dependent Cushing syndrome and adrenal hyperplasia.

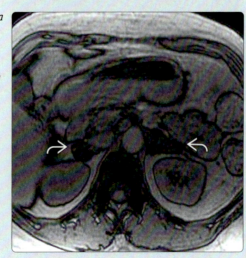
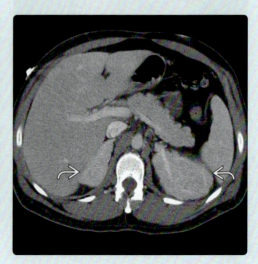

(Left) Out-of-phase T1 MR of a patient with Cushing syndrome shows signal suppression of enlarged, nodular adrenal glands ⤴. Work-up for causes of cortisol excess (exogenous steroids, ACTH-dependent and -independent Cushing syndrome) includes patient history, a battery of lab tests, and, potentially, imaging. Here, cortisol excess was due to pituitary adenoma. (Right) CECT of a young male patient shows massively enlarged adrenals ⤴, a characteristic feature of congenital adrenal hyperplasia.

Adrenal Insufficiency

TERMINOLOGY

- Addison disease
- Inadequate secretion of corticosteroids resulting from partial or complete destruction of adrenal glands

IMAGING

- Acute: Addisonian crisis, adrenal apoplexy
  o Heterogeneous, hyperdense, enlarged (hemorrhagic) adrenals
- Subacute
  o Enlarged glands with decreased density (caseation or necrosis)
- Chronic
  o Small, atrophic glands (autoimmune)
  o Dense, chunky calcifications (infection)

PATHOLOGY

- Idiopathic autoimmune disorders (80% of cases in developed countries)

- Granulomatous diseases: Tuberculosis (most common cause in underdeveloped nations), sarcoidosis
- Neoplasms: Metastases (e.g., lung, ovary, breast, kidney), lymphoma, leukemia
- Adrenal hemorrhage, necrosis, or thrombosis: Stress after surgery, shock, anticoagulation, sepsis (e.g., Waterhouse-Friderichsen syndrome), coagulation disorders, antiphospholipid syndrome
- Central adrenal insufficiency due to ↓ production/action of adrenocorticotrophic hormone (from either pituitary or hypothalamic disease)

CLINICAL ISSUES

- Chemistry: Hyponatremia, hyperkalemia, azotemia, hypercalcemia, hypoglycemia
- Acute symptoms: Fever, abdominal or back pain, hypotension, weakness
- Chronic symptoms: Progressive lethargy, weakness, cutaneous pigmentation, weight loss

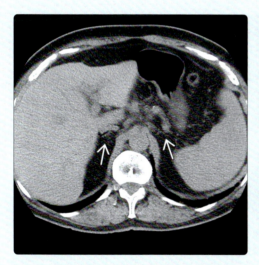
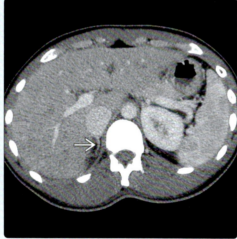

(Left) NECT of a 71-year-old woman with autoimmune polyendocrine syndrome (adrenal insufficiency, hypothyroidism) shows diminutive adrenals ➡. Interestingly, this patient also had a longstanding history of sarcoid, an additional cause for both primary and secondary (pituitary, hypothalamic) adrenal insufficiency. (Right) CECT of a young male with acute adrenal insufficiency shows a barely perceptible right adrenal gland ➡. A serum cortisol after cosyntropin stimulation was undetectable.

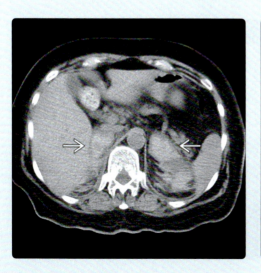
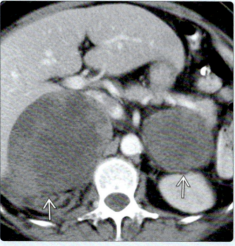

(Left) NECT of an elderly woman performed for evaluation of hypotension, hyponatremia, hypoglycemia, and sepsis post knee replacement shows bilateral adrenal hemorrhage ➡, a rare cause for acute adrenal insufficiency. (Right) Axial CECT of a male patient with advanced lung carcinoma shows massive necrotic adrenal metastases ➡. Lab data (↓ Na, ↑ K) and an ACTH stimulation test confirmed profound adrenal insufficiency, which was treated with steroid maintenance therapy.

Neonatal Adrenal Hemorrhage

TERMINOLOGY

- Perinatal bleeding into normal adrenal gland
  - Associated with many perinatal stressors: Asphyxia, sepsis, birth trauma, coagulopathies
  - ↑ frequency in full-term & large infants

IMAGING

- Right > left; bilateral in 5-10%
- US: Echogenic avascular mass replacing or expanding newborn adrenal gland
  - Appearance varies with timing of imaging
    - Acute: Hemorrhage appears echogenic & mass-like
    - Subacute: Blood products liquefy & contract, creating mixed echotexture mass
    - Chronic: Adrenal resumes normal size, ± Ca^{2+} or cyst
- CT, MR: Nonenhancing ± rim of enhancing adrenal
  - MR may show high T1 signal intensity &/or "blooming" on GRE, depending on age of blood products

- Radiographs (months to years later): Small unilateral or bilateral adreniform Ca^{2+}

TOP DIFFERENTIAL DIAGNOSES

- Neuroblastoma
- Congenital adrenal hyperplasia
- Extralobar bronchopulmonary sequestration

CLINICAL ISSUES

- Newborns may present with anemia, dropping hematocrit, jaundice, palpable mass, or adrenal insufficiency
  - Medical therapy for adrenal insufficiency rarely needed

DIAGNOSTIC CHECKLIST

- In neonate: Follow-up US in 2-6 weeks to confirm expected evolution with ↓ size
  - If larger or more solid, work-up for neuroblastoma
- In older child with incidental radiographic paraspinal Ca^{2+}
  - If morphology & extent unclear, start with abdominal ultrasound to exclude neuroblastoma

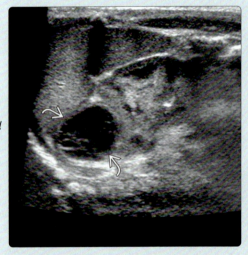
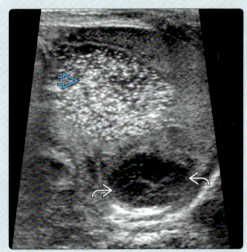

(Left) Longitudinal oblique ultrasound shows a complex cystic lesion ➥ in the adrenal gland of a neonate. There are many thin internal septations in this case of subacute neonatal adrenal hemorrhage. Adrenal hemorrhages are fairly common in neonates who are stressed by congenital heart disease, surgery, ECMO, sepsis, acidosis, etc. (Right) Transverse ultrasound of the same lesion shows fine internal septations ➥ in this evolving, partially liquefied hemorrhage. Note the tiny gas bubbles in the stomach ➥.

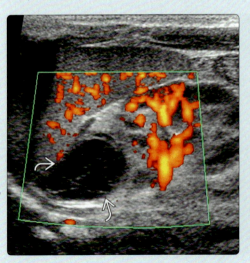
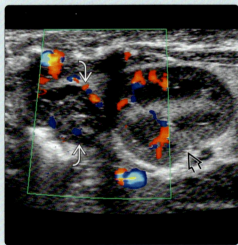

(Left) Longitudinal oblique power Doppler ultrasound of the same neonatal adrenal hemorrhage shows absence of blood flow in the lesion ➥ with normal perfusion of the adjacent kidney and spleen. (Right) Transverse oblique color Doppler ultrasound performed 2 months later shows partial resorption of the same hematoma with improved blood flow in the adrenal gland ➥. Mass effect on the left renal upper pole ➥ has resolved.

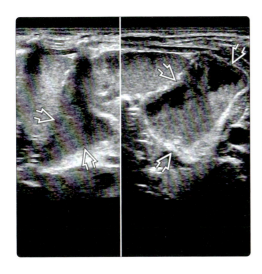

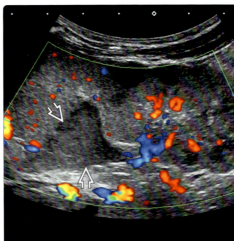

(Left) *Longitudinal (left) & transverse (right) images of the left suprarenal region in a 9-day-old infant with congenital heart disease show a mixed echogenicity lesion ➡ with well-defined margins between the spleen & kidney.* (Right) *Color Doppler US in the same patient shows absence of blood flow in the lesion ➡, typical of adrenal hemorrhage.*

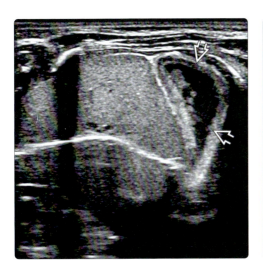

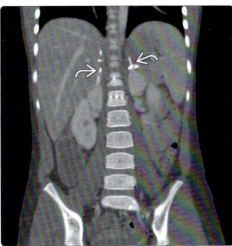

(Left) *Transverse ultrasound of the same lesion a week later shows progressive liquefaction ➡, consistent with evolving hemorrhage & confirming the benign nature of the "mass."* (Right) *Coronal CECT in an elementary school age patient (who had been a premature infant) shows Ca²⁺ in both adrenal regions ➡, likely due to remote neonatal adrenal hemorrhages.*

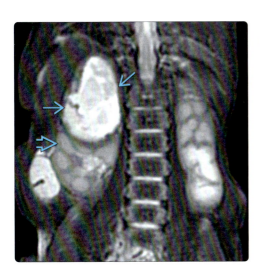

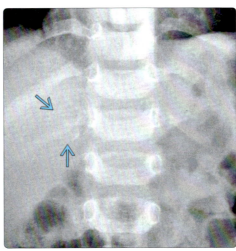

(Left) *Coronal T2 FS MR in a 20 day old with left prenatal hydronephrosis shows a heterogeneous right suprarenal mass ➡ deforming the right kidney ➡. The mass was T1 bright with a few foci of "blooming" on GRE (not shown). Serial ultrasounds showed progressive decrease in the size of the mass over the next 5 weeks.* (Right) *AP radiograph in the same patient 18 months later shows a small residual suprarenal Ca²⁺ ➡, consistent with a remote adrenal hemorrhage.*

IMAGING

- Relatively uncommon condition but potentially catastrophic event seen in patients of all ages
- More common in neonates than children and adults
- Nontraumatic hemorrhage (often bilateral): Causes are classified into 5 categories
  o Stress, hemorrhagic diathesis or coagulopathy, neonatal stress, adrenal tumors, idiopathic
- Manifest with adrenal insufficiency when 90% of adrenal tissue is destroyed
- Round or oval mass of high attenuation (50-90 HU)
  o Asymmetric enlargement of adrenal glands

PATHOLOGY

- Bilateral adrenal hemorrhage
  o Anticoagulation therapy (most common)
  o Stress: Surgery, sepsis, burns, hypotension, steroids
- Unilateral adrenal hemorrhage
  o Blunt abdominal trauma (right gland > left gland)

- Pathogenesis (nontraumatic)
  o Stress or adrenal tumor → increased adrenocorticotropic hormone → increased arterial blood flow + limited venous drainage → hemorrhage

CLINICAL ISSUES

- Waterhouse-Friderichsen syndrome: Skin rash, cough, headache, dizziness, arthralgias, and myalgias
  o Due to septicemia, especially with meningococcal organisms

DIAGNOSTIC CHECKLIST

- Check for history of trauma, anticoagulant therapy, coagulopathies, malignancies, stress, adrenal tumor
- NECT: Hyperdense lesion within adrenal gland
- MR: Varied signal intensity based on age of hematoma

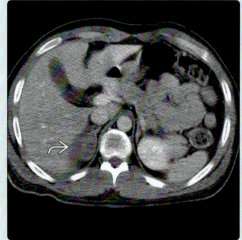
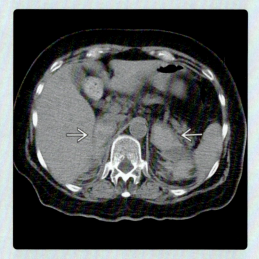

(Left) CECT of a young male patient post blunt trauma shows an isolated right adrenal hematoma ➘. Traumatic adrenal hemorrhage is typically associated with other abdominal visceral injuries and high injury severity scores. The presumed mechanism for this adrenal hemorrhage was an acute rise in adrenal venous pressure. (Right) NECT of an elderly female patient with adrenal insufficiency and overwhelming pneumococcal sepsis shows bilateral adrenal hemorrhage ➘.

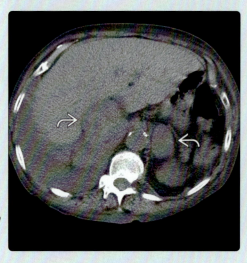
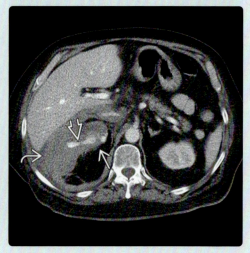

(Left) NECT of a hypotensive female patient with known metastatic non-small cell carcinoma shows bilateral adrenal hematomas ➚. Small preexisting adrenal metastases were shown on a prior staging CT. (Right) CECT of an anticoagulated patient shows right adrenal hemorrhage ➘, surrounding perinephric hemorrhage ➘, and active extravasation ➘. Although most adrenal hemorrhage can be managed conservatively, active extravasation and hypotension prompted angiography and embolization.

IMAGING

- "Adrenal cyst" is descriptive term, not pathological diagnosis
- True adrenal cysts
  - Majority are endothelial cysts (lymphangiomas)
  - Epithelial cysts exceedingly rare
  - Simple or minimally complex adrenal cyst, thin rim calcification, no enhancement
- Pseudocysts
  - Prior hemorrhage inferred
  - Nonenhancing but complex contents and wall calcification
  - Relevant history (extraadrenal malignancy, rapid growth), biochemical evaluation (cortisol, metanephrines): Consider underlying adrenal neoplasm
- Parasitic (echinococcal) cyst

TOP DIFFERENTIAL DIAGNOSES

- Adrenal adenoma

- CECT: Enhancing mass without visible wall or peripheral calcifications
- Gastric diverticulum
  - Air-, fluid-, or contrast-filled mass with no enhancement of contents
- Adrenal myelolipoma
  - Macroscopic fat
- Necrotic adrenal tumor
- Retroperitoneal bronchogenic cyst

CLINICAL ISSUES

- No treatment required usually
- Imaging surveillance performed, although intensity and length of follow-up not defined

DIAGNOSTIC CHECKLIST

- Complicated cyst has high attenuation, thick enhancing wall, &/or septations

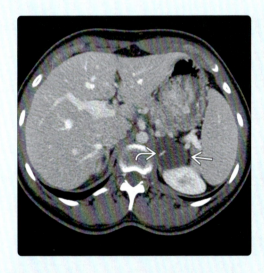
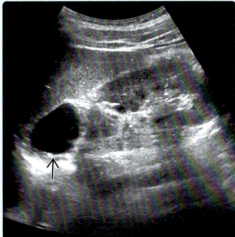

(Left) Axial CECT in a 28-year-old woman with abdominal pain shows an incidental left adrenal cystic lesion ➡. Note thin cyst septation ➡, a finding characteristic of an endothelial adrenal cyst. (Right) Ultrasound in the same patient confirms an anechoic left suprarenal-adrenal cyst ➡. The simple appearance of the cyst and the lack of additional relevant clinical history (malignancy, hypertension, etc.) prompted surveillance rather than resection for this incidental, benign endothelial cyst.

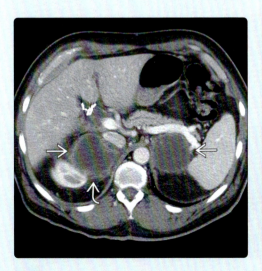
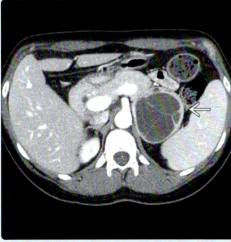

(Left) Staging CT examination in a 66-year-old man with metastatic lung carcinoma shows large bilateral necrotic adrenal metastases ➡. The clinical history and an enhancing rind ➡ prevent an erroneous diagnosis of benign adrenal cysts. (Right) Axial CECT in a hypertensive 36-year-old woman shows a peripherally enhancing, septated 7-cm left adrenal pheochromocytoma ➡. Enhancing soft tissue should prompt testing for an underlying adrenal neoplasm.

Adrenal Adenoma

KEY FACTS

IMAGING

- Well-circumscribed, uniform, low-attenuation, small adrenal mass
  - Low attenuation at NECT due to abundant intracytoplasmic lipid
  - Imaging features of typical lipid-rich adenomas
    - NECT: < 10 HU (71% sensitivity, 98% specificity)
    - MR: Significant decrease in signal intensity at out-of-phase T1W imaging (due to intravoxel lipid and water)
  - Lipid-poor adenomas (10-40% of cases): Utilize relative or absolute CT contrast washout kinetics for diagnosis (website calculators are readily available)
- Accounts for vast majority of adrenal "incidentalomas"
  - Imaging and lab intensive algorithm suggested for incidental adrenal lesions, though overwhelming majority are benign and hormonally inactive
  - Primary hyperaldosteronism (Conn syndrome): 80% due to unilateral, typically small (< 2-cm) adenoma
  - Cushing syndrome: 80-85% due to adrenal hyperplasia

TOP DIFFERENTIAL DIAGNOSES

- Adrenal metastases and lymphoma
- Adrenal myelolipoma
- Adrenal (macronodular) hyperplasia
- Pheochromocytoma
- Adrenal carcinoma
- Gastric diverticulum
- Adrenal cyst

DIAGNOSTIC CHECKLIST

- Asymptomatic mass
  - Usually nonfunctioning adenoma, even in patients with known cancer
- NECT and MR are equally accurate for diagnosis of lipid-rich adenoma
- Utilize dedicated CECT adrenal protocol for diagnosis of potential lipid-poor adenomas

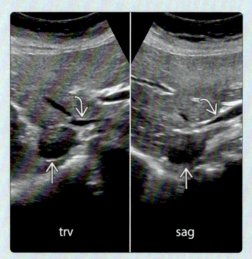
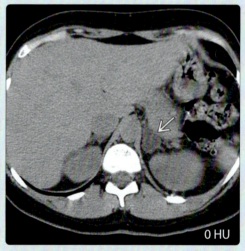

(Left) Transverse and sagittal ultrasounds of a 70-year-old woman with elevated liver function tests show an incidental solid right adrenal lesion ➡ posterior to the IVC ➡. Although statistically an adenoma, the ultrasound appearance is nonspecific. NECT confirmed a lipid-rich adenoma. (Right) Axial NECT of a 45-year-old man shows a uniform, 2-cm, low-attenuation (0 HU) left adrenal lesion ➡. NECT is typically the initial imaging modality of choice for adrenal mass characterization, but a follow-up MR was performed.

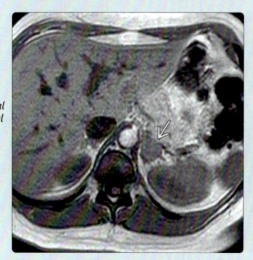
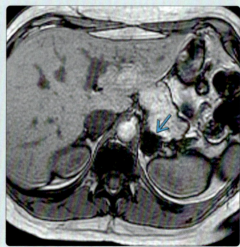

(Left) Axial T1 in-phase MR performed on the same patient shows a well-circumscribed, intermediate signal intensity left adrenal lesion ➡. (Right) The corresponding out-of-phase T1WI MR shows uniform signal suppression of the left adrenal gland ➡. Low attenuation (< 10 HU) at NECT and signal dropout at chemical shift MR are characteristic features of lipid-rich adenomas.

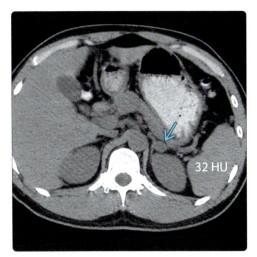
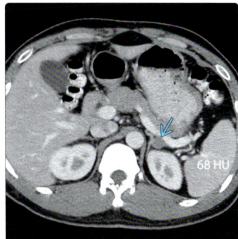

(Left) *A dedicated adrenal washout CT examination was performed in this 28-year-old man with an incidental, 1.5-cm, left adrenal nodule. The attenuation of the nodule before contrast administration was 32 HU ➡.* (Right) *The attenuation of the same left adrenal nodule ➡ increased to 68 HU during the portal venous phase of enhancement. The portal venous phase occurs ~ 70 seconds after initiation of an IV contrast bolus.*

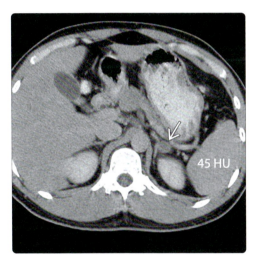
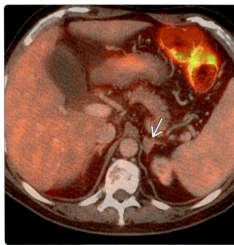

(Left) *Axial CECT of the same patient obtained 15 minutes post contrast administration shows nodule ➡ deenhancement to 45 HU. The absolute washout of > 60% is diagnostic of a lipid-poor adenoma. Adrenal CECT is utilized for indeterminate lesions at NECT or chemical shift MR.* (Right) *PET/CT examination of a 54-year-old man with a history of lymphoma shows a 1.8-cm left adrenal lesion ➡ with FDG uptake similar or less than the liver, a characteristic appearance of an incidental adrenal adenoma.*

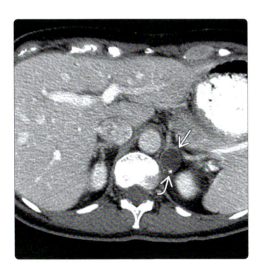
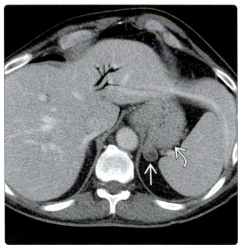

(Left) *Axial CECT shows a 3-cm, low-attenuation (2 HU) left adrenal mass ➡. No enhancement was shown relative to a baseline NECT. Note rim calcification ➡. Both are features of an adrenal (pseudo) cyst, a mimic of a lipid-rich adenoma.* (Right) *Axial CECT shows a low (6 HU) left suprarenal lesion ➡. Its location adjacent to the gastric fundus ➡ indicates a gastric diverticulum. Identification of gas or contrast within the "mass" and coronal images may prevent an erroneous diagnosis of a lipid-rich adenoma.*

Adrenal Myelolipoma

TERMINOLOGY

- Uncommon benign tumor composed of mature fat tissue and hematopoietic elements (myeloid and erythroid cells)

IMAGING

- Uncommon, benign, nonfunctioning adrenal tumor
- Accounts for 7-15% of incidental adrenal masses, usually in older population
- Typically unilateral and very rarely bilateral
- Large tumors can mimic retroperitoneal lipomas, liposarcomas
- Asymptomatic, though larger tumors may hemorrhage
- CT
  - Lesion containing fat attenuation (-30 to -90 HU): Fat within tumor is diagnostic
  - Usually well-defined mass with recognizable pseudocapsule (remaining adrenal)
  - Punctate calcifications seen (24% of cases)
  - Coronal reconstruction helpful to differentiate from exophytic renal angiomyolipoma
- MR
  - Tumor with major fat component
  - T1WI in phase: Typically hyperintense
  - Fat-suppression sequences: Loss of signal

TOP DIFFERENTIAL DIAGNOSES

- Adrenal adenoma
  - Intracellular lipid vs. macroscopic fat
- Adrenal metastases and lymphoma
- Retroperitoneal liposarcoma
- Pheochromocytoma
- Adrenal carcinoma
- Renal angiomyelolipoma
  - Coronal CT reconstruction or MR useful to determine organ of origin

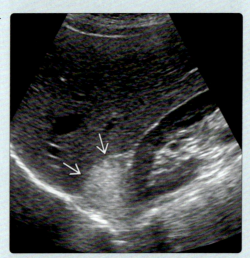
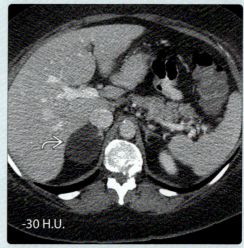

(Left) Ultrasound of a 52-year-old woman with right upper quadrant pain shows a subtle echogenic right suprarenal mass ➡. Even large myelolipomas may not be perceived at ultrasound given their isoechogenicity relative to retroperitoneal fat. (Right) Axial CECT of the same patient shows a fat-attenuation right adrenal lesion ➡. Macroscopic fat is the hallmark of myelolipomas, though the fat may be interspersed with soft tissue myeloid elements and hemorrhage.

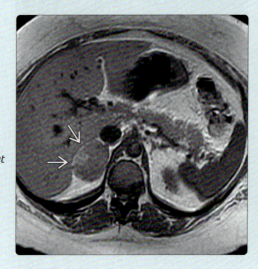
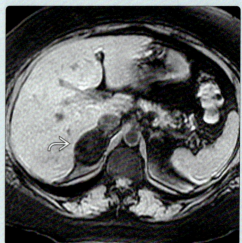

(Left) Follow-up T1WI MR shows a relatively intense right adrenal lesion ➡. No significant signal loss was demonstrated at out-phase imaging (not shown). (Right) Axial T1WI MR with fat saturation confirms that the right adrenal lesion ➡ is composed of fat, a finding pathognomonic of a myelolipoma. Macroscopic fat indicates a myelolipoma (as opposed to the intracellular lipid that is characteristic of adrenal adenomas).

Pheochromocytoma

TERMINOLOGY

- Tumor arising from chromaffin cells of adrenal medulla or extraadrenal paraganglia

IMAGING

- Adrenal medulla (90%)
- Extraadrenal (10%)
  - Along sympathetic chain: Anywhere from neck to urinary bladder
  - Subdiaphragmatic (98%); thorax (1-2%)
  - Organ of Zuckerkandl and near urinary bladder are relatively common sites
- Hereditary pheochromocytomas
  - Small, bilateral adrenal lesions in younger patient
- Sporadic pheochromocytoma
  - Large (> 3 cm) unilateral adrenal mass in older patient
- Ultrasound: Hypoechoic suprarenal lesion
  - Cystic components may be identified
- NECT: > 10 HU

- CECT
  - Delayed washout kinetics typically similar to adrenal carcinoma and metastases, but rapid washout (like adenoma) is possible
  - Heterogeneous enhancement: Necrosis, cystic degeneration, hemorrhage
- MR
  - Traditional, classic imaging feature: T2 ("light bulb") hyperintensity
    - Not specific or sensitive: Variable signal intensity due to hemorrhage, necrosis
  - Hypervascular solid components
- MIBG: For ectopic, recurrent, and metastatic tumors

DIAGNOSTIC CHECKLIST

- Pheochromocytoma is not distinguished from other tumors by imaging appearance alone
  - Clinical history and lab values are necessary for diagnosis

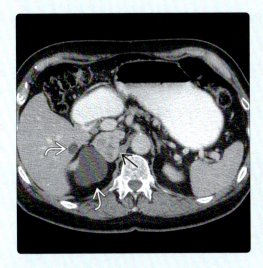

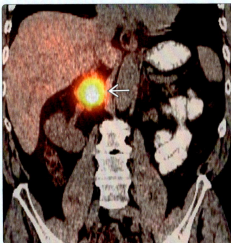

(Left) CECT performed on a 72-year-old man with right upper quadrant pain shows a vascular right adrenal lesion ➡. Vascularity and minimal washout prompted an evaluation for a pheochromocytoma. Note the adjacent right renal and hepatic cysts ➡. (Right) A 24-hour urine metanephrine evaluation of the same patient was positive. I-123 MIBG CT-SPECT exam (performed to exclude metastases) confirms a solitary 4-cm right adrenal pheochromocytoma ➡.

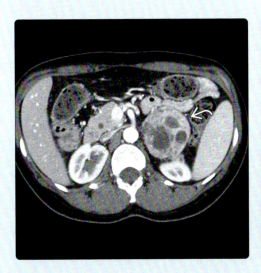

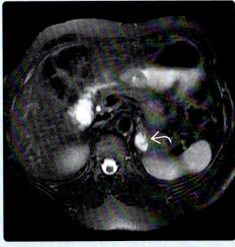

(Left) CECT shows a 7-cm left adrenal mass ➡. The DDx includes adrenal carcinoma, pheochromocytoma, or a metastasis. Urinary metanephrines were ↑. Laparoscopic resection (after a and β blockade) confirmed a pheochromocytoma. (Right) T2WI MR shows a T2-intense ("light bulb") left adrenal lesion ➡. Although this appearance was historically thought to be characteristic of pheochromocytomas, it is neither sensitive nor specific. ↑ 24-hour urine metanephrines confirmed a pheochromocytoma.

TERMINOLOGY

- Malignant tumor of sympathetic chain primitive neural crest cells
- Increasing degrees of cellular differentiation/benignity along spectrum: Neuroblastoma (malignant) → ganglioneuroblastoma → ganglioneuroma (benign)

IMAGING

- Location
  - Adrenal (35-48%)
  - Extraadrenal retroperitoneum (25-35%)
  - Posterior mediastinum (16-20%)
- Small round solitary mass vs. large multilobulated lesion
- Aggressive tumor with tendency to invade adjacent tissues
- Frequently engulfs & displaces adjacent vascular structures (rather than just displacing)
- Ca^{2+} in up to 90% by CT
- Metastases in 50-60% at diagnosis, most commonly to bone, lymph nodes, liver, soft tissues

TOP DIFFERENTIAL DIAGNOSES

- Wilms tumor
- Neonatal adrenal hemorrhage
- Less common adrenal tumors
- Other cystic/solid suprarenal lesions

CLINICAL ISSUES

- Most common extracranial solid malignancy in children
- Median age at diagnosis: 15-17 months
- Wide variety of clinical presentations; most commonly presents as palpable abdominal mass
- Features associated with better prognosis
  - Age at diagnosis < 18 months
  - Stage 4S/MS
  - Localized tumor not involving vital structures
  - Absent *MYCN* (N-myc) oncogene amplification

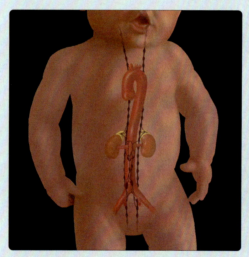
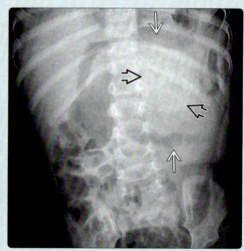

(Left) *This graphic shows the anatomic extent of the sympathetic chain ganglia (including the adrenal glands) from the cervical region to the pelvis. Neuroblastoma (NBL) can arise anywhere along the sympathetic chain.* (Right) *Supine AP abdominal radiograph in a 1-year-old boy with a palpable abdominal mass shows displacement of bowel loops ➡ by a large, heterogeneously calcified mass ➡ in the left abdomen.*

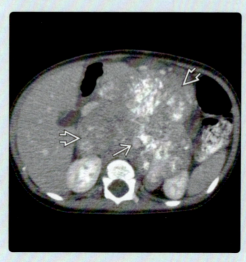
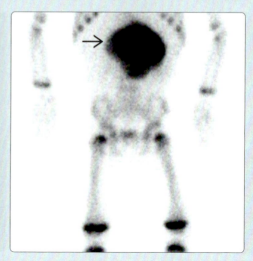

(Left) *Axial CECT in the same patient shows the large, lobulated, calcified mass ➡ crossing the midline. The mass encases & lifts the aorta ➡ off of the spine. These features are typical of NBL.* (Right) *Anterior Tc-99m nuclear medicine bone scan in the same patient shows radiotracer uptake ➡ throughout the heavily calcified abdominal mass. No cortical bone metastases were detected in this study. Note the intense (but normal) radiotracer uptake at the primary growth centers of the visualized bones.*

TERMINOLOGY

Definitions

- Malignant tumor of sympathetic chain primitive neural crest cells
- Increasing degrees of cellular differentiation/benignity along spectrum: Neuroblastoma [(NBL), malignant] → ganglioneuroblastoma (GNBL) → ganglioneuroma [(GN), benign]

IMAGING

General Features

- Best diagnostic clue
  - Partially calcified, lobulated suprarenal/paraspinal mass in infant
- Location
  - Anywhere along sympathetic chain from neck to pelvis
    - Adrenal (35-48%)
      - 90% adrenal in prenatally detected cases
    - Extraadrenal retroperitoneum (25-35%)
    - Posterior mediastinum (16-20%)
    - Pelvis (2-3%)
    - Neck (1-5%)
    - Metastatic disease with no primary identified (1%)
- General imaging features
  - Small, round, solitary suprarenal/paraspinal mass vs. large, lobulated lesion crossing midline
  - Aggressive tumor, may invade adjacent tissues
    - Intraspinal invasion via neural foramina
    - Kidney, muscle
  - Frequently engulfs & displaces adjacent vascular structures (rather than just displacing/compressing)
  - Ca^{2+} in up to 90% by CT
  - Metastases in 50-60% at diagnosis, most commonly to bone, lymph nodes, liver, soft tissues
    - Liver: Well-defined focal vs. extensive poorly defined lesions with hepatomegaly
    - Bone: Focally destructive cortical &/or well-defined or confluent intramedullary lesions
    - Soft tissues: Cutaneous/subcutaneous lesions may be visible on physical exam & imaging

Radiographic Findings

- Often occult or subtle by radiographs
  - Ca^{2+} in only 30% by radiography
- Displacement of bowel by soft tissue mass
- Widening of inferior thoracic paraspinal soft tissues
  - May be only finding of retrocrural extension of upper abdominal mass
- Subtle bony clues of soft tissue mass
  - Splaying/remodeling of adjacent ribs
  - Vertebral body scalloping, small pedicle
- Bone metastasis
  - May be extensive with little radiographic presence (especially marrow disease)
  - May be only presenting clinical/imaging finding

CT Findings

- Mass often heterogeneous from necrosis, hemorrhage
  - Ca^{2+} in up to 90% by CT

MR Findings

- Generally intermediate to high T2/intermediate to low T1 signal intensity
  - Heterogeneity from Ca^{2+}, hemorrhage, necrosis
- Variable enhancement from none to intermediate
- Excellent depiction of intraspinal extension
- High sensitivity/specificity for marrow disease (but ↓ specificity post therapy)

Ultrasonographic Findings

- Grayscale ultrasound
  - Mass often heterogeneous
    - Ca^{2+} causing echogenic foci ± posterior acoustic shadowing
  - Suprarenal location displaces/distorts kidney
- Color Doppler
  - Variable internal tumor vascularity
  - Vessels engulfed/lifted by tumor

Nuclear Medicine Findings

- Bone scan
  - Tc-99m MDP
  - ↑ uptake in bony metastasis (cortical > marrow)
  - May be useful in follow-up of non-MIBG-avid NBL
  - Uptake in primary mass in up to 74% of cases
- PET
  - 18-FDG remains primary radiotracer
  - High sensitivity for soft tissue & bony NBL, though generally < MIBG
    - Select populations may benefit from PET, particularly non-MIBG-avid disease
- MIBG scintigraphy
  - I-123 MIBG for diagnosis, staging, follow-up imaging
  - MIBG related to norepinephrine; therefore, avid uptake in catecholamine production process
  - ↑ uptake at any site of active NBL
    - Sensitivity, specificity: ~ 90% in NBL
  - Evaluates bony cortical & marrow disease
  - In MIBG-avid tumors, posttherapy evaluation more specific than MR or FDG-PET

Imaging Recommendations

- Best imaging tool
  - US excellent 1st-line modality for palpable abdominal mass in child
  - MR increasingly used over CT for characterizing tumor & defining extent at diagnosis & follow-up
  - MIBG remains favored nuclear medicine study for diagnosis, staging, follow-up

DIFFERENTIAL DIAGNOSIS

Wilms Tumor

- Mean age: 3 years
- Ca^{2+} uncommon
- Grows like ball, displacing vessels
- Arises from kidney: Claw sign of residual renal parenchyma along tumor
- Lung metastases in 20%
- Invasion of renal vein + inferior vena cava

Neonatal Adrenal Hemorrhage

- Cystic &/or solid-appearing avascular suprarenal mass
- Serial US show gradual ↓ in size with ↑ Ca^{2+}

Less Common Adrenal Tumors

- Pheochromocytoma (uncommon in young children)
- Adrenal cortical neoplasms (usually hormonally active)

Other Cystic/Solid Suprarenal Lesions

- Congenital adrenal hyperplasia
- Extralobar bronchopulmonary sequestration
- Foregut duplication cyst
- Lymphatic malformation

PATHOLOGY

General Features

- Genetics
  - Increased copies of *MYCN* oncogene (*MYCN* or N-myc amplification): Poorer prognosis (even stage MS)
  - Deletion of 1p, 11q alleles: Poorer prognosis
  - DNA index (measure of ploidy): Better prognosis from 1.26-1.76 (near triploid)
  - Only 1-2% of cases familial, often with multiple primary tumors in infants
- Associated abnormalities
  - Neurofibromatosis type 1, Beckwith-Wiedemann syndrome, Hirschsprung disease
  - Most NBL cases occur in children without associations

Staging, Grading, & Classification

- International NBL Staging System
  - Original 1-4S system based on resection, pathology (1988, 1993)
  - Used for risk groups by Children's Oncology Group (COG)
- International NBL Risk Group Staging System
  - More comprehensive, imaging-based system (2009)
  - Utilizes modifying image-defined risk factors
    - L1: Tumor in 1 body compartment, no vital structures involved
    - L2: Tumor in 2 body compartments **or** encasing/invading major structures
    - M: Distant metastases
    - MS: Age < 18 months; metastases confined to skin, liver, bone marrow
      - Bones (including marrow) must be clear by MIBG to qualify for stage 4S/MS (with marrow disease limited to less than 10% involvement by biopsy)
  - Used to stratify as very low, low, intermediate, or high risk in conjunction with age, genetics, histology
    - May replace COG risk stratification

Microscopic Features

- Malignant tumor of primitive neural crest cells
- Composed of neuroblastic cells (small round blue cells) + schwannian stroma cells
  - Shimada classification combines histology + age
- Homer Wright rosettes: Circular orientation of NBL cells around neuropil

CLINICAL ISSUES

Presentation

- Most common signs/symptoms
  - Painless abdominal mass
- Other signs/symptoms
  - Malaise, irritability, weight loss, limping, opsoclonus-myoclonus, Horner syndrome, cerebellar ataxia, neurologic symptoms related to compression, hypertension, watery diarrhea with hypokalemia
  - Classic presentations
    - Skin metastases: Blueberry muffin syndrome
    - Skull base metastases: "Raccoon eyes"
    - Massive liver metastases: Pepper syndrome
  - 90-95% of NBL patients have elevated levels of catecholamines/metabolites (VMA, HVA) in urine

Demographics

- Age
  - Median age at presentation: 15-17 months
  - 95% diagnosed by 7 years
- Epidemiology
  - Most common extracranial solid malignancy in children
    - Most common malignancy of infancy

Natural History & Prognosis

- COG risk stratification
  - Low risk (30% of all NBL, 70% of neonatal NBL): 5-year survival > 95% with observation (select cases) or surgery
    - Spontaneous regression most likely in
      - Newborns with small adrenal lesions
      - Non-*MYCN* amplified infants with localized disease or asymptomatic 4S/MS disease
  - Intermediate risk (20% of all NBL): 5-year survival > 90% with surgery + chemotherapy
  - High risk (50% of all NBL): 5-year survival of 30-40% with intensive multimodality therapy
    - May include myeloablative therapy with stem cell rescue, biologic agents, I-131 MIBG therapy, especially for refractory/recurrent disease

SELECTED REFERENCES

1. Irwin MS et al: Neuroblastoma: paradigm for precision medicine. Pediatr Clin North Am. 62(1):225-56, 2015
2. Maki E et al: Imaging and differential diagnosis of suprarenal masses in the fetus. J Ultrasound Med. 33(5):895-904, 2014
3. Sharp SE et al: Functional-metabolic imaging of neuroblastoma. Q J Nucl Med Mol Imaging. 57(1):6-20, 2013
4. Fisher JP et al: Neonatal neuroblastoma. Semin Fetal Neonatal Med. 17(4):207-15, 2012
5. Nour-Eldin NE et al: Pediatric primary and metastatic neuroblastoma: MRI findings: pictorial review. Magn Reson Imaging. 30(7):893-906, 2012
6. Brisse HJ et al: Guidelines for imaging and staging of neuroblastic tumors: consensus report from the International Neuroblastoma Risk Group Project. Radiology. 261(1):243-57, 2011
7. McCarville MB: Imaging neuroblastoma: what the radiologist needs to know. Cancer Imaging. 11 Spec No A:S44-7, 2011
8. Sharp SE et al: Pediatrics: diagnosis of neuroblastoma. Semin Nucl Med. 41(5):345-53, 2011
9. Cohn SL et al: The International Neuroblastoma Risk Group (INRG) classification system: an INRG Task Force report. J Clin Oncol. 27(2):289-97, 2009
10. Lonergan GJ et al: Neuroblastoma, ganglioneuroblastoma, and ganglioneuroma: radiologic-pathologic correlation. Radiographics. 22(4):911-34, 2002

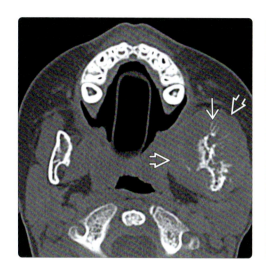

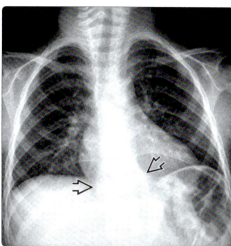

(Left) Axial bone CT in a 3-year-old boy with a hard left facial mass shows a soft tissue tumor ⇨ arising from an abnormal left mandibular ramus. Note the cortical destruction & permeation of the ramus with an aggressive periosteal reaction of radiating perpendicular spicules ⇨. This finding is commonly seen in NBL metastases to the skull. (Right) AP chest radiograph in the same patient shows widening of the lower thoracic paraspinal stripes ⇨, a common finding in NBL due to its sympathetic chain origin.

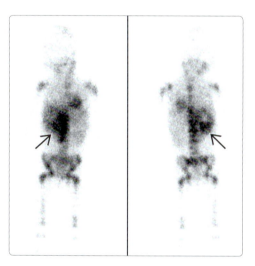

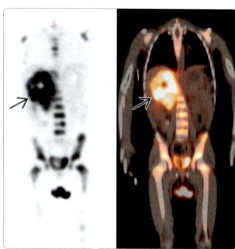

(Left) Anterior & posterior I-123 MIBG scans in a 2-year-old NBL patient show uptake throughout the primary tumor ⇨ in the right abdomen as well as numerous foci of skeletal metastases. Note that the skeleton is not normally visualized with MIBG, making all foci of bony uptake in these images consistent with metastatic disease. (Right) F-18 FDG-PET & fused PET/CT images in the same patient show increased metabolic activity within the primary tumor ⇨ as well as numerous sites of skeletal disease.

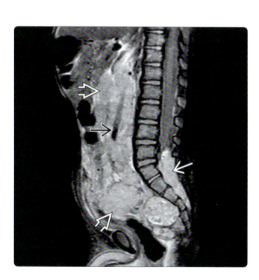

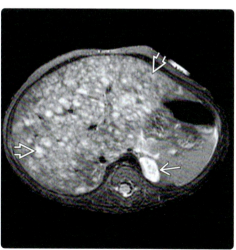

(Left) Sagittal STIR MR in a 2-year-old NBL patient shows a large retroperitoneal mass ⇨ encasing & displacing the aorta ⇨. Intraspinal extension ⇨ is also seen distally. (Right) Axial T2 FS MR in a 2-month-old boy with hepatomegaly shows innumerable hyperintense lesions ⇨ throughout the liver. The hyperintense left suprarenal mass ⇨ essentially confirms metastatic NBL, though specific histologic tumor analysis is required for complete determination of diagnosis, staging, & therapy.

Adrenal Carcinoma

IMAGING

- Best tool: CT or MR, including multiplanar views
- CECT shows most important aspects of tumor
  - Large, solid, unilateral adrenal mass with invasive margins (bilateral in 10%)
  - Functioning tumors: Usually 5 cm at presentation
  - Nonfunctioning tumors: ≥ 10 cm
  - Washout kinetics similar to adrenal metastases
- May contain hemorrhagic or cystic areas
  - Calcification within tumor seen in 30% of cases
- ± venous invasion, renal vein and inferior vena cava (IVC)
- ± invasion into adjacent renal parenchyma
- Metastases to lung bases, liver, or retroperitoneal nodes
  - Best shown on CT
- MR optimal for characterizing abdominal extent
  - T1 C+: Heterogeneous enhancement (tumor necrosis)
  - Renal vein, IVC, and adjacent renal parenchymal invasion well depicted on MR
  - Sagittal imaging helps to evaluate IVC invasion
  - Delineate tumor-liver interface if tumor on right
- PET/CT: Marked FDG uptake

TOP DIFFERENTIAL DIAGNOSES

- Adrenal adenoma
- Adrenal metastases and lymphoma
- Adrenal myelolipoma
- Pheochromocytoma
- Upper pole of renal cell carcinoma
- Adrenal hemorrhage (hematoma)
- Ganglioneuroma

DIAGNOSTIC CHECKLIST

- Typical: Large, unilateral adrenal mass with invasive margins, venous nodal invasion, and lung metastases

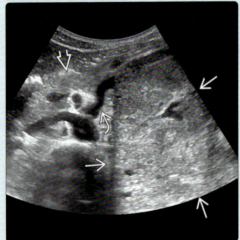 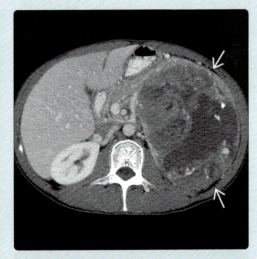

(Left) *Ultrasound performed on a 34-year-old man shows a huge solid left retroperitoneal mass ⮞ that displaces the left renal vein ⮞ and pancreas ⮞ anteriorly. The mass was separate from the left kidney at real-time sonography.* (Right) *CECT of the same patient shows a huge vascular and necrotic left upper quadrant mass ⮞. An endocrine evaluation was negative, and an oncocytic adrenal carcinoma was resected. Nonfunctional adrenal carcinomas are typically large and invasive at presentation.*

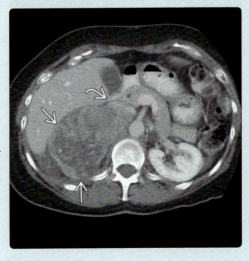 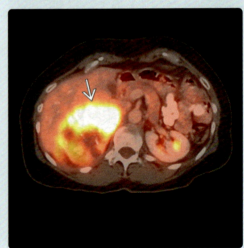

(Left) *CECT of a 55-year-old woman shows a 13-cm vascular, necrotic, right suprarenal mass ⮞ that displaces and is inseparable from the inferior vena cava ⮞. An endocrine work-up was positive for ↑ urinary cortisol and metanephrines.* (Right) *PET/CT examination of the same patient shows marked FDG uptake in the nonnecrotic portions of the mass ⮞. An adrenal carcinoma was resected. Marked FDG uptake and venous invasion are characteristic features of this aggressive tumor.*

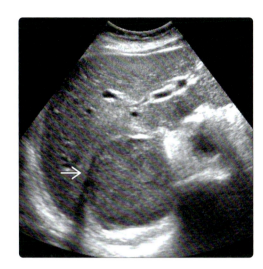

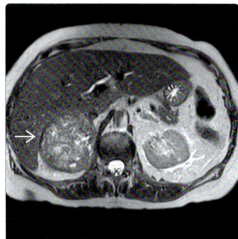

(Left) *Ultrasound shows a solid right suprarenal mass* ➡. *The DDx of large, hypoechoic solid adrenal lesions is nonspecific but it includes metastases, pheochromocytomas, and adrenal carcinomas.* (Right) *T2 MR of the same patient shows a mixed-intensity right adrenal mass* ➡. *An adrenal carcinoma adherent to the liver was identified during a debulking attempt. The prognosis for most adrenal carcinomas is dismal, and chemotherapeutic options are limited.*

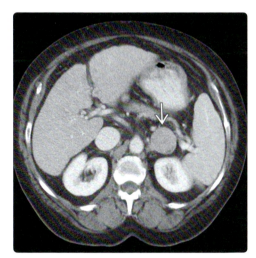

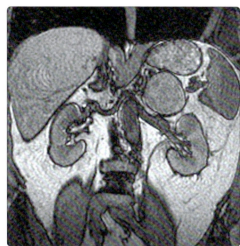

(Left) *Surveillance CECT of a 59-year-old woman with cirrhosis shows growth of an enhancing 4-cm indeterminate left adrenal mass* ➡. *A follow-up adrenal CT showed that relative washout of the lesion was < 40%.* (Right) *T1 opposed-phase MR of the same patient shows no loss of signal from the left adrenal lesion. Growth and imaging features ruling out either a lipid-rich or -poor adenoma prompted resection. A low-grade T1 stage adrenal carcinoma with vascular invasion was resected.*

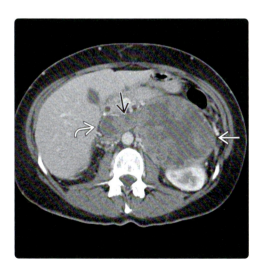

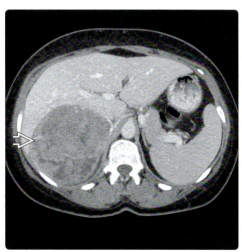

(Left) *CECT shows a huge left suprarenal mass* ➡ *with tumor thrombus in left renal vein* ➡ *and cava* ➡. *Renal cell carcinoma (RCC) was suspected at both imaging and surgery, but invasive adrenal carcinoma was identified at pathology.* (Right) *CECT shows a huge right suprarenal mass* ➡. *Nonfunctioning adrenal carcinoma was suspected at both CT and surgery, but clear cell RCC was identified within en bloc specimen. Both cases demonstrate the difficulty of differentiating adrenal carcinoma from upper pole RCC.*

T | Definition of Primary Tumor (T)

T Category	T Criteria
TX	Primary tumor cannot be assessed
T0	No evidence of primary tumor
T1	Tumor ≤ 5 cm in greatest dimension, no extraadrenal invasion
T2	Tumor > 5 cm, no extraadrenal invasion
T3	Tumor of any size with local invasion but not invading adjacent organs (adjacent organs include kidney, diaphragm, great vessels, pancreas, spleen, and liver)
T4	Tumor of any size with invasion of adjacent organs (kidney, diaphragm, pancreas, spleen, or liver) or large blood vessels (renal vein or vena cava)

Adapted with permission from AJCC Cancer Staging Manual 8th ed., 2017.

N | Definition of Regional Lymph Node (N)

N Category	N Criteria
NX	Regional lymph nodes cannot be assessed
N0	No regional lymph node metastasis
N1	Metastasis in regional lymph node(s)

Adapted with permission from AJCC Cancer Staging Manual 8th ed., 2017.

M | Definition of Distant Metastasis (M)

M Category	M Criteria
M0	No distant metastasis
M1	Distant metastasis

Adapted with permission from AJCC Cancer Staging Manual 8th ed., 2017.

AJCC | Prognostic Stage Groups

When T is...	And N is...	And M is...	Then the stage group is...
T1	N0	M0	I
T2	N0	M0	II
T1	N1	M0	III
T2	N1	M0	III
T3	Any N	M0	III
T4	Any N	M0	III
Any T	Any N	M1	IV

Adapted with permission from AJCC Cancer Staging Manual 8th ed., 2017.

T1

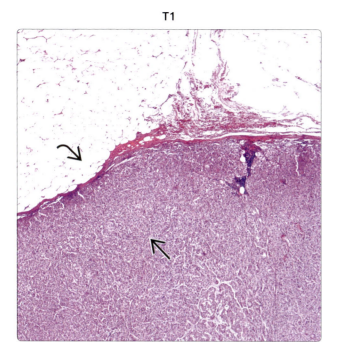

Low-power magnification of an H&E section shows sheets of adrenal cortical neoplastic cells ➡ that are limited to the adrenal gland (T1). Adipose tissue ➡ surrounding the adrenal gland is negative for tumor. (Original magnification: 40x.)

T2

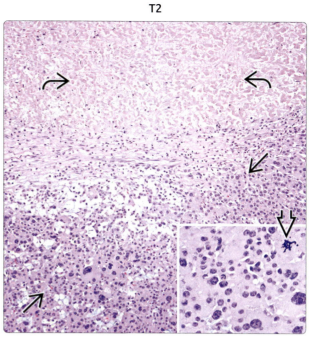

Photomicrograph shows an H&E section from adrenal cortical carcinoma ➡ with large areas of necrosis in the upper aspect of the slide ➡. The inset shows the particularly striking nuclear pleomorphism (large vs. small nuclei) as well as a mitotic figure ➡. (Original magnification: 400x.)

T3

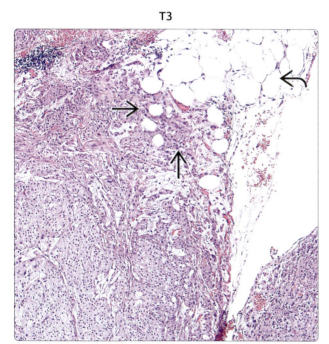

H&E stain shows a tumor with local invasion but no extension into the adjacent organs, consistent with T3 disease. The adrenal cortical carcinoma invades ➡ locally into the surrounding adrenal fat ➡. (Original magnification: 100x.)

T4

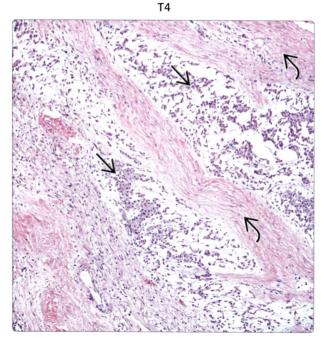

In T4 disease, a tumor invades into the adjacent organs. This tumor extends to involve the diaphragm. This photomicrograph shows the neoplastic tumor cells ➡ extending into surrounding fibrotic connective tissue ➡. (Original magnification: 400x.)

T1

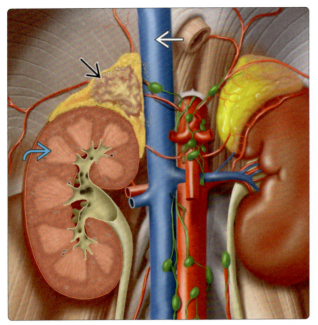

Coronal graphic demonstrates T1 disease. The primary tumor ➡️ is ≤ 5 cm in greatest dimension without invasion of the adjacent organs, including kidney ➡️ or inferior vena cava (IVC) ➡️.

T2

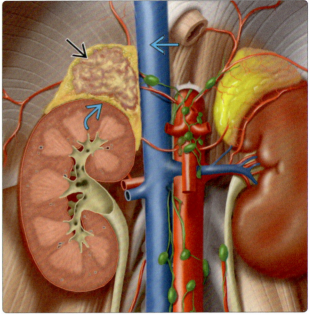

Coronal graphic demonstrates T2 disease. The primary tumor ➡️ is > 5 cm in greatest dimension without invasion of the adjacent organs, including kidney ➡️ or IVC ➡️.

T3

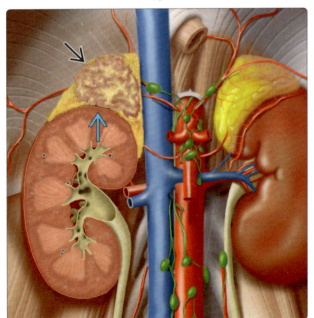

Coronal graphic demonstrates T3 disease. The primary tumor may be any size with local invasion beyond the confines of the adrenal capsule, shown in the superolateral margin ➡️, but no involvement of the adjacent organs, such as the kidney ➡️.

T4

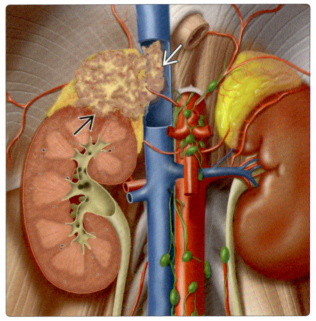

Coronal graphic demonstrates T4 disease. The primary tumor can be any size with local invasion beyond the confines of the adrenal capsule and into the adjacent organs, including the kidney ➡️. Direct extension into the IVC is illustrated ➡️.

T4

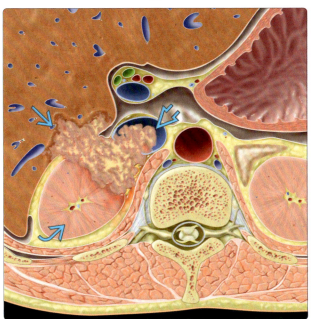

N1 and M1

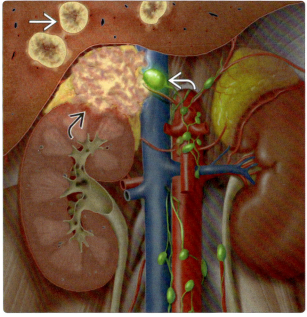

Axial graphic demonstrates right-sided adrenal cortical carcinoma invading the adjacent organs, including the right kidney ➡, liver ➡, and IVC ➡.

Coronal graphic shows primary adrenal cortical carcinoma with invasion into the adjacent kidney ➡. N1 and M1 disease with an enlarged paraaortic lymph node ➡ and multifocal hepatic metastases ➡ are also illustrated.

Metastases, Organ Frequency

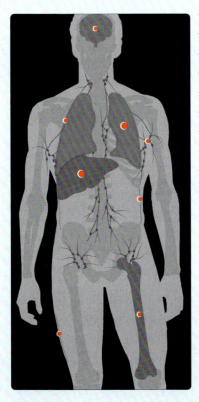

Liver	11%
Lung	9%
Bone	3%
Distant lymph nodes	2%
Peritoneum	1%
CNS	< 1%
Pleura	< 1%
Skin	< 1%

Data from Bilimoria KY et al: Adrenocortical carcinoma in the United States: treatment utilization and prognostic factors. Cancer. 113(11):3130-6, 2008.

IMAGING

- CT: Mild enhancement of bilateral adrenal masses
- MR: T2-intense, T1-isointense (to muscle), bulky adrenal masses
- Ultrasound: Hypoechoic suprarenal lesions
- PET/CT: Hypermetabolic adrenal tumor

TOP DIFFERENTIAL DIAGNOSES

- Adrenal metastases
  - Heterogeneous adrenal masses
  - Clinical history, identification of primary lesion aids diagnosis
  - Adrenal insufficiency rare despite size
- Adrenal hemorrhage
  - High attenuation at NECT in acute setting
  - Predisposing history: Sepsis, anticoagulation
- Adrenal adenoma
  - Typically incidental finding
  - Attenuation < 10 HU at NECT, contrast kinetics (rapid washout)
- Adrenal tuberculosis and fungal infection
  - May also present with adrenal insufficiency
  - Necrotic adrenal masses in acute setting
  - Chronic infection: Adrenal calcification

PATHOLOGY

- Majority are diffuse large B-cell lymphoma
- Little or no extraadrenal visceral, nodal involvement

CLINICAL ISSUES

- B symptoms (fever, night sweats, weight loss), adrenal insufficiency
- Poor prognosis

DIAGNOSTIC CHECKLIST

- Consider if large bilateral adrenal masses, in elderly male patient with adrenal insufficiency, and no known primary malignancy

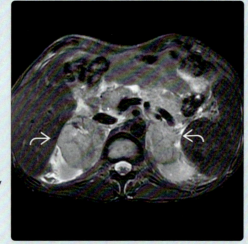
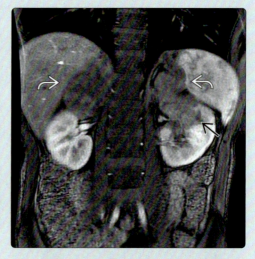

(Left) Axial T2 TSE performed on a 36-year-old male patient with malaise and adrenal insufficiency shows bilateral bulky T2-intense adrenal masses ➡. (Right) Coronal GD-enhanced T1 C+ MR in the same patient shows both adrenal masses ➡ mildly enhanced. Note the direct extension of tumor into the upper pole of the left kidney ➡. The differential diagnosis includes adrenal metastases, although adrenal insufficiency and lack of a history of an extra-adrenal primary suggests an alternative diagnosis.

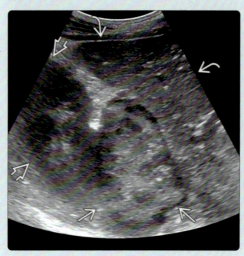
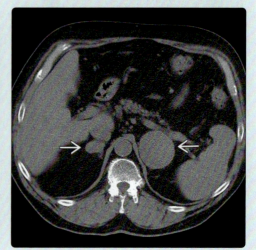

(Left) Ultrasound performed prior to biopsy on the same patient shows a large mixed echogenicity mass ➡ adjacent to the kidney ➡ and liver ➡. The biopsy revealed B-cell lymphoma. Complete remission was achieved after CHOP and rituximab. (Right) NECT performed on an elderly male patient with fatigue and adrenal insufficiency shows large adrenal masses ➡. No additional nodal or visceral disease was identified. A diagnosis of primary large B-cell lymphoma was confirmed after ultrasound-guided biopsy.

TERMINOLOGY

- Refers to 2 adjacent but histologically different tumors within same adrenal gland (no histologic admixture at interface)
  - Not a composition tumor (i.e., tumor containing admixture of 2 different cell types)
  - Adenoma and myelolipoma reported to be most common adrenal collision tumor, though adenomas may contain small foci of macroscopic fat

IMAGING

- Both tumors may be malignant, both may be benign, or 1 malignant and 1 benign
- FDG-avid mass suggests malignant tumor
- CT to recognize adrenal mass
- PET/CT to characterize mass
  - Most practical noninvasive means of making diagnosis
  - Histologic verification by percutaneous biopsy with imaging guidance

TOP DIFFERENTIAL DIAGNOSES

- Adrenal adenoma
- Adrenal carcinoma
- Adrenal metastases and lymphoma
- Adrenal myelolipoma
- Adrenal hemorrhage

DIAGNOSTIC CHECKLIST

- Adenomas may contain foci of fat and be indistinguishable from adenoma/myelolipoma collision tumor
- Metastasis and adenoma collision tumor is most clinically relevant
- 2 distinct masses with differing attenuation or signal attenuation
- PET/CT useful for diagnosis of adenoma-metastasis collision tumor

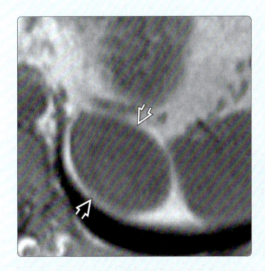
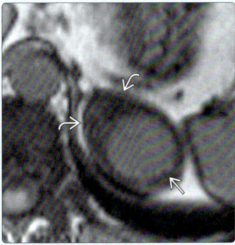

(Left) Axial in-phase T1WI MR shows an indeterminate, 4-cm, left adrenal lesion ⇨. (Right) Corresponding out-of-phase MR shows that the adrenal mass is actually composed of 2 distinct lesions. Signal suppression of the peripheral lesion ⇨ indicates a lipid-rich adenoma. The higher signal intensity central lesion ⇨ is a metastasis. Collision tumors such as this may be due simply to chance, given the high prevalence of adenomas and metastases in the oncologic patient population. (Courtesy E. Caoili, MD.)

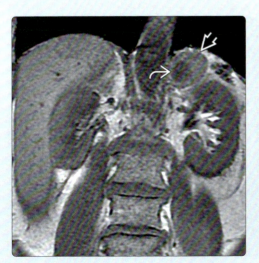
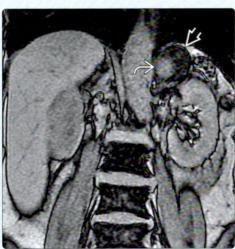

(Left) Coronal T1WI in-phase MR performed to evaluate an adrenal lesion in an elderly woman with pulmonary fibrosis shows a 3-cm left adrenal mass ⇨. Note the well-circumscribed, ↓ signal central component ⇨. (Right) Out-of-phase image again shows peripheral signal suppression ⇨ (indicating a lipid-rich adenoma) and a separate, indeterminate lesion ⇨. Growth of the mass prompted resection. A collision tumor composed of an adenoma and a schwannoma (a rare benign adrenal lesion) was shown at pathology.

IMAGING

- Likelihood of adrenal metastasis at imaging depends upon clinical history
  - Increased likelihood of adrenal metastasis if history of extrarenal malignancy
  - Imaging needed to differentiate between isolated benign adrenal lesion (typically adenoma) and metastasis during initial staging and surveillance
    - NECT attenuation < 10 HU or signal loss at out-phase gradient-echo MR: Lipid-rich adenoma
    - Rapid washout at CECT (> 60% at 15 minutes): Likely lipid-poor adenoma
      - Caveat: Rapid washout observed with hypervascular metastases from HCC, RCC
    - FDG PET/CT: Uptake in adrenal mass significantly greater than liver suggests metastasis
  - Comparison to prior studies critical: New adrenal mass in patient with known (active) extraadrenal malignancy indicates metastasis

- Biopsy rarely needed for diagnosis but may be performed for equivocal lesions, particularly if surgery or ablation considered for potential isolated adrenal metastasis
- Incidental adrenal lesions ("incidentaloma") are rarely metastases

TOP DIFFERENTIAL DIAGNOSES

- Adrenal adenoma
- Adrenal carcinoma
- Adrenal hemorrhage

CLINICAL ISSUES

- Common target organ for metastases from lung, breast, melanoma
- Typically implies late-stage disease
- Adrenal insufficiency if large, bilateral metastases

DIAGNOSTIC CHECKLIST

- Clinical setting usually indicates correct diagnosis

(Left) *Ultrasound of a patient with lung carcinoma shows a solid right adrenal lesion* ➡. *The appearance is nonspecific, but the history suggests an adrenal metastasis. Biopsy performed because of equivocal findings at PET/CT confirmed a metastasis.* (Right) *CECT shows hepatic metastases* ➡, *abdominal adenopathy* ➡, *and adrenal lesions* ➡ *in a patient with esophageal carcinoma. The imaging appearance of the adrenal lesions is nonspecific, but clinical history and widespread disease confirm adrenal metastases.*

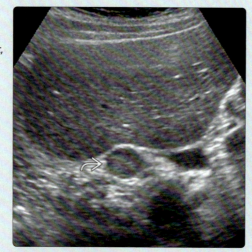
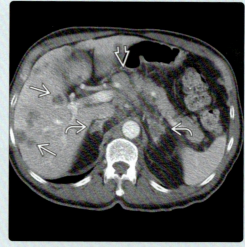

(Left) *Axial T2WI MR of an elderly male patient with a history of non-small cell lung carcinoma shows large, bilateral adrenal masses* ➡. *Rapid growth from a prior staging CT (not shown) and the clinical history indicate adrenal metastases.* (Right) *Axial PET/CT shows an isolated FDG-avid right adrenal metastasis* ➡ *in a patient with a history of T2N0 esophageal carcinoma post esophagectomy. An adrenalectomy was performed given the initial stage and absence of other metastases.*

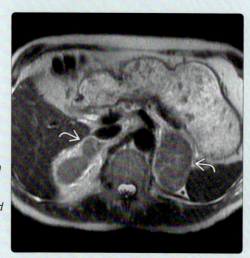
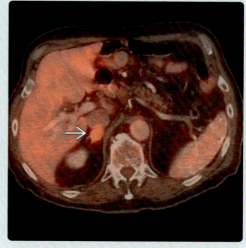

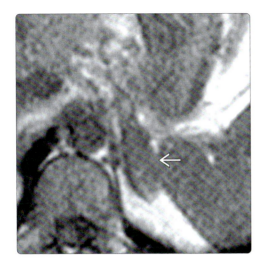 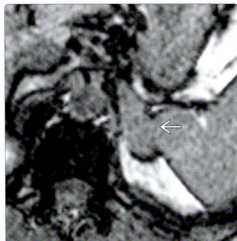

(Left) Axial T1WI in-phase MR shows a left adrenal mass ➡ in this case of metastatic lung cancer. (Right) Axial T1WI opposed-phase MR of the same patient shows no signal "dropout" from the adrenal mass ➡. A lipid-poor adenoma may have a similar appearance. Growth from a prior comparison study indicates a metastasis.

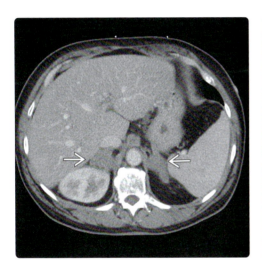 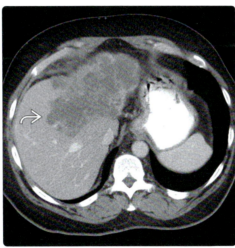

(Left) CT performed on a patient with colon carcinoma shows enlarged, nodular adrenals ➡. In isolation, the appearance is nonspecific: Considerations include adenomas, hyperplasia, or lymphoma, but interval development indicates metastases. (Right) An image from the same patient shows a new hepatic metastasis ➡. Definitive characterization of adrenal metastases in oncologic patients is usually unnecessary, though ancillary tests (NECT, washout CT, or biopsy) may be employed in select circumstances.

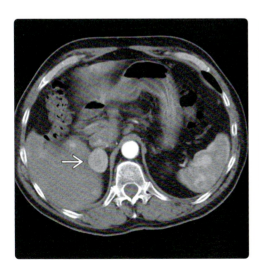 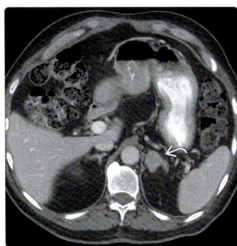

(Left) CECT of a patient with multifocal HCC shows a briskly enhancing right adrenal lesion ➡. Rapid washout (not shown) might suggest an adenoma, but interval growth indicates a vascular metastases. Adrenal metastases from vascular primaries (HCC, RCC) may mimic lipid-poor adenomas at wash-out CT. (Right) Axial CECT of a patient with a history of lung cancer shows a new adrenal mass ➡. Although a relative washout of 42% might suggest a lipid-poor adenoma, biopsy confirmed a metastasis.

SECTION 4
Kidney and Renal Pelvis

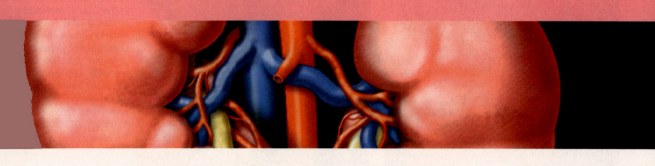

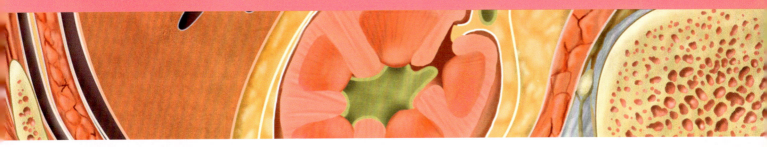

Renal Failure and Medical Renal Disease

Vascular Disorders

Trauma

Transplantation

Treatment Related

Imaging Anatomy

The kidneys are bean-shaped, paired, retroperitoneal organs. The renal parenchyma has 2 major components: The cortex (outer portion) and the medulla (inner portion). The renal parenchyma is divided in multiple lobes (8-18), each of which is composed of medulla (pyramid) and cortex. Each pyramid drains into a minor calyx. Multiple (2-3) minor calyces converge into a major calyces. The renal pelvis, an extension of the ureter, collects urine from multiple calyces.

The functional unit is the nephron. It is composed of the renal corpuscle (glomerulus and Bowman capsule) and tubules (proximal and distal convoluted tubules and loop of Henle). The filtrate from the distal convoluted ducts passes into collecting ducts that extend to the tip of the medulla (papilla).

Principles of Renal Physiology

The main functions of the kidneys are the maintenance of homeostasis, removal of metabolic waste products, and production of urine. The functions are carried out with a combination of glomerular filtration, tubular reabsorption, and tubular secretion. Filtration is conducted in the renal corpuscle (glomerulus, Bowman capsule) in the cortex, while reabsorption and secretion occur in the different tubular components (proximal, distal convoluted tubule, loop of Henle, collecting ducts) located in the cortex and medulla.

Glomerular filtration rate (GFR) is the volume of fluid filtered in the glomerulus per unit of time per unit of body surface area. It is determined by the net filtration rate, capillary permeability, and surface area of the capillary bed. Estimated GFR, an indicator of renal function, can be calculated using the Modification of Diet in Renal Disease equation based on serum creatinine, age, gender, and race.

Iodinated Contrast Media

Iodinated contrast media (ICM) are hydrophilic chemical compounds excreted from the kidneys by glomerular filtration alone. Enhancement (i.e., increased attenuation) after injection of ICM is based on several agent-related (e.g., concentration, volume, rate of injection), patient-related (weight, height, cardiac output), and technical-related (scan delay for CT acquisition) factors. ICM are described based on their dissociation in solution (ionic, nonionic), osmolarity compared to plasma (high, iso-, low osmolar), and number of triiodinated benzene groups (monomer, dimer).

Contrast-induced nephropathy (CIN) is an acute kidney injury (absolute increase in serum creatinine of 0.5 mg/dL or relative 25% increase from baseline value) occurring within 24-48 hours following intravascular administration of contrast material. The most important risk factor for CIN is underlying renal dysfunction (GFR < 60 mL/minute/1.73m²). In patients at risk for CIN but still requiring injection of contrast media, the following prophylactic measures should be taken: Intravenous hydration, lower dose of hypo- or isoosmolar contrast media, and no nephrotoxic drugs.

MR Contrast Media

Gadolinium-based MR contrast agents (GBCA) are paramagnetic compounds that increase signal intensity (SI) (i.e., enhancement) by increasing the T1 relaxation rate. The evaluation of the genitourinary tract is conducted using extracellular agents, preferably with high relaxivity.

Approved extracellular GBCAs include gadoterate meglumine, gadobutrol, gadopentetate dimeglumine, gadodiamide, gadoversetamide, gadoteridol, and gadobenate dimeglumine. Extracellular GBCAs are 100% excreted by the kidneys with the exception of gadobenate dimeglumine, which has a 95% renal excretion and a 5% hepatobiliary excretion.

Adverse Reactions to Contrast Media

Adverse reactions to contrast media can be classified as allergic-like and physiologic and have an overall low incidence rate. The most significant risk factor for an allergic-like reaction is a documented allergic reaction to prior exposure. The majority of the reactions can be classified as mild and are not life threatening (e.g., limited urticaria, nausea/vomiting). Moderate (e.g., facial edema, vasovagal reaction) and severe (e.g., laryngeal edema with hypoxia, hypertensive emergency) adverse reactions need to be recognized and managed promptly. For prophylaxis measures and management of adverse reactions to contrast media, consult the most recent guidelines (version 10.2, 2016) from the American College of Radiology.

Imaging Techniques and Indications

Ultrasound

Ultrasound is an important imaging modality for the assessment of the kidneys. In patients with acute or chronic kidney injury, ultrasound represents the modality of choice to exclude hydronephrosis and assess renal size.

It is ideally suited for differentiating cystic from solid masses. A simple cystic lesion is anechoic with a sharp posterior border and increased through transmission. While ultrasound can confidently diagnose simple cysts, complicated cysts should be further evaluated with dedicated contrast-enhanced CT and MR.

Most renal cell carcinomas (RCC) have a heterogeneous hypo- to mildly hyperechoic appearance; however, 20% may have a more uniform hyperechoic appearance and be confused with an angiomyolipoma (AML). It is imperative that all solid masses be further evaluated with either CT or MR to differentiate AML from RCC.

CT

Contrast-enhanced multiphase CT is the preferred imaging modality for the characterization of renal lesions.

Unenhanced scan: An unenhanced scan should be performed routinely in a renal mass work-up to evaluate baseline density in the assessment of lesion enhancement and presence of intralesional fat, hemorrhage, and calcifications.

Corticomedullary phase (20-80 seconds postcontrast injection): While this phase is helpful for the evaluation of renal vasculature, it is fraught with pitfalls for the evaluation of renal masses. In this phase, RCC may be missed.

Nephrographic phase (80-120 seconds postcontrast injection): In this phase, the kidney has a homogeneous uniform nephrogram. This is the best phase for the detection and evaluation of renal masses.

Excretory phase (3-5 minutes postcontrast injection): In this phase, the contrast is excreted into the renal collecting system. 3D reconstructions in the excretory phase allow evaluation of the collecting system, including the renal pelvis, ureter, and bladder.

MR

MR imaging can be used as an alternative to CT or as a problem-solving tool to characterize indeterminate lesions detected on CT (e.g., confirmation of cystic nature of small lesions). The renal mass protocol usually consists of the following sequences.

T2-weighted imaging (T2WI): Simple cysts have high, homogenous SI on T2WI, similar to the cerebrospinal fluid, whereas complicated, hemorrhagic cysts vary in SI depending on the stage of hemorrhage. Among solid lesions, papillary RCC and fat-poor AML have low SI on T2WI, whereas clear cell and chromophobe RCC, as well as oncocytoma, usually show moderately high SI on T2WI.

T1-weighted imaging (T1WI): In-phase and opposed-phase gradient-echo (GRE) ("chemical shift") imaging and frequency-selective fat-suppressed imaging are helpful for the detection of intralesional fat. Intralesional "bulk fat" is a diagnostic feature of classic AML and manifests as a loss of SI on frequency-selective fat-suppressed images and "India ink artifact" (signal loss at the interface of lesion and surrounding renal parenchyma) on opposed-phase T1WI. Loss of SI within the lesion on opposed-phase images compared with in-phase images indicates a small amount of fat (intravoxel), which can be seen with few fat cells of fat-poor AML or intracellular fat of clear cell-type RCC.

3D fat-saturated GRE T1WI: This sequence is performed in the axial or coronal plane before and after the intravenous administration of an extracellular GBCA to assess organ and lesion enhancement. Similar to CT, images can be obtained during the corticomedullary, nephrographic, and excretory phase. Enhancement is commonly assessed qualitatively.

Approach to Renal Mass

The following questions helps in the characterization of a renal lesion.

Is Mass Cystic or Solid?

Knowing if a mass is cystic or solid is the single most important question for the evaluation of a renal mass. The key imaging feature for the differentiation is the presence of enhancement. A cystic mass is a lesion composed of nonenhancing fluid.

Cystic lesions: The vast majority of simple unilocular cystic lesions are benign cysts. The Bosniak classification groups cystic lesions into 5 categories based on their imaging appearance; the more complex the lesion, the higher the risk of malignancy. The classification is used to determine management of cystic lesion. While simple or minimally complicated cysts (Bosniak classes I and II) are considered benign and need no treatment or imaging follow-up, complicated cysts with thick septations or enhancing nodules (Bosniak classes III and IV) are usually considered surgical lesions. Bosniak class IIF category includes complicated cysts requiring imaging follow-up. Clinical information is also helpful in further differentiating cystic masses. For example, a multilocular cystic nephroma (a benign cyst renal neoplasm) is seen in young boys and middle-aged women. Hematoma and abscess should also be suspected based on clinical history.

Lesions measuring < 20 HU or > 70 HU on unenhanced CT are considered benign, representing simple and hemorrhagic cysts, respectively. Lesions measuring 20-70 HU on unenhanced CT (i.e., hyperdense lesions) are indeterminate and require contrast administration to assess for enhancement. If the patient cannot tolerate IV contrast, ultrasound or MR can be used for characterization. At ultrasound, hyperdense lesions on CT may often appear as anechoic, benign cysts.

Solid lesions: An enhancing mass is considered a solid lesion. On CT, enhancement is considered present when there is at least a 20-HU increase in attenuation after contrast injection. An increment of 10-20 HU is considered indeterminate and requires further evaluation with additional imaging, biopsy, or imaging follow-up. "Pseudoenhancement" refers to the artificial increase in attenuation of a simple fluid-containing cystic lesion on postcontrast images. On MR, subtraction images (postcontrast minus precontrast) are commonly used to qualitatively assess intralesional enhancement. While clear cell and chromophobe RCC usually show avid enhancement, papillary RCC is characterized by minimal enhancement. Benign renal lesions, such as oncocytoma and fat-poor AML, may show avid enhancement.

Is Growth Pattern Expansile or Infiltrative?

If a mass is solid, the next step is to evaluate the growth pattern. Renal masses tend to have 2 growth patterns: (1) Expansile, circumferential and (2) infiltrative.

Over 90% of RCCs have a spherical, expansile, ball-shaped growth pattern and commonly extend beyond the cortex of the kidney. Other solid lesions, including oncocytomas and AMLs, also have this growth pattern.

An infiltrative pattern can be seen in both inflammatory (e.g., acute pyelonephritis) and neoplastic conditions, and, hence, clinical history is important in differentiating this group. The renal neoplasm most commonly presenting with an infiltrative growth pattern is transitional cell carcinoma. A minority of RCCs will have an infiltrative growth pattern, usually with aggressive histologic tumor types, including medullary carcinoma and sarcomatoid tumors. Finally, renal lymphoma may appear with either growth pattern.

Does Mass Contain Fat?

If a solitary renal mass measures soft tissue density, the diagnosis is RCC until proven otherwise. Features, such as a central scar, may suggest oncocytoma as an alternative diagnosis, but RCC cannot be excluded without histologic evaluation.

A renal mass containing macroscopic fat is overwhelmingly likely to be an AML, although RCC may rarely contain fat. This generally occurs when large tumors have engulfed fat or have undergone osseous metaplasia; the presence of dense calcification and fat within a renal mass is highly suspicious for RCC.

A small percentage of AMLs (~ 5%) contain only a few fat cells and are named fat-poor AMLs and cannot be confidently differentiated from other solid lesions. The small amount of fat is not confidently detected at CT, and these lesions commonly appear homogeneously hyperattenuating on unenhanced CT.

Is Mass Solitary or Are There Multiple Masses?

When multiple solid renal masses are seen, one should consider syndromes. Multiple RCCs and cysts occur in von Hippel-Lindau disease. Multiple AMLs should raise the index of suspicion for tuberous sclerosis. Lymphoma and metastases can also present with multiple masses.

(Left) *Graphic shows renal anatomy and its 2 major components: Cortex (outer portion)* ➡️ *and medulla (inner portion)* ⇉. *The renal filtrate from each pyramid of the medulla is collected into minor and major calyces and passes into the renal pelvis* ➡️ *and ureter* ⇨. **(Right)** *Table summarizes different generations of iodinated contrast media with their corresponding iodine content and osmolarity.*

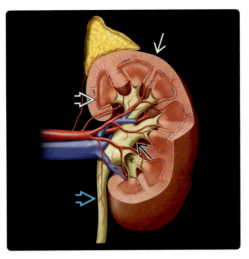

1st Generation: Ionic High-Osmolar Contrast Media		
Name	Iodine Content	Osmolality
Diatrizoate *(Hypaque 50)*	300 mg/mL	1550 mOsm/kg
Metrizoate *(Isopaque 370)*	370 mg/mL	2100 mOsm/kg
2nd Generation: Nonionic Low-Osmolar Contrast Media		
Name	Iodine Content	Osmolality
Iopamidol *(Isovue 370)*	370 mg/mL	800 mOsm/kg
Iohexol *(Omnipaque 350)*	350 mg/mL	880 mOsm/kg
Iopromide *(Ultravist 370)*	370 mg/mL	770 mOsm/kg
Ioxilan *(Oxilan 350)*	350 mg/mL	700 mOsm/kg
3rd Generation: Nonionic Iso-Osmolar Contrast Media		
Name	Iodine Content	Osmolality
Iodixanol *(Visipaque 320)*	320 mg/mL	290 mOsm/kg

(Left) *Longitudinal ultrasound of the right kidney shows an anechoic lesion* ➡️ *with imperceptible walls and posterior acoustic enhancement* ⇉, *compatible with a simple renal cyst.* **(Right)** *Axial CECT shows a Bosniak class III cystic mass (multilocular cystic nephroma) with thick, calcified septa. The Bosniak classification groups cystic lesions into 5 categories based on the CT imaging appearance; the more complex the lesion, the higher the risk of malignancy.*

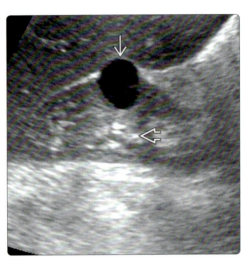
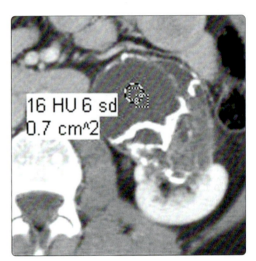

16 HU 6 sd
0.7 cm^2

(Left) *Axial CECT shows a small, low-attenuation lesion* ➡️ *in the cortex of the right kidney. The lesion measures 31 HU, and it is therefore indeterminate. It may represent a small cyst with "pseudoenhancement" or a small solid lesion.* **(Right)** *Axial FS T2 MR in the same patient shows a simple-appearing, high signal intensity (similar to the cerebrospinal fluid) lesion* ➡️, *proving the cystic nature of the indeterminate right renal lesion seen on CT. The increased attenuation of the lesion on CECT is related to "pseudoenhancement."*

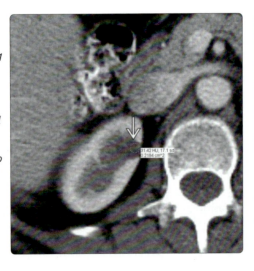
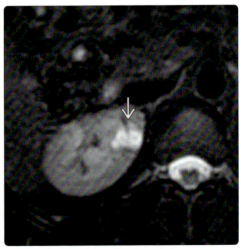

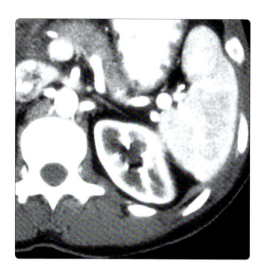
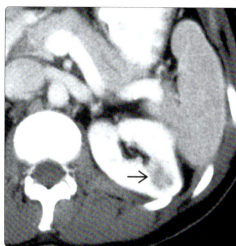

(Left) Axial CECT acquired in the corticomedullary phase shows a normal left kidney. (Right) Axial CECT in the same patient acquired in the nephrographic phase shows an abnormal hypoenhancing area ⇨ in the medullary portion of the kidney. This patient had an elevated white count and pyuria, and this proved to be a focal area of pyelonephritis. Low-attenuation abnormalities in the medullary portion of the kidney are easily missed in the corticomedullary phase.

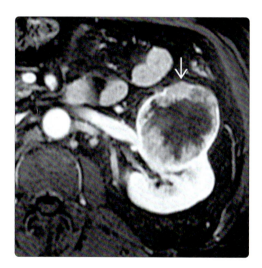
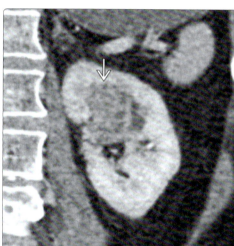

(Left) Axial gadolinium-enhanced MR of a 57-year-old man with renal cell carcinoma shows a typical expansile growth pattern. The mass ⇨ has heterogeneous enhancement, and it is partially exophytic. (Right) Coronal CECT of the left kidney in a 63-year-old woman with transitional cell carcinoma presenting with hematuria is shown. The tumor ⇨ shows an infiltrative growth pattern with obliteration of the calyces and the sinus fat of the upper pole of the left kidney. The renal shape is preserved.

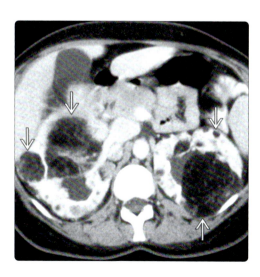
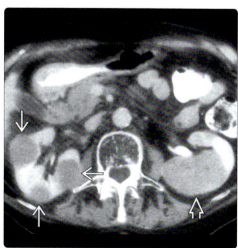

(Left) Axial CECT shows multiple bilateral, renal fat-containing masses ⇨ of varying size, consistent with multiple classic (fat-rich) angiomyolipomas in a patient with tuberous sclerosis. (Right) Axial CECT shows multiple renal lesions with 2 patterns of growth. Within the right kidney are 3 well-defined, round, ball-shaped masses ⇨, while on the left there is a larger infiltrating mass ⇨. When there are multiple masses displaying both types of growth, lymphoma is the primary consideration.

TERMINOLOGY

- Synonym: Fetal lobulation, persistent fetal lobulation
- Normal variant anatomy with indentations of renal surface caused by incomplete fusion of renal lobes

IMAGING

- US
  - Color Doppler shows normal flow and cortical thickness separated by thin echogenic cleft
  - Lobations are clefts of echogenic capsule and perirenal fat invaginating between normal-thickness renal cortex
- CECT during corticomedullary phase shows normal-thickness cortex, invaginated by thin, hypodense surface cleft
- Morphology
  - Sharp, shallow indentations along renal surface
  - Indentations extend between renal pyramids and calyces

TOP DIFFERENTIAL DIAGNOSES

- Cortical scar
  - Loss or thinning of cortex due to ischemia or infection
  - Often **overlies** distorted calyx (lobation clefts are between calyces)

PATHOLOGY

- Fetal human kidney consists of numerous separate renal lobes (reniculi)
  - Each lobe consists of 1 renal pyramid surrounded by cortex and supplied by single calyx, artery, and vein
  - Each lobe marked by surface indentations (lobations)
- Lobes usually disappear by end of childhood, resulting in smooth surface of most adult kidneys
  - Fetal lobation present in > 10% of children, 4% of adults
  - Lobation is often prominent on sonography of newborns

CLINICAL ISSUES

- More common in infants and children

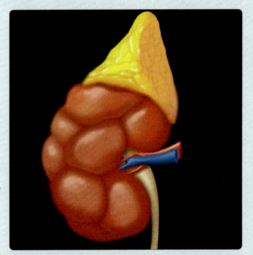
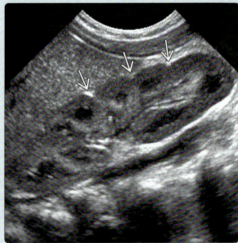

(Left) Graphic depicts the typical lobulated appearance of the kidney in fetal life, reflecting the development of the kidney from numerous lobes, each consisting of a renal pyramid and its associated cortex. Note that the adrenal gland is relatively large compared to the kidney in fetal life and childhood. (Right) Sagittal US in this 6-week-old infant shows fetal lobation (clefts ➡). Note echogenicity of the cortex and paucity of renal sinus fat, which are normal findings in infants and children.

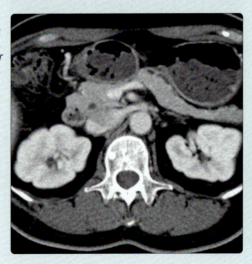
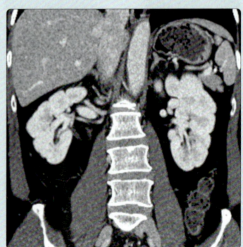

(Left) Axial CECT in the corticomedullary phase shows classic bilateral fetal lobation. Note that each surface cleft or indentation extends into a column of normal-thickness renal cortex. (Right) Coronal reformation of CECT in the same patient shows classic bilateral fetal lobation with each renal lobe and its cortex demarcated by surface clefts.

TERMINOLOGY

- Normal-variant line at plane of embryologic fusion off embryologic elements forming kidneys (renunculi)
- a.k.a. junctional parenchymal defect (JPD)

IMAGING

- Classically seen in anterosuperior aspect of kidney (at junction of upper and middle 1/3 of kidney)
  - Less commonly seen in posteroinferior aspect (at junction of middle and lower 1/3 of kidney)
- Right > left (~ 2x more common on right side)
- Runs obliquely from anterosuperior toward posteroinferior surface; usually extends to renal sinus
- Better seen on US, due to higher spatial resolution and multiplanar imaging (better seen on parasagittal planes)
- US
  - Echogenic line running obliquely from anterosuperior to posteroinferior surface of kidney (junctional line)
  - Peripheral wedge-shaped echogenicity along plane of fusion of renunculi (caused by Invagination of perirenal fat)

TOP DIFFERENTIAL DIAGNOSES

- Renal scar
  - Lack of cortical thinning and classic location of JPD helps to differentiate these entities
- Angiomyolipoma (AML)
  - Classic location, preservation of renal contour, and extension toward renal sinus help to differentiate JPD from AML

PATHOLOGY

- Based on concept that kidneys develop from fusion of 2 sub kidneys (renunculi)
  - Posterosuperior and anteroinferior renunculi fuse to form kidney
- Invagination of perirenal fat into defect results in its wedge-shaped appearance

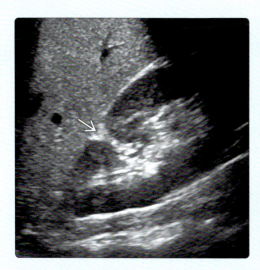
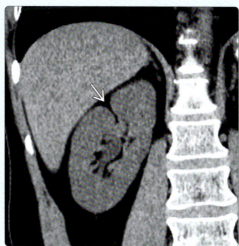

(Left) Sagittal oblique US through the right kidney in 55-year-old man shows triangular echogenicity ➡ in the anterior aspect of the upper pole, which extends into the renal sinus, compatible with junctional parenchymal defect. (Right) Coronal CT in the same patient better shows the fat-density notch ➡ and the defect through the upper pole, which extends to the sinus fat.

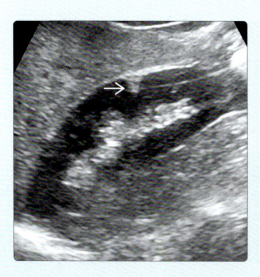
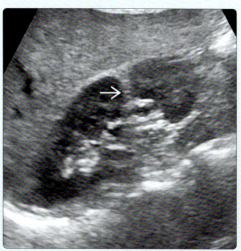

(Left) Sagittal oblique US through the right kidney in a 48-year-old woman shows an echogenic wedge-shaped defect ➡ in the anterior aspect of the lower pole. (Right) Slightly different section through the right kidney in the same patient shows extension of the defect ➡ into the renal sinus. The anterior aspect of the lower pole is a less common location for junctional parenchymal defect. Note increased hepatic echogenicity due to steatosis.

KEY FACTS

TERMINOLOGY

- Congenital anomaly in which kidneys are fused by isthmus at lower poles

IMAGING

- Ectopic kidneys, lying lower than normal kidneys
- Isthmus usually anterior to aorta, caudal to confluence of iliac veins, and below inferior mesenteric artery
- CT: Better defines structural abnormalities, complications, and associated abnormalities
- 2 types of fusion
  - Midline or symmetrical fusion (90% of cases)
  - Lateral or asymmetrical fusion (10% of cases)
- Variant arterial supply
  - Multiple, bilateral renal arteries
  - Arteries arising from aorta or iliacs
- Posterior calyces are located more inferior, posterior, and medially than in normal kidneys: Relevant for percutaneous nephrolithotomy

TOP DIFFERENTIAL DIAGNOSES

- Renal ectopia
- Renal displacement

PATHOLOGY

- Other anomalies of kidneys and other organs are common, such as
  - Ureteropelvic junction (UPJ) obstruction
  - Vesicoureteral reflux

CLINICAL ISSUES

- Complications
  - Traumatic injury (more prone)
  - Recurrent infections: Due to concurrent vesicoureteral reflux and UPJ obstruction
  - Urolithiasis: 75% metabolic calculi, 25% struvite calculi
  - Wilms tumor: 2-8x ↑ risk in pediatric population with horseshoe kidney
  - Primary renal cell carcinoma: ↑ prevalence

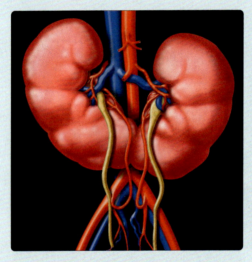
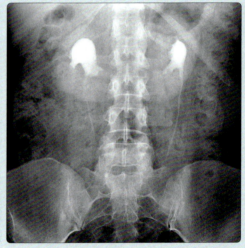

(Left) Graphic shows a horseshoe kidney. Note the multiple renal arteries arising from the aorta and iliac arteries. (Right) Frontal projection from IVP shows a horseshoe kidney. Note the U-shaped nephrogram and low-lying kidneys. The lower pole calyces converge toward the midline near the isthmus.

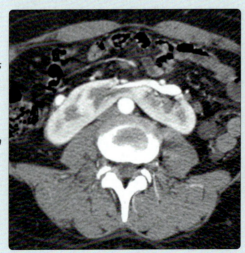
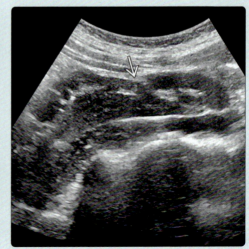

(Left) Axial CECT shows fusion of the lower poles of the kidneys across the midline below the level of the inferior mesenteric artery. The isthmus contains functioning enhancing parenchyma. Note the forward-facing calyces. (Right) Axial oblique US through the midline abdomen shows a horseshoe kidney with midline isthmus ➡ in contiguity with the lower poles.

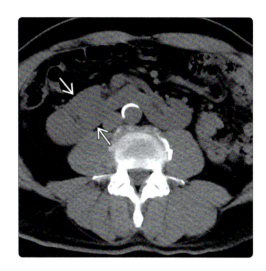

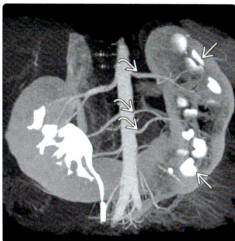

(Left) Axial NECT in 63-year old man shows an asymmetric-type horseshoe kidney with lateral fusion (a less common variant). The right kidney has a normal position, while the left kidney is horizontally positioned across the midline. Note the isthmus ➡. (Right) Coronal CECT volumetric reformat demonstrates multiple renal arteries ➡, some of which have probably crossed and partially obstructed the infundibula on the left side. The left side calyces are dilated ➡, and the cortex is thinned.

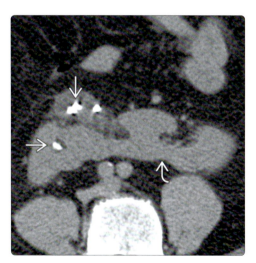

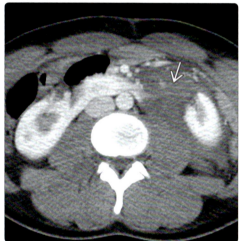

(Left) Axial NECT shows a horseshoe kidney with multiple calculi ➡ and cortical scarring ➡. (Right) Axial CECT shows a large laceration ➡ of the left moiety of a horseshoe kidney with surrounding hematoma.

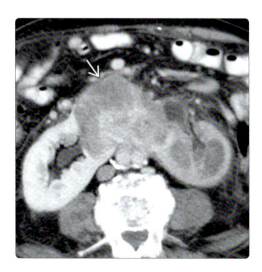

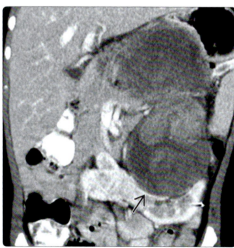

(Left) Axial CECT shows a large mass ➡ replacing most of the isthmus and left moiety of a horseshoe kidney. The mass proved to be renal cell carcinoma. (Right) Coronal CECT in a 3-year-old boy shows a large, heterogeneous mass ➡ arising from the left moiety of a horseshoe kidney. The mass proved to be Wilms tumor.

Kidney and Renal Pelvis

TERMINOLOGY

- Renal tissue in abnormal location
  - Anywhere from presacral to intrathoracic; may cross midline; may involve 1 or both kidneys
- Includes horseshoe or pancake kidney; crossed fused ectopia; pelvic, iliac/pelvic (ptotic/mobile), & thoracic kidneys
- Results from abnormal ascent & rotation of fetal kidney
  - Kidneys form at sacral level, ascend to L1, & rotate 90° by term
  - High incidence of multiple renal arteries & veins (vessels normally obliterate during renal ascent)

IMAGING

- Ultrasound typically sufficient to document location & morphology of ectopic & fused kidneys
  - Accurate lengths often difficult to obtain due to less reniform shape, ± poorly defined margin with contralateral kidney

- Other modalities reserved for specific questions as needed: Function, stones, vasculature, ureteral course
  - Bladder insertion of ureter is usually on side where kidney initially formed
  - Isthmus of horseshoe kidney may contain functioning renal tissue or fibrotic nonfunctional tissue

CLINICAL ISSUES

- Most asymptomatic, incidentally discovered at imaging
- Horseshoe kidney most common: 1 in 400 births
- M > F for all types of ectopia
- Associated abnormalities
  - Ectopic kidney more susceptible to traumatic or iatrogenic injury, obstruction, infection, stasis, & stones
  - Contralateral renal dysplasia (4%), cryptorchidism (5%), hypospadias (5%), hypertension (15%), vesicoureteral reflux (20-30%)
  - Horseshoe kidneys associated with chromosomal abnormalities, including Turner syndrome

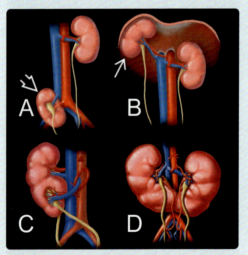
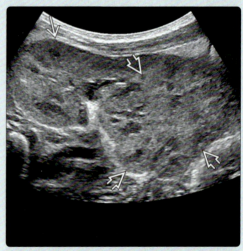

(Left) Graphic shows variations of renal ectopia & fusion: (A) Pelvic kidney ➡, (B) subdiaphragmatic/thoracic kidney ➡, (C) crossed fused renal ectopia, & (D) horseshoe kidney. (Right) Longitudinal US shows a crossed fused renal ectopia in the left abdomen with a relatively normal upper moiety ➡ & a malrotated, globular lower moiety ➡. Note that the long axis of each moiety is different, which helps distinguish this entity from a duplication. Also, no renal tissue will be seen in the contralateral renal fossa in this setting.

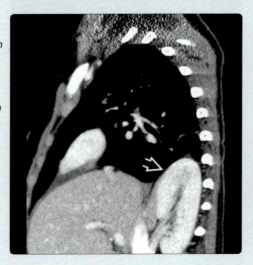
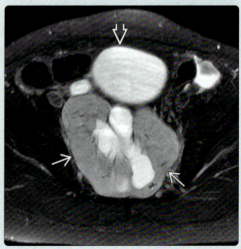

(Left) Sagittal CECT shows a right kidney ➡ bulging into the posterior right lung base in this patient with a subdiaphragmatic or thoracic kidney. (Right) Axial T2 FS MR in the same patient shows a dilated renal collecting system just posterior to the urinary bladder ➡ in this pelvic pancake kidney ➡.

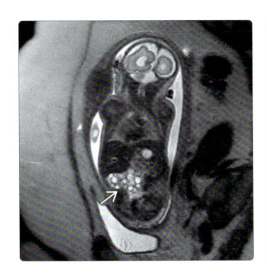

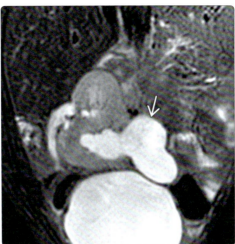

(Left) *Coronal SSFSE T2 fetal MR shows multiple varying sized cysts in a crossed fused kidney* ➡ *in this patient who was subsequently shown to have a multicystic dysplastic kidney with a minimally functional upper pole.* (Right) *Coronal T2 FS MR urography shows a dilated collecting system & tortuous ureter* ➡ *in this case of a pelvic kidney.*

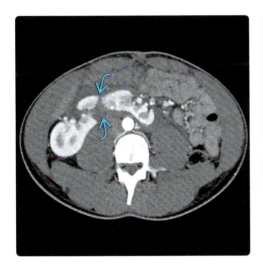

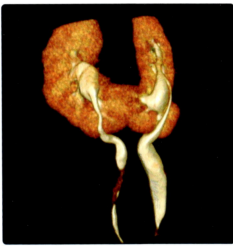

(Left) *Axial CECT shows a crossed fused ectopic kidney with renal laceration near the junction of the right & left moieties* ➡ *in this 14-year-old patient with blunt trauma to the abdomen while playing soccer.* (Right) *3D reformation from a CECT scan in a patient with multiple congenital anomalies shows a horseshoe kidney with fused lower poles & anteriorly directed renal pelves.*

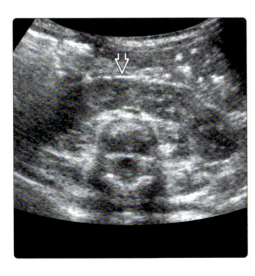

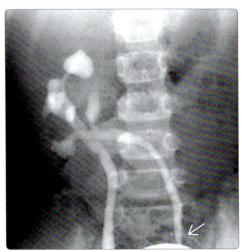

(Left) *Transverse US in a patient with a horseshoe kidney shows a band of renal parenchyma* ➡ *crossing over the spine.* (Right) *Frontal fluoroscopic image during a VCUG shows reflux into a crossed fused kidney with the lower moiety ureter crossing the midline to the left side of the bladder* ➡ *(since this kidney initially formed as a left kidney).*

KEY FACTS

TERMINOLOGY

- Congenital absence of functioning renal tissue
- Congenital abnormality of kidney and urinary tract

IMAGING

- Complete absence of 1 or both kidneys
  - No ectopia or fusion anomaly
  - Left-sided predominance
- Bowel fills renal fossa
- Linear configuration of ipsilateral adrenal gland
  - "Lying down adrenal" rarely mistaken for abnormal kidney in neonate
- ± compensatory hypertrophy of remaining kidney
- Best modality: Ultrasound (pre- or postnatal)

TOP DIFFERENTIAL DIAGNOSES

- Involuted multicystic dysplastic kidney
- Ectopic kidney, including crossed fused ectopia
- Prior nephrectomy

PATHOLOGY

- Unilateral renal agenesis associated with
  - Contralateral renal anomalies in 31-48%
    - Vesicoureteral reflux most common in 24% (screening suggested)
  - Chromosomal abnormalities
  - Extrarenal anomalies in up to 30%
  - Müllerian abnormalities
    - **O**bstructed **h**emi**v**agina, **i**psilateral **r**enal **a**genesis (OHVIRA syndrome)
  - Zinner syndrome (wolffian duct anomaly)

CLINICAL ISSUES

- Unilateral usually asymptomatic; associated with medical renal disease later in life
- Bilateral renal agenesis results in Potter sequence if no intervention (amnioinfusion): Anhydramnios, lung hypoplasia, bell-shaped chest, dysmorphic facies, fetal demise

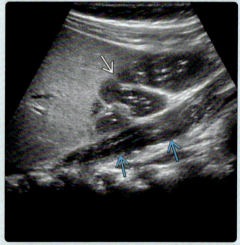
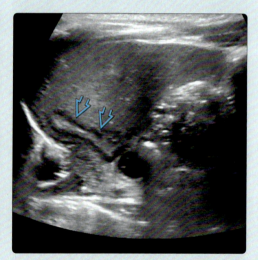

(Left) Longitudinal US of the right renal fossa in a 1-day-old girl with right renal agenesis shows absence of the kidney in the expected location along the right psoas muscle ➡. There are normal, fluid-filled bowel loops in the right renal fossa ➡. (Right) Oblique US of the right renal fossa in a 1-day-old boy with right renal agenesis shows an elongated, linear adrenal gland (lying down adrenal) ➡.

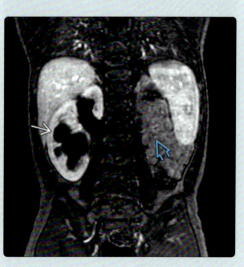
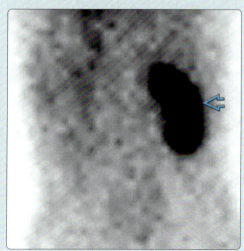

(Left) Coronal T1 C+ MR with fat saturation in a 3 year old with left renal agenesis shows an absence of renal tissue in the left renal fossa, which is filled with decompressed bowel ➡. The right renal collecting system is dilated ➡ secondary to a ureteropelvic junction obstruction. (Right) Posterior coronal image from a Tc-99m DTPA renal scan in a 2 year old with left renal agenesis shows normal radiotracer uptake in the right kidney ➡ with no radiotracer uptake on the left.

Ureteropelvic Junction Obstruction

KEY FACTS

TERMINOLOGY

- Functional or anatomic obstruction to urine flow from renal pelvis into ureter at their anatomic junction
  - If left untreated, may result in symptoms, renal damage, or it may spontaneously resolve

IMAGING

- Pyelocaliectasis with abrupt ureteropelvic junction (UPJ) narrowing
- Imaging recommendations
  - To quantitate relative obstruction and function
    - Diuretic renography: Tc-99m-labeled mercaptoacetyltriglycine (MAG3)
  - To assess anatomy and etiology: Neonates and children: Ultrasonography
    - Neonates and children: Ultrasonography
    - Adults: CT urography and CTA
      - □ Depiction of relation of UPJ obstruction to vessels is important for planning endoluminal surgery

TOP DIFFERENTIAL DIAGNOSES

- Extrarenal pelvis
- Urolithiasis (renal calculi)
- Tumor

CLINICAL ISSUES

- Most common signs/symptoms
  - Neonates: Prenatal screening; palpable mass
  - Children and adults: Abdominal pain, hematuria
  - Dietl crisis: Acute onset of flank pain/nausea with diuresis
    - Symptoms during MAG3 Lasix administration is highly suggestive of UPJ obstruction
- Demographics
  - Any age; less commonly presents in adults

DIAGNOSTIC CHECKLIST

- Diuretic renogram defines function
- CT and MR defines altered morphology

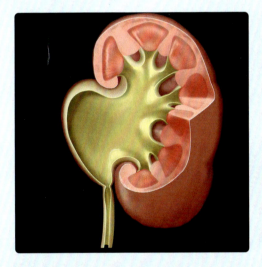

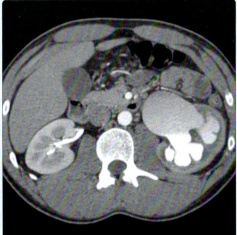

(Left) Graphic shows a congenital ureteropelvic junction (UPJ) obstruction with abrupt narrowing and angulation at the UPJ with resulting pelvocaliectasis and mild cortical atrophy. (Right) A split bolus CT urogram shows marked left renal hydronephrosis, a delayed nephrogram, and slight cortical thinning. The left ureter was normal, and no intrinsic or extrinsic masses or obstructing processes were identified. The relationship among the renal hilar structures is not displayed optimally.

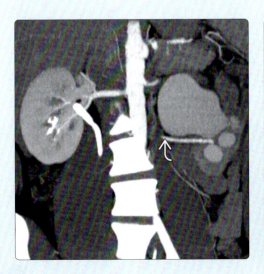

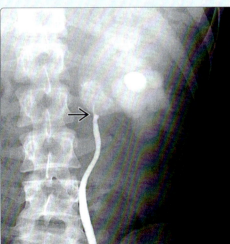

(Left) Coronal CT in the same patient shows an "accessory" lower pole renal artery ➡ that appears to lie close to the UPJ. Assessment of renal vasculature is important when planning for surgical or endoluminal repairs to the UPJ. (Right) Retrograde pyelogram in the same patient shows an abrupt transition from normal-caliber ureter to the dilated renal pelvis at the UPJ ➡. Note the dilution of injected contrast as it streams into the pelvis as a jet.

KEY FACTS

TERMINOLOGY

- Retrograde flow of urine from bladder toward 1 or both kidneys

IMAGING

- International Reflux Study Committee grading system of vesicoureteral reflux (VUR)
  - I: Reflux into ureter but not reaching renal pelvis
  - II: Reflux reaching pelvis without blunting of calyces
  - III: Mild calyceal blunting
  - IV: Progressive calyceal & ureteral dilation
  - V: Very dilated & tortuous collecting system
  - ± intrarenal reflux as modifier to grades II+
- Voiding cystourethrogram (VCUG) or contrast-enhanced voiding urosonogram (ceVUS) preferred when anatomic detail of upper tracts & urethra needed
- Nuclear cystogram, VCUG, or ceVUS for follow-up

CLINICAL ISSUES

- Affects up to 2% of general population
- VUR seen in 25-40% of children with acute pyelonephritis
- VUR seen in 5-50% of asymptomatic siblings of children with documented reflux
- 80% outgrow VUR before puberty
- ↑ grade or longer standing VUR, more numerous urinary tract infections, & possible renal scarring
- VUR in lower pole of duplicated collecting system
- Treatment options
  - Prophylactic antibiotic therapy (medical management)
  - Ureteral reimplantation surgery (surgical management)
  - Endoscopic periureteral injections (minimally invasive endoscopic management)
    - Treatment-induced hydroureteronephrosis following endoscopic procedures uncommon & usually self-limited

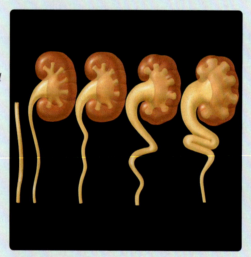
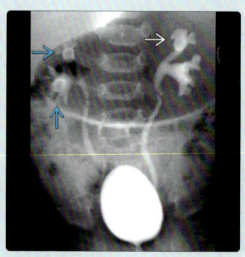

(Left) Graphic depiction of the International Reflux Study Committee grading system is shown. Note the progressive level of reflux, dilatation, calyceal blunting, and ureteral tortuosity from grade I on the left to grade V on the right. (Right) Voiding cystourethrogram (VCUG) in an infant shows bilateral vesicoureteral reflux (VUR). On the right, the calyces are sharp ➡ (grade II). On the left, the calyces are slightly blunted ➡, and the ureter is mildly dilated and tortuous, making this grade III VUR.

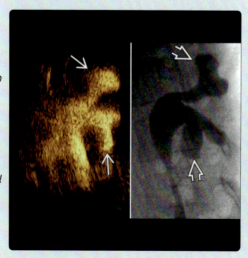
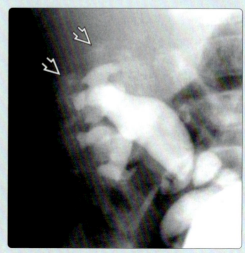

(Left) An 11-year-old boy with long-standing VUR with refluxed contrast in the kidney, calyceal dilatation, and rounded fornices on ceVUS (rotated for comparison purposes) ➡ and fluoroscopic VCUG ➡ is shown. Grade IV reflux was confirmed on both imaging modalities. (Right) Frontal VCUG shows grade V VUR into the right kidney with a dilated tortuous ureter, blunted calyces, and intrarenal reflux into the tubules ➡.

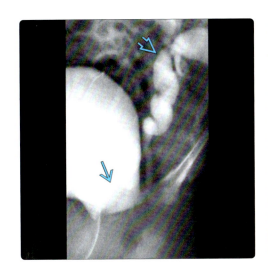

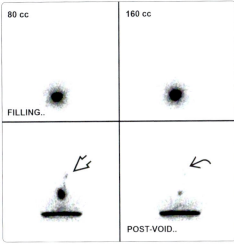

(Left) VCUG shows high-grade VUR ⇨ on the left and a globular filling defect in the bladder base ⇨ corresponding to a ureterocele. (Right) Posterior nuclear cystogram images show refluxed radiotracer extending into the right ureter and reaching the intrarenal collecting system ⇨. Note that reflux occurs only during voiding and drains well on the postvoid image in this patient ⇨.

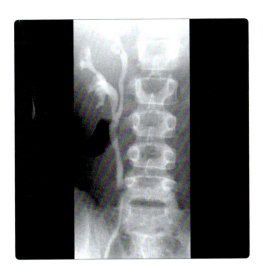

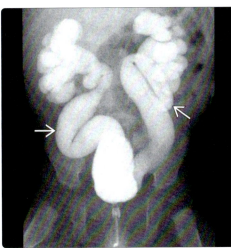

(Left) VCUG shows VUR into a partially duplicated collecting system, which resembles the letter Y. VUR can sometimes be seen fluoroscopically entering one limb of the Y 1st, receding, and then filling the other limb, the so-called yo-yo reflux. (Right) VCUG shows large-volume VUR into both kidneys, which have very dilated and tortuous collecting systems ⇨. Bilateral grade V reflux was diagnosed in this 3-month-old boy with febrile urinary tract infection.

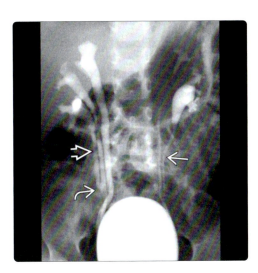

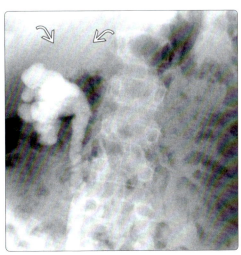

(Left) Frontal VCUG shows high-grade VUR into a triplicated ureter ⇨ on the right plus lower grade reflux into a duplicated ureter on the left ⇨. Two of the 3 right ureters join inferiorly ⇨. (Right) VCUG shows grade IV VUR into the lower pole of a duplicated right kidney. Note that no upper pole calyces are seen ⇨, and there are 10 calyces visualized. Also, the long axis points abnormally to the ipsilateral shoulder. US can confirm a duplication as the cause for this "drooping lily" rather than a cyst or mass.

KEY FACTS

TERMINOLOGY

- Presence of 2 separate pelvicalyceal collecting systems in 1 kidney
  - Partial duplication: Ureters join above urinary bladder
    - Most common, often of no consequence
  - Complete duplication: Ureters have separate bladder insertions

IMAGING

- Central renal sinus fat separated by band of cortical tissue
  - Renal parenchyma otherwise normal unless complications of VUR &/or obstruction present
- Separate renal pelves often visible on either side of cortical band ± separate proximal ureters
- Duplicated kidneys tend to be larger than nonduplex kidneys, even without hydronephrosis
- With complete duplication, ureter draining upper pole of kidney inserts in bladder inferior & medial to ureter draining lower pole of kidney (Weigert-Meyer rule)

- Lower pole ureter inserts in trigone & tends to have VUR
  - VUR may be present without ureter & collecting system dilatation
- Upper pole ureteral orifice ectopic in location, often associated with ureterocele, & tends to obstruct
- Drooping lily sign: Classic appearance of opacified lower pole collecting system on IVP or VCUG, displaced by mass-like upper pole hydronephrosis
  - Renal collecting system axis deviated, points to ipsilateral shoulder (normal points to contralateral shoulder)
  - Correlation with US critical to confirm upper pole obstruction rather than other mass lesion

CLINICAL ISSUES

- Incidence of 12-15% in general population
- Treatment depends on extent of anomalies & complications

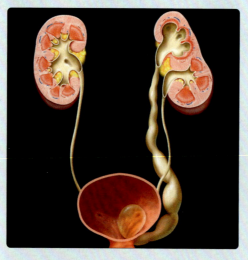
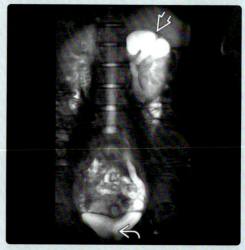

(Left) Coronal graphic shows a normal right kidney and completely duplicated left kidney with a poorly draining upper pole ectopic ureterocele seen in the bladder medial and inferior to the lower pole ureteral orifice. The lower pole ureter on the left inserts into bladder orthotopically at the trigone. (Right) Coronal MR urogram in a teenager shows a duplicated left kidney and obstructed upper pole moiety ➡, which drains ectopically into the vagina ➡. Note the cortical thinning of the left upper pole from chronic injury.

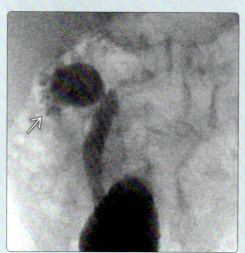
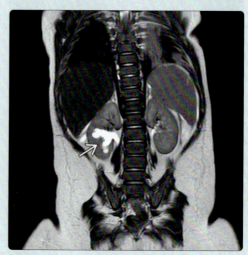

(Left) Frontal VCUG in a patient with a duplicated right kidney shows grade 4 vesicoureteral reflux (VUR) into the lower pole moiety ➡. Upper pole moieties tend to obstruct, and lower poles tend to reflux. (Right) Coronal T2WI MR in a 4 month old shows a duplicated right kidney with moderate pelvocaliectasis affecting only the lower pole ➡. The left kidney is not duplicated.

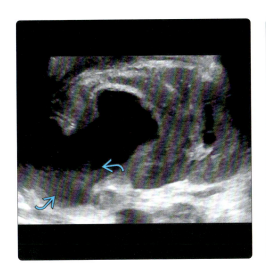

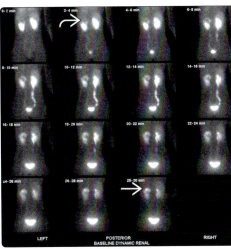

(Left) Sagittal US in an 18 month old with fever shows a duplicated right kidney with hydronephrosis of the upper pole moiety collecting system, which contains echogenic layering material ➘, compatible with pyonephrosis. (Right) Posterior images from a Tc-99m MAG3 renogram in the same patient show delayed uptake by the upper pole of the left kidney ➚ with poor function and excretion ➘. The postdiuretic washout curve for the left upper pole was flat (not shown).

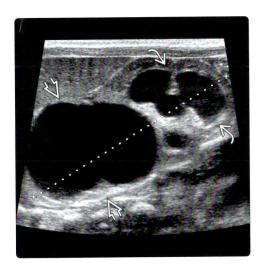

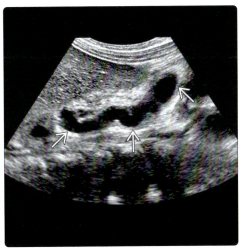

(Left) Longitudinal oblique US in a patient with a duplicated right kidney shows severe dilation of the upper pole moiety ➘ with marked parenchymal thinning. There is also mild to moderate dilation of the lower pole moiety ➘. Cursors mark the length of the kidney. (Right) Longitudinal oblique US in the same patient shows the tortuous course of the dilated right upper pole ureter ➘.

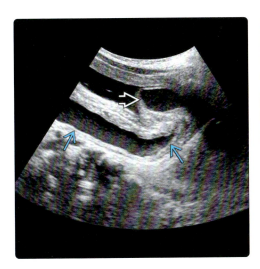

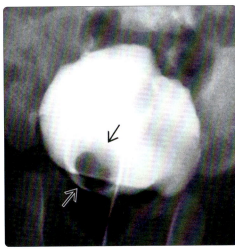

(Left) Longitudinal oblique US in the same patient follows the right upper pole dilated ureter ➘ into the bladder base, where the ureter ends in an ectopic ureterocele ➘. This patient has a completely duplicated right kidney with an obstructed upper pole moiety. (Right) Frontal VCUG shows a round filling defect ➘ in the bladder base from an ectopic ureterocele. Ureteroceles can be very large and occasionally prolapse during voiding, causing bladder outlet obstruction.

TERMINOLOGY

- Congenital cystic dilatation of distal submucosal portion of ureter within urinary bladder
- Intravesical: Completely contained within bladder
- Extravesical: Partially extends to bladder neck, urethra, or perineum
- Orthotopic (simple): Orifice located in bladder trigone
- Ectopic: Orifice located anywhere else; almost always associated with upper pole of duplicated system

IMAGING

- Voiding cystourethrogram and contrast-enhanced voiding urosonogram
  - Round/ovoid filling defect in urinary bladder
  - Early filling image important: Full bladder may compress or efface ureterocele
- Ultrasound, MR Urogram
  - Thin-walled, round/ovoid cystic structure
    - May collapse with ureter peristalsis

- May be large, occupy entire bladder
- Intravenous urography: "Cobra head" sign of contrast filling orthotopic ureterocele with thin peripheral halo

TOP DIFFERENTIAL DIAGNOSES

- Pseudoureterocele: Acquired dilatation of distal ureter from partial ureteral obstruction, usually caused by malignancy or calculus
  - Thicker, less-defined wall or halo of pseudoureterocele

CLINICAL ISSUES

- Ectopic extravesical > orthotopic intravesical by 3:1 ratio
- Cecoureterocele: Ectopic ureterocele where intravesical portion dissects submucosally below trigone and urethra
  - If obstructs becomes surgical emergency
- Typical treatment: Endoscopic incision of ureterocele, especially if infected or obstructed in neonate
  - May change bladder trigone configuration, causing new vesicoureteral reflux

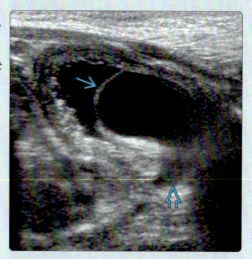

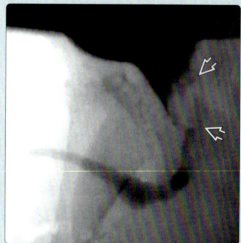

(Left) Longitudinal ultrasound of the urinary bladder in an 18 day old with prenatally detected hydronephrosis shows a large, thin-walled cyst ➡️ filling much of the bladder lumen, typical of a ureterocele. The cyst connects to a dilated distal left ureter ➡️. (Right) Oblique voiding cystourethrogram shows prolapse of a ureterocele into the posterior urethra ➡️ as voiding begins. Voiding stopped seconds later due to urethral obstruction.

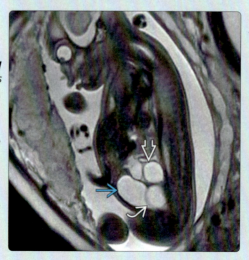

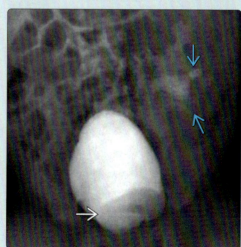

(Left) Sagittal T2 SSFSE MR from a fetal MR shows a thin-walled ureterocele ➡️ within the urinary bladder ➡️ with a tortuous and dilated ureter ➡️ superiorly. (Right) VCUG shows grades 2-3 vesicoureteral reflux into the left lower pole collecting system ➡️. The drooping lily configuration of contrast within the lower pose strongly suggests obstruction of an upper pole moiety (as confirmed on the ultrasound). The upper pole ureterocele ➡️ remains visible in the contrast-filled bladder.

Congenital Megacalyces and Megaureter

KEY FACTS

TERMINOLOGY

- Megacalyces: Dilatation of calyces with normal-sized renal pelvis and ureter
- Megaureter: Enlarged ureter (diameter > 7 mm); 3 types
  - Obstructing
  - Refluxing
  - Nonobstructing, nonrefluxing

IMAGING

- Megacalyces
  - Caliectasis, normal renal pelvis, no evidence of obstruction
  - Narrow, crescent-shaped medulla; absent papillae
  - Numerous calyces, polygonal (not usual cup shape)
- Megaureter
  - Dilated ureter (> 7 mm) tapers to normal caliber just proximal to bladder
  - Left side more common
  - Varying degrees of hydronephrosis

TOP DIFFERENTIAL DIAGNOSES

- Obstructive hydronephrosis
- Vesicoureteral reflux

PATHOLOGY

- Megacalyces
  - Hypoplastic medullary pyramids
- Megaureter
  - Adynamic distal ureteral segment, which has normal caliber (primary obstructed)

CLINICAL ISSUES

- Ranges from mild stable ureterectasis to severe progressive hydroureteronephrosis
  - Rarely progresses to renal failure
- Surgery performed in cases of recurrent urinary tract infections or worsening renal function
  - Ureteral reimplant ± tapering

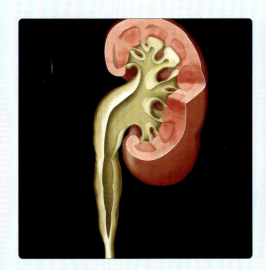

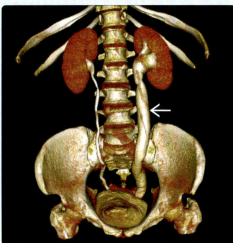

(Left) Graphic shows megacalyces. The calyces and proximal ureter are grossly dilated, and the calyces are increased in number in some cases. There is only mild atrophy of the papillae and renal cortex. (Right) Coronal volume-rendered CECT shows pelvocaliectasis and a dilated left ureter ➡. No intrinsic or extrinsic obstructing process was found. The right ureter is normal. A radionuclide renogram showed almost normal and equal function in both kidneys.

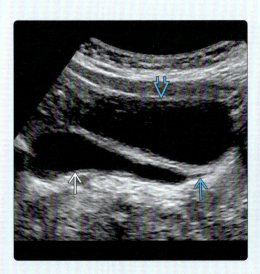

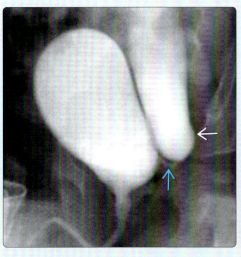

(Left) Longitudinal ultrasound at the left ureterovesical junction of a male infant shows a dilated left ureter ➡ tapering distally to a normal caliber aperistaltic juxtavesical segment ➡ that shows urothelial thickening. The urinary bladder ➡ is seen anteriorly. (From DI: Pediatrics, 3e.) (Right) Oblique fluoroscopic image from a voiding cystourethrogram in the same patient shows vesicoureteral reflux into the normal caliber juxtavesical segment ➡ with transition to the proximally dilated ureter ➡. (From DI: Pediatrics, 3e.)

KEY FACTS

TERMINOLOGY

- Megaureter-megacystis syndrome (MMS)
  - Marked vesicoureteral reflux (VUR) with repetitive large volume urine recycling
  - Leads to enlarged urinary bladder

IMAGING

- Voiding cystourethrogram (VCUG)
  - Large urinary bladder with smooth, thin wall
    - > 2x estimated normal bladder capacity
  - Unilateral or bilateral high-grade VUR
    - VUR into single collecting system or lower pole of duplex system
  - Voiding demonstrates complete bladder emptying
  - However, bladder rapidly refills by drainage of refluxed contrast from dilated collecting systems
    - Termed aberrant micturition, though bladder neck & urethra normal

TOP DIFFERENTIAL DIAGNOSES

- Mechanical bladder outlet obstruction
  - Posterior urethral valves
  - Extrinsic/intrinsic mass
  - Obstructing ureterocele
- Functional bladder outlet obstruction
  - Neurogenic bladder
- Megacystis of unclear etiology
  - Prune-belly (Eagle-Barrett) syndrome
  - Megacystis-microcolon-hypoperistalsis syndrome
  - Megalourethra

CLINICAL ISSUES

- Most commonly presents with urinary tract infections or hydronephrosis on prenatal ultrasound
- Bladder function may deteriorate if VUR does not improve
- With spontaneous resolution or surgical correction of VUR, bladder function usually improves

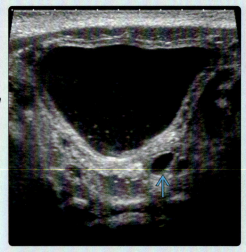
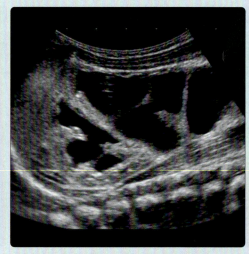

(Left) Transverse ultrasound in a 3-day-old boy with a history of prenatal hydronephrosis shows a large thin-walled bladder & left hydroureter ➡ with urothelial thickening. (Right) Longitudinal ultrasound of the left kidney in the same patient shows asymmetric upper pole (UP) vs. lower pole (LP) pelvocaliectasis & cortical thinning, suggesting collecting system duplication. As no ureterocele was seen in the bladder, this finding suggests an obstructed ectopic UP ureter & high-grade LP vesicoureteral reflux (VUR).

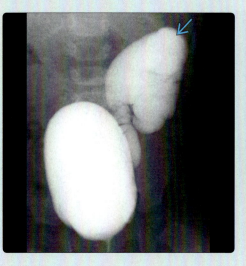
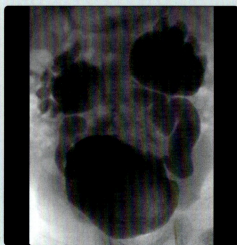

(Left) Frontal VCUG in the same patient shows grade V left lower pole VUR ➡ with a large bladder. (The orientation of the visualized collecting system long axis towards the ipsilateral shoulder suggests duplication.) The bladder capacity was > 2x the estimated normal capacity. (Right) Frontal fluorospot during VCUG in a 7-day-old boy with prenatal hydronephrosis shows massive bilateral VUR & large bladder. The urethra was normal and the bladder emptied completely during voiding, typical of MMS.

Megacystis-Microcolon-Intestinal Hypoperistalsis Syndrome

KEY FACTS

TERMINOLOGY

- Megacystis-microcolon-intestinal hypoperistalsis syndrome: Rare disease of smooth muscle dysfunction resulting in poor motility of GI & GU tracts
- Synonyms: Berdon syndrome & familial visceral myopathy

IMAGING

- Very dilated urinary bladder with poor or no emptying
  - Polyhydramnios with megacystis on prenatal imaging suggests diagnosis
- Nonobstructive urinary tract dilatation
  - Variable degree of pelvocaliectasis & hydroureter, present in ~ 50%
  - Bladder decompression improves urinary tract dilatation
- Variably dilated, featureless small bowel with malrotation on upper GI
  - Poor/absent peristalsis; pseudoobstruction
- Unused ahaustral microcolon on contrast enema
- If severe abdominal distention → pulmonary compromise

TOP DIFFERENTIAL DIAGNOSES

- Posterior urethral valves
- Prune-belly syndrome
- Cloacal malformation
- Hirschsprung disease

PATHOLOGY

- Mutation in *ACTG2* gene → abnormal smooth muscle actin filaments
- Autosomal dominant, often de novo mutation

CLINICAL ISSUES

- Female > > male
- Clinical triad: Abdominal distention, bilious emesis, failure to pass meconium or urine
- Previously lethal within 1 year
- Survival improved with total parenteral nutrition & small bowel or multivisceral transplant

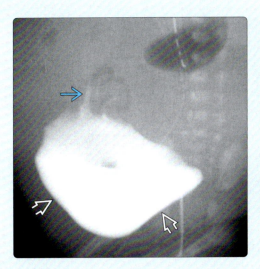

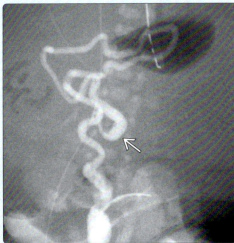

(Left) Anterior oblique view of the urinary bladder during a VCUG shows an enlarged, smooth-walled bladder ⇥ in this newborn with MMIHS. Contrast in a tubular projection ⇥ from the bladder dome likely represents a urachal remnant. (Right) Frontal contrast enema in a newborn with MMIHS shows a very small caliber, unused microcolon without haustrations positioned in the midline abdomen. The cecum ⇥ is overlying the spine. Marked hydronephrosis is displacing the bowel.

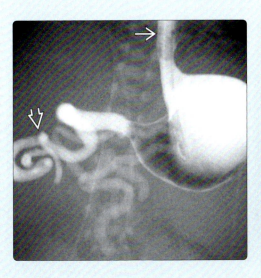

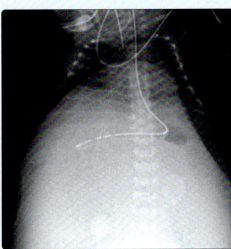

(Left) Frontal upper GI image performed through a nasogastric tube shows full-column gastroesophageal reflux into the lower esophagus ⇥ with distal passage of contrast into featureless small bowel ⇥ malpositioned in the right upper abdomen, consistent with malrotation. (Right) Frontal view of the chest in a newborn with MMIHS shows marked abdominal distention causing mass effect on the lungs. Pulmonary function and development may be compromised both in utero and postnatally in MMIHS.

TERMINOLOGY

- Congenital triad of
  - Urinary tract dilatation
  - Cryptorchidism
  - Abdominal wall muscle deficiency/laxity (with thin wrinkled skin resembling prune)

IMAGING

- Radiographs: Large abdomen with laterally bulging flanks
  - ± undulation or "wrinkling" of redundant skin
  - ± centralization of bowel gas due to markedly dilated ureters &/or renal collecting systems
  - Pulmonary hypoplasia with small, bell-shaped thorax ± pneumothorax
- VCUG: Marked bilateral vesicoureteral reflux
  - Dilated posterior urethra but true mechanical obstruction uncommon
- US: Dilated bladder and ureters; ± pelvocaliectasis, cystic renal dysplasia, urachal anomalies

- Empty scrotum (cryptorchidism)
- MR urography can help delineate complex anatomy and assess renal drainage and dysplasia

TOP DIFFERENTIAL DIAGNOSES

- Posterior urethral valves
- Severe vesicoureteral reflux
- Primary megaureter
- Megacystis microcolon intestinal hypoperistalsis syndrome

CLINICAL ISSUES

- Etiology unknown
- 1 in 30,000 to 40,000 live births; 95-99% male
- Variable renal impairment and pulmonary hypoplasia determine prognosis
- Many survivors but usually with chronic health issues
  - Dialysis or renal transplant in 10-20%

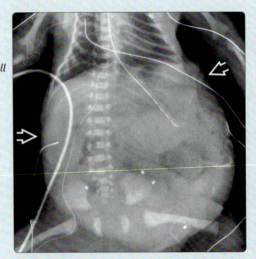
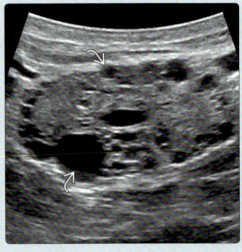

(Left) *Frontal abdominal radiograph in a newborn shows an enlarged abdomen with a flaccid, undulating abdominal wall ⇒ and a small thorax, typical of Prune-Belly (or Eagle-Barrett) syndrome (PBS or EBS).* (Right) *Longitudinal US in the same newborn with PBS shows numerous cysts ⇒ scattered through the echogenic renal parenchyma with poor corticomedullary differentiation. The findings are typical of cystic dysplasia of the kidneys, likely due to longstanding bladder outlet obstruction.*

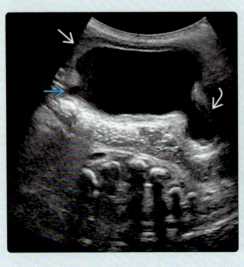
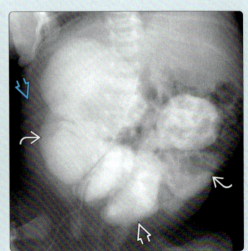

(Left) *Longitudinal US of the pelvis in newborn male with PBS shows a keyhole appearance of the bladder with posterior urethral dilatation ⇒, bladder wall thickening ⇒, and a bladder diverticulum ⇒. No obstructing urethral anomaly was seen on VCUG.* (Right) *Frontal VCUG in a patient with PBS shows infused contrast filling the bladder and rapidly refluxing into markedly dilated, tortuous ureters bilaterally ⇒. The ureters hold several times the volume of the bladder ⇒. Note the wrinkled abdominal wall ⇒.*

KEY FACTS

TERMINOLOGY

- Developmental malformation resulting in cystic mass in perirenal and peripelvic area

IMAGING

- Uni- or multilocular cystic mass in perirenal or peripelvic area
- Best imaging tool: CT or MR
- CT and MR imaging findings
  - Subcapsular mass with fluid attenuation on CT and high signal intensity on T2WI MR
- Ultrasonographic findings
  - Cystic mass, uni- or multilocular

TOP DIFFERENTIAL DIAGNOSES

- Renal and perirenal abscess
  - Complex fluid collections with enhancing septa
- Urinoma
  - Fluid collection filling with contrast on delayed images
- Renal cell carcinoma
  - Uni- or multilocular cystic mass with thick wall
  - Enhancing, smooth or nodular septa
- Perinephric lymphoma
  - Soft tissue perinephric mass with mild homogeneous enhancement

PATHOLOGY

- Failure of development of normal lymphatic tissue in perirenal &/or peripelvic area
- Thin-walled cysts with single layer of endothelium

CLINICAL ISSUES

- Asymptomatic; dull flank pain; palpable mass; hypertension; hematuria
- Seen in any age
- Conservative management in asymptomatic cases

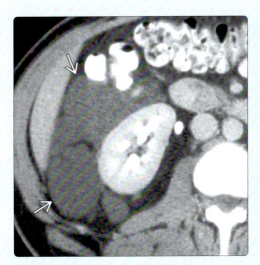

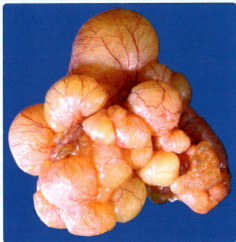

(Left) Axial CECT shows a fluid-attenuation multilocular mass ➡ within the right perirenal space, abutting the renal capsule. The fluid attenuation and multilocular appearance make lymphangioma the most likely diagnosis. (Right) Gross photograph from the same patient shows multiple, well-defined cysts, correlating with the CT appearance and compatible with renal lymphangiomatosis.

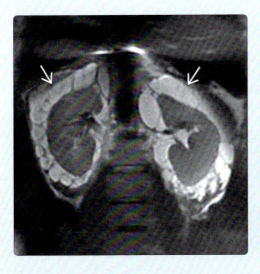

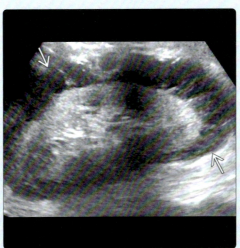

(Left) Coronal T2 FS MR shows bilateral hyperintense, multilocular collections ➡ in the perinephric space compatible with lymphangiomatosis. (Right) Ultrasound of the right kidney acquired on the longitudinal plane in the same patient shows lymphangiomatosis as multiple anechoic perinephric collections ➡ with thin internal septations.

KEY FACTS

IMAGING

- Voiding cystourethrogram or contrast-enhanced voiding urosonogram
  - Abrupt transition from dilated posterior urethra to small bulbar urethra at level of valvular tissue; actual valve tissue may not be visible
  - Bladder enlargement, trabeculation, muscular hypertrophy, diverticula, ± patent urachus
  - Vesicoureteral reflux (50-70%)
  - Ejaculatory duct reflux
- Ultrasound
  - Bilateral hydroureteronephrosis
  - Echogenic, dysplastic kidneys with poor corticomedullary differentiation ± cortical cysts, urinomas, ascites
  - Lobular bladder with thickened, irregular wall ± diverticula
  - Keyhole sign of dilated posterior urethra

PATHOLOGY

- Varying degrees of chronic urethral obstruction due to fusion &/or prominence of plicae colliculi (concentric folds in posterior urethra)

CLINICAL ISSUES

- Severity and duration of obstruction determines age of presentation and clinical symptoms, which include
  - Perinatally: Oligohydramnios, hydronephrosis, anuria, urinary ascites, urinoma, pulmonary hypoplasia
  - In infancy: Urinary tract infection, sepsis, urinary retention, poor urinary stream, failure to thrive
  - In childhood: Abnormal voiding patterns, hesitancy, straining, poor stream, large postvoid residual, renal insufficiency/failure
- 30-40% will eventually develop end-stage renal disease
- 75% have long-term urinary bladder dysfunction, likely due to myogenic failure
- Fertility issues common in long-term survivors

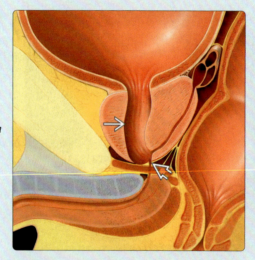
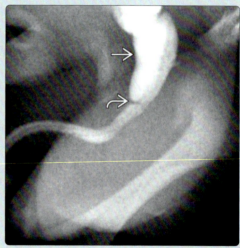

(Left) *Sagittal graphic shows an enlarged posterior urethra* ➡ *extending through the prostate with an abrupt change in urethral caliber* ➡ *just distal to the verumontanum at a typical level of valve tissue.* (Right) *Lateral oblique voiding cystourethrogram (VCUG) in a newborn with posterior urethral valves (PUV) shows the same anatomy from the previous graphic. There is a dilated posterior urethra* ➡ *with an abrupt change in urethral caliber just distal to the valve tissue* ➡.

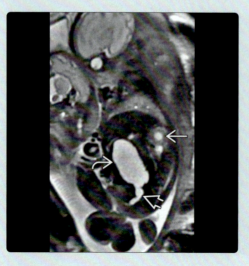
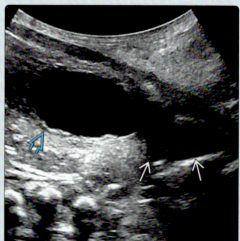

(Left) *Sagittal SSFSE T2 MR in a 3rd trimester twin gestation shows a fetus with an elongated, mildly thick-walled urinary bladder* ➡, *hydronephrosis* ➡, *and a dilated posterior urethra* ➡ *(keyhole sign) typical of PUV.* (Right) *Longitudinal US in a newborn with PUV shows a dilated posterior urethra* ➡ *inferior to the bladder base (postnatal keyhole sign equivalent). Note the irregular bladder wall thickening* ➡.

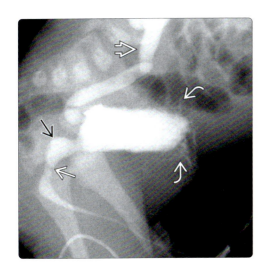
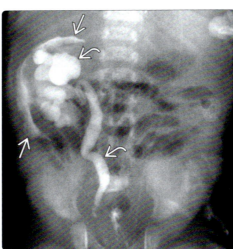

(Left) *Lateral VCUG in a newborn with PUV shows the thin valvular tissue* ➡ *at the inferior margin of the dilated posterior urethra* ➡. *The urinary bladder wall is markedly thickened with contrast extending between the trabeculations* ➡. *High-grade unilateral vesicoureteral reflux (VUR)* ➡ *is noted.* (Right) *Frontal VCUG in the same patient after voiding shows contrast pooling around the kidney* ➡. *This urinoma is due to high-pressure VUR* ➡ *causing a forniceal rupture in the setting of a chronic bladder outlet obstruction.*

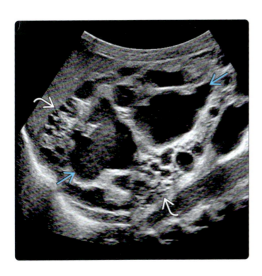
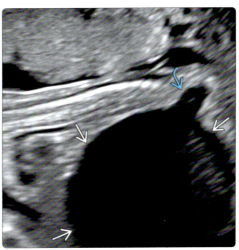

(Left) *Longitudinal US of the left kidney in a newborn with PUV shows marked pelvocaliectasis* ➡ *and cystic dysplastic changes of the renal cortex* ➡ *due to chronic obstruction in utero.* (Right) *Prenatal US shows the dilated posterior urethra* ➡ *at the base of the large urinary bladder* ➡, *the so-called keyhole sign. PUV is the most common cause of lower urinary tract obstruction in a male fetus. (From DI: Obstetrics, 3e.)*

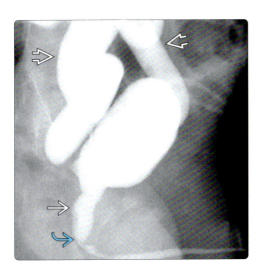
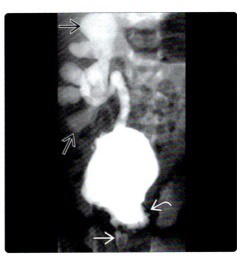

(Left) *Oblique VCUG in a newborn shows PUV* ➡, *dilated posterior urethra* ➡, *and large-volume bilateral VUR* ➡. (Right) *Frontal VCUG in an infant shows high-grade VUR into the right kidney* ➡ *with irregular bladder wall thickening* ➡ *and a dilated posterior urethra* ➡. *High-grade unilateral VUR is protective of the contralateral renal function.*

KEY FACTS

TERMINOLOGY

- Acute infection of renal parenchyma

IMAGING

- Best diagnostic clue: Wedge-shaped, striated areas of decreased enhancement and renal swelling on CECT
- CT findings
  - Wedge-shaped or rounded areas of poor/streaky enhancement
    - Striated nephrogram: Best identified on nephrographic &/or excretory phase
    - Inflammatory changes in perirenal fat
- MR findings
  - ↑ signal intensity on T2WI and DWI of affected areas
  - Wedge-shaped or rounded areas of poor/streaky enhancement
- Ultrasound findings
  - Often negative

- ↓ perfusion in areas of pyelonephritis at color Doppler and power Doppler evaluation

TOP DIFFERENTIAL DIAGNOSES

- Renal infarction
- Renal cell carcinoma
- Renal lymphoma
- Vasculitis

PATHOLOGY

- Ascending infection (most common)
  - *Escherichia coli*

CLINICAL ISSUES

- ↑ incidence in women < 40 years and men > 65 years
- Cyclical fever, flank pain, vomiting, leukocytosis, pyuria

DIAGNOSTIC CHECKLIST

- Diagnosis of acute pyelonephritis is usually based on combination of clinical and laboratory presentation

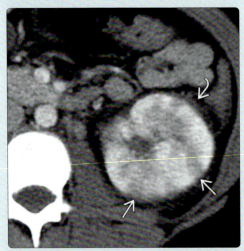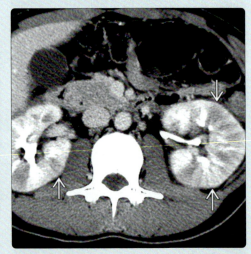

(Left) *Axial CECT shows "striated" nephrogram ➡ and trace perinephric fluid ➡ compatible with acute pyelonephritis in a patient presenting with urinary tract infection, fever, and abdominal pain.* (Right) *Axial CECT shows bilateral, wedge-shaped areas of renal parenchymal hypoenhancement ("striated" nephrograms) from pyelonephritis ➡.*

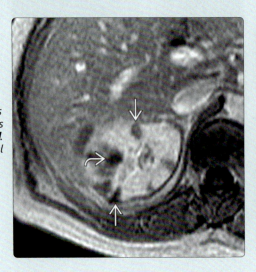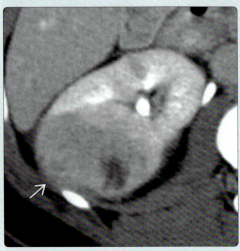

(Left) *Axial gadolinium-enhanced T1WI MR through the right kidney shows multiple wedge-shaped areas of hypoenhancement ➡ compatible with pyelonephritis. Small intraparenchymal round focus of hypoenhancement suggests a developing microabscess ➡.* (Right) *Axial CECT shows focal severe pyelonephritis with mass-like swelling and a "striated" nephrogram ➡.*

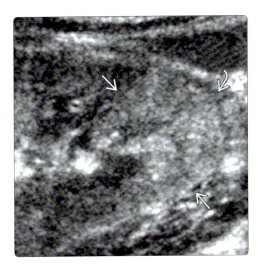
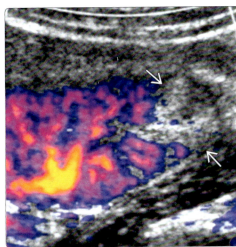

(Left) Sagittal grayscale sonogram of acute hemorrhagic pyelonephritis shows the wedge-shaped area of increased echogenicity within the lower pole ➡ and the thin rim of adjacent perinephric fluid ➡. (Right) Sagittal power Doppler ultrasound in the same patient demonstrates absence of flow in the area of pyelonephritis ➡.

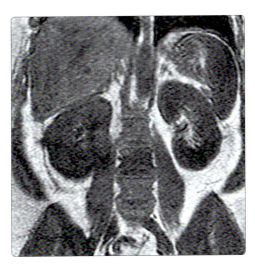
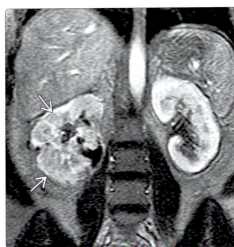

(Left) Coronal T1WI MR of the kidneys demonstrates no clear abnormality. (Right) Coronal gadolinium-enhanced T1WI MR in the same patient reveals diminished perfusion throughout the right kidney from severe pyelonephritis ➡.

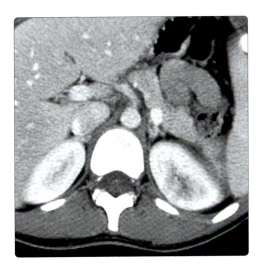
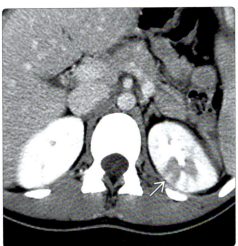

(Left) Axial CECT of the left kidney during corticomedullary phase demonstrates no abnormality. (Right) Axial CECT in the same patient during excretory phase shows decreased perfusion to the upper pole of the left kidney from pyelonephritis ➡.

TERMINOLOGY

- Renal scarring and atrophy secondary to multiple episodes of acute pyelonephritis during early childhood
  - Most cases are secondary to vesicoureteral reflux (VUR)

IMAGING

- Deep cortical scars overlying deformed calyces
- Scarring is often seen in poles of kidney
  - Upper pole > lower pole
- Typically asymmetric, segmental, and unilateral
- Hypertrophy of residual normal tissue
  - May mimic mass
- Blunting, dilating of calyces
  - Secondary to retraction of papilla
- Dystrophic calcification
- Compensatory hypertrophy of contralateral kidney when unilateral

TOP DIFFERENTIAL DIAGNOSES

- Renal tuberculosis
- Renal infarction
- Radiation nephritis
- Chronic renal failure

PATHOLOGY

- Etiology: Reflux of infected urine from bladder > urinary obstruction, calculi, foreign body
- In some cases, disease may progress in absence of any bacteriuria or obstruction
- Acute pyelonephritis in adults resolves and does not lead to scarring

CLINICAL ISSUES

- Time of resolution of VUR depends on grade
- Management of VUR includes prophylactic antibiotics and surgery

(Left) Graphic shows the grading system for vesicoureteric reflux, showing progressive levels of reflux, calyceal blunting, and renal cortical injury from grade 1 on the left to grade 5 on the right. (Right) Axial CECT obtained during the excretory phase shows marked and deep cortical scarring ⇨ consistent with chronic pyelonephritis.

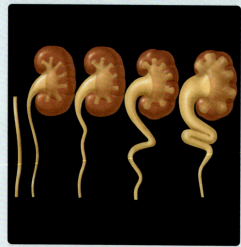
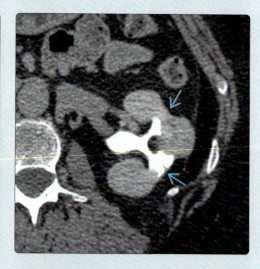

(Left) Supine frontal view during voiding cystourethrogram (VCUG) shows grade 4 vesicoureteral reflux (VUR) on the right ⇨ and grade 3 VUR on the left ⇨ in this 6-year-old boy with chronic recurrent pyelonephritis. (Right) Prone spot view from Tc-99m dimercaptosuccinic acid (DMSA) scan in the same patient shows marked right kidney atrophy with patchy decreased cortical uptake ⇨. Split function was 93.5% left kidney and 6.5% right, consistent with multifocal scarring & reflux nephropathy.

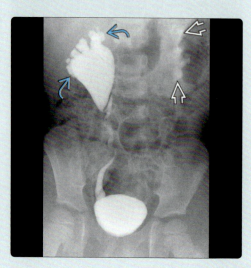
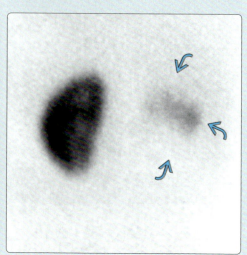

Xanthogranulomatous Pyelonephritis

KEY FACTS

TERMINOLOGY

- Chronic infection of kidney and surrounding tissues characterized by destruction of renal parenchyma and replacement by lipid-laden macrophages

IMAGING

- Best imaging tool: CECT
- Findings on CT
  - Enlarged kidney with preserved reniform morphology
    - Focal form is less common (10-27% of cases)
  - Low-attenuation renal &/or perirenal lesions (xanthomas)
  - Diffuse or focally absent nephrogram
  - Centrally obstructing calculus; staghorn
  - Contracted pelvis; dilated calyces
- Findings on US
  - Multiple anechoic or hypoechoic masses (xanthomas)
  - Acoustic shadowing from central staghorn calculus

TOP DIFFERENTIAL DIAGNOSES

- Renal abscess
- Pyonephrosis
- Renal cell carcinoma

PATHOLOGY

- Accumulation of lipid-laden macrophages (xanthoma cells) and granulomatous infiltrate
- Pathogens: *Escherichia coli*; *Proteus mirabilis*

CLINICAL ISSUES

- Age: 45-65 years (more frequent in women)
- Symptoms/signs: Dull flank pain, fever, palpable mass
- Treatment: Nephrectomy usually required

DIAGNOSTIC CHECKLIST

- Difficult to distinguish from other infections or neoplasms
  - Histologic diagnosis required, not based solely on imaging studies

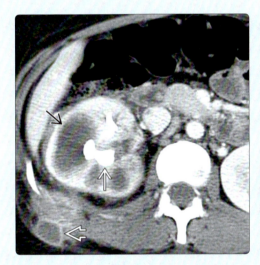
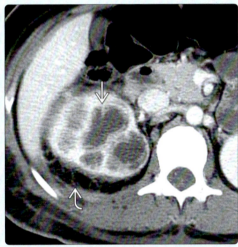

(Left) *Axial CECT in a 65-year-old woman who presented with pyuria, fever, and right flank pain demonstrates a central stone in the renal pelvis ➡ with surrounding low-attenuation lesions ➡. Note the extension of the inflammatory process through the perirenal space, resulting in an abdominal wall abscess ➡. (Right) Axial CECT in the same patient reveals perirenal stranding ➡ and multiple low-attenuation, necrotic renal lesions ➡ corresponding to debris-filled calyces and xanthoma collections.*

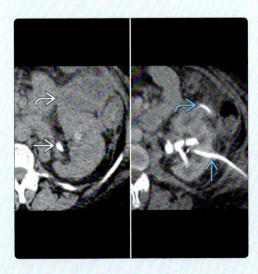
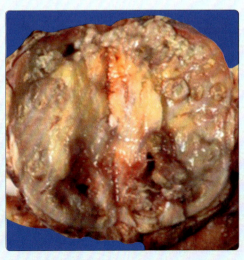

(Left) *Axial NECT (left) of the left kidney in a 55-year-old woman with xanthogranulomatous pyelonephritis shows a staghorn pelvic calculus ➡ and a perinephric xanthoma ➡. Axial CECT (right) obtained after percutaneous drainage of perinephric xanthoma ➡ and placement of a nephrostomy tube ➡ is shown. (Right) Gross pathology of the left kidney in the same patient shows xanthogranulomatous pyelonephritis with prominent suppurative and acute inflammatory exudate.*

Emphysematous Pyelonephritis

IMAGING

- Best imaging tool: CT
- CT findings
  - Intraparenchymal gas ± perirenal extension
  - ± renal or perirenal fluid collections
  - Classification systems based on distribution of gas and fluid collections
- Ultrasound findings
  - Nondependent echogenic foci in renal parenchyma &/or collecting system
  - "Dirty shadowing"; ring-down artifacts

TOP DIFFERENTIAL DIAGNOSES

- Emphysematous pyelitis
- Perforated duodenal ulcer
- Iatrogenic

PATHOLOGY

- Most common pathogen
  - *Escherichia coli*

CLINICAL ISSUES

- Life-threatening infection
- Prognosis affected by clinical/lab presentation and gas extension
- Overall mortality: 11-50%
- Highest mortality rates if bilateral &/or parenchymal destruction is not associated with fluid components
- Treatment
  - Fluid and electrolyte resuscitation; antibiotic therapy
  - Percutaneous drainage of gaseous parenchymal collection
  - Nephrectomy

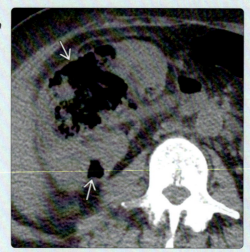
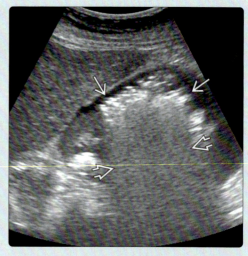

(Left) Axial NECT shows a large amount of gas ➡ within the right kidney, compatible with emphysematous pyelonephritis. No fluid collections are present. CT is the best imaging modality for diagnosis and assessment of gas extension. (Right) Sagittal ultrasound of the right kidney in the same patient reveals nondependent echoes within the renal parenchyma ➡ associated with "dirty shadowing" ➡.

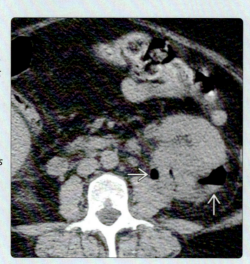
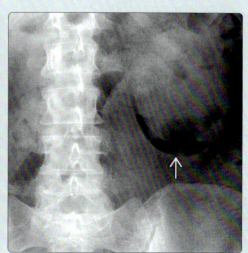

(Left) Axial NECT in a 69-year-old diabetic woman who presented with a fever and flank pain demonstrates large gas-fluid collections in the left renal parenchyma ➡, diagnostic of a gas-forming abscess from emphysematous pyelonephritis. (Right) Anteroposterior radiography in the same patient demonstrates a curvilinear gas collection ➡ outlining the lower pole of the left kidney.

TERMINOLOGY

- Localized collection of pus due to suppurative necrosis in kidney

IMAGING

- Best imaging tool
  - CECT and Gd-enhanced MR for diagnosis
  - US to provide guidance for percutaneous sampling or drainage
- Findings at CECT and gadolinium-enhanced MR
  - Renal &/or perirenal fluid collection usually with thick enhancing wall (rim or ring enhancement)
  - ± gas within collection
  - Usually with perinephric fat stranding
- Findings at ultrasound
  - Anechoic or hypoechoic collection
  - ± internal septations
  - ± low-level echoes (debris)
  - ± "dirty shadowing" (gas)

TOP DIFFERENTIAL DIAGNOSES

- Infected or hemorrhagic cyst
- Renal cell carcinoma
- Metastases and lymphoma

CLINICAL ISSUES

- Most common signs/symptoms
  - Fever, flank or abdominal pain, chills, dysuria
- Treatment
  - Antibiotic therapy
  - Antibiotic therapy + percutaneous drainage via US or CT
  - Surgery

DIAGNOSTIC CHECKLIST

- Consider clinical history and urinalysis to diagnose and differentiate from malignancy
- On CECT, presence of ring enhancement is key finding for differentiating abscess from solid lesion

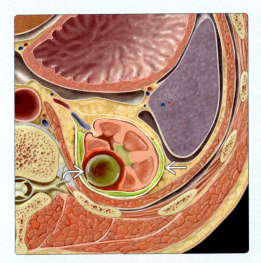 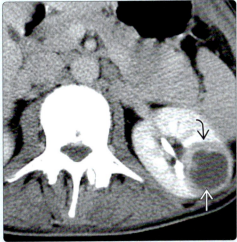

(Left) Illustration shows a left renal abscess with a thick peripheral rim ➡ and adjacent infected perinephric fluid ➡. (Right) Axial CECT in a 46-year-old woman with a history of diabetes, now presenting with left flank pain and fever, demonstrates a nonenhancing fluid collection in the left kidney compatible with an abscess ➡. Note the thick, irregular wall of the abscess capsule ➡.

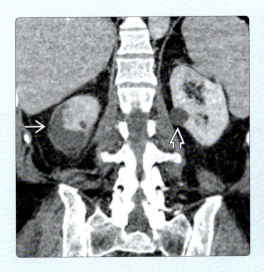 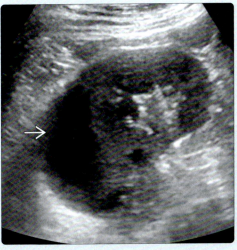

(Left) Image shows a 70-year-old man with right subcapsular rim-enhancing fluid collection ➡ compatible with a renal abscess. Note contralateral small, simple left renal cyst ➡. (Right) Longitudinal ultrasound of the right kidney in the same patient shows the renal abscess as an elongated, subcapsular anechoic collection ➡. US-guided fluid aspiration revealed the presence of Enterococcus faecalis.

TERMINOLOGY

- Infection of obstructed renal collecting system

IMAGING

- CT
  - Dilated renal collecting system
  - Fluid-debris level ± gas in renal pelvis
  - Thickened urothelial lining of renal pelvis and proximal ureter
- Ultrasound
  - Dilated renal collecting system
    - Low-level echoes
    - Fluid-debris levels

TOP DIFFERENTIAL DIAGNOSES

- Hydronephrosis
- Transitional cell carcinoma

PATHOLOGY

- Purulent fluid in dilated renal collecting system
  - Causes of renal collecting system obstruction
    - Stone, tumor, postsurgical stricture, congenital anomalies

CLINICAL ISSUES

- Medical emergency
- If left untreated → sepsis → death
- Must be treated emergently
  - Antibiotics + urgent drainage of pus
  - Percutaneous nephrostomy or ureteral catheterization

DIAGNOSTIC CHECKLIST

- Consider ultrasound or CT-guided aspiration of fluid in dilated collecting system to confirm diagnosis

(Left) Axial NECT in pyonephrosis shows severe dilatation of the right renal collecting system ➡. The attenuation of the fluid within the dilated renal pelvis is higher than water. Note perinephric inflammatory changes ➡. (Right) Renal ultrasound shows a dilated collecting system ➡ filled with low-level echoes ➡; the combination of imaging findings is diagnostic for pyonephrosis. Pyonephrosis is a medical emergency that can lead to severe sepsis if left untreated.

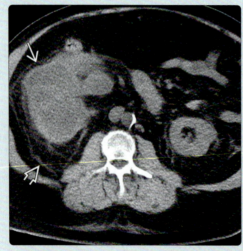 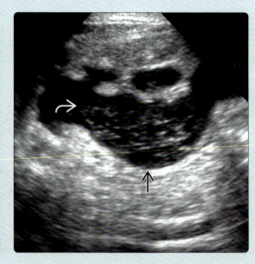

(Left) Axial CECT of the pelvis in a patient with fever and a left lower quadrant renal transplant demonstrates severe pyonephrosis of the renal allograft. Note severe dilatation of the renal pelvis ➡ with gas ➡ and fluid with attenuation higher than water. (Right) Longitudinal ultrasound through the left lower quadrant renal allograft in the same patient with severe pyonephrosis reveals severe dilatation of the renal collecting system with echogenic material ➡. Nephrostomy drainage was performed emergently.

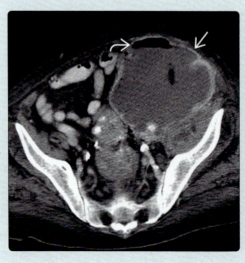 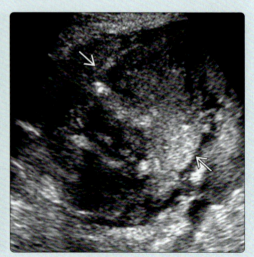

KEY FACTS

TERMINOLOGY

- Renal involvement by unusual infections in immunocompromised or debilitated host

TOP DIFFERENTIAL DIAGNOSES

- Candidiasis
  - Kidney is major target organ in candidemia
  - Nonenhancing filling defect within dilated collecting system on CT
  - Focal abscess/microabscess within parenchyma; may extend into perirenal space
- *Pneumocystis jirovecii*
  - Most common opportunistic infection in HIV/AIDS patients (CD4 < 200)
  - Punctate cortical calcifications in healing phase
- Aspergillosis
  - Immunocompromised patients (rare)
  - Etiology: *Aspergillus fumigatus* and *Aspergillus flavus*
  - Filling defects ("fungus balls") within dilated collecting system
  - Renal aspergilloma (pseudotumor)
- Cytomegalovirus
  - Common opportunistic infection in HIV/AIDS patients
  - Renal infection noted in widespread disease
  - Renal microabscess on CT
- Tuberculosis
  - Hematogenous spread of *Mycobacterium tuberculosis*
    - 4-8% of patients with pulmonary disease
  - Strictures (ureter, infundibulum, pelvis)
  - Calcifications (punctate, linear, curvilinear, diffuse)
    - "Putty kidney": End-stage infection associated with diffuse calcifications (autonephrectomy)

DIAGNOSTIC CHECKLIST

- Serologic studies are very helpful to establish diagnosis as imaging findings are often nonspecific

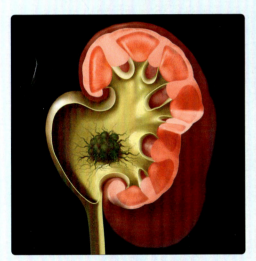 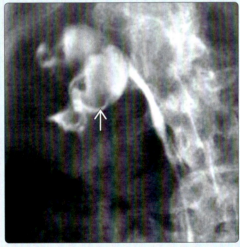

(Left) *Graphic shows a hydronephrotic kidney with a "fungus ball" in the dilated pelvis. Renal fungal infections may result from Candida albicans or Aspergillus and usually occur in debilitated patients. They may result from or cause ureteral obstruction.* (Right) *Retrograde pyelogram of the right kidney shows filling defects* ➡ *in a mildly dilated collecting system corresponding to a "fungus ball" in a patient with Candidiasis.*

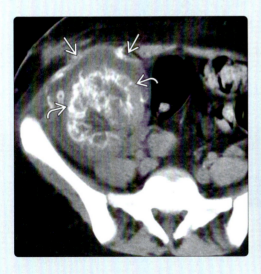 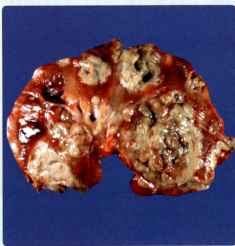

(Left) *NECT of a young patient with a failed transplant and fever shows amorphous calcification throughout the allograft* ➚ *and a rim of perinephric fluid* ➡. *Aspergillus infection was confirmed after biopsy and nephrectomy. The diagnosis of renal aspergillosis is difficult given its rarity and nonspecific appearance, but a history of immunosuppression is typical.* (Right) *Gross pathology image of the renal allograft shows multiple abscesses.*

KEY FACTS

TERMINOLOGY

- Fluid-filled renal lesion

IMAGING

- **Bosniak classification**
  - Imaging-based classification of renal cystic lesions
    - Class I: Benign cysts
    - Class II: Minimally complicated cysts; benign
    - Class IIF: Requires CT/MR imaging follow-up
    - Class III: More complicated cysts; usually managed surgically (biopsy controversial)
    - Class IV: Malignant lesions; require surgery
- Simple cyst
  - US: Simple, uncomplicated cyst; spherical or ovoid, anechoic content, sharply defined, imperceptible wall, and acoustic enhancement
  - NECT: Sharply marginated, round, smooth, homogeneous, hypodense (< 20 HU) mass

- MR: ↓ signal intensity on T1WI and ↑ signal intensity on T2WI
- Neoplastic cystic masses: Enhancing soft tissue component

TOP DIFFERENTIAL DIAGNOSES

- Renal cell carcinoma
- Renal abscess
- Autosomal dominant polycystic kidney disease
- Uremic cystic disease

CLINICAL ISSUES

- Asymptomatic or palpable mass and flank pain
- Present in 20-30% of middle-aged adults, incidence increases with age

DIAGNOSTIC CHECKLIST

- Image evaluation and classification of cystic masses are key to management

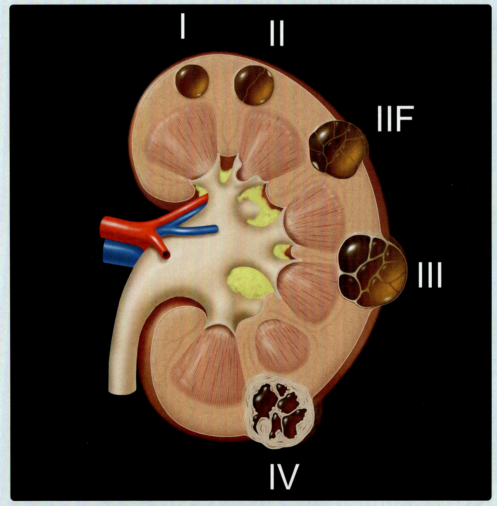

Medical illustration shows cystic lesions categorized according to the Bosniak classification. The Bosniak system classifies complexity of cystic lesions based imaging features on CT and MR. The classification provides indications on the risk of malignancy and helps guiding management and treatment. Note the following: Class I = simple cyst; class II = minimally complicated; class IIF (F = follow-up) = more complex than a class II cyst requiring imaging follow-up to confirm benignity; class III = more complicated cyst usually managed surgically (biopsy controversial); class IV = high risk of malignancy, requires surgery.

TERMINOLOGY

Definitions

- Fluid-filled renal lesion

IMAGING

General Features

- **Bosniak classification**
  - Imaging-based classification of renal cystic lesions
    - Used with CT and MR imaging
  - 5 categories
    - Class I: Benign cysts
      - □ Well-defined, rounded, homogeneous, lucent (0- to 20-HU, near-water-density) mass with thin or imperceptible, nonenhancing wall and contents; no septa or calcifications
    - Class II: Minimally complicated cysts; benign
      - □ Thin (< 1 mm) septations, smooth, ± perceived (not measurable) enhancement
      - □ Calcification of short segment of wall or septa
      - □ Hyperdense cyst (> 20 HU), no enhancement, spherical, partially exophytic, usually ≤ 3 cm in diameter
    - Class IIF: Requires CT/MR imaging follow-up
      - □ Multiple thin septations ± perceived (not measurable) enhancement
      - □ Minimal wall or septal thickening ± perceived (not measurable) enhancement
      - □ Thick calcifications
      - □ Hyperdense, intraparenchymal cysts > 3 cm
      - □ No enhancing nodules
    - Class III: More complicated cysts; usually managed surgically (biopsy controversial)
      - □ Irregular and thickened septa &/or wall + measurable enhancement
      - □ ± thickened and irregular calcification
      - □ Benign lesions: Hemorrhagic cysts, renal abscess, mixed epithelial and stromal tumor, complicated benign septated cysts
      - □ Malignant lesions: Cystic nephroma, multiloculated cystic renal cell carcinoma
    - Class IV: Malignant lesions; require surgery
      - □ Enhancing component, irregular wall thickening

Ultrasonographic Findings

- Grayscale ultrasound
  - Simple, uncomplicated cyst: Spherical or ovoid, anechoic content, sharply defined, imperceptible wall, and acoustical enhancement
  - Hemorrhagic cyst: Internal echoes (clot); thick calcified wall ± multiloculated (chronic)

CT Findings

- NECT
  - Simple, uncomplicated cyst
    - Sharply marginated, round, smooth, homogeneous, hypodense (< 20 HU) mass; thin imperceptible wall
  - Complicated cysts
    - Due to hemorrhage, infection, ischemia, proteinaceous fluid
    - May show ↑ density (> 20 HU on NECT), septations, wall thickening, calcifications
    - Classification & management based on Bosniak classes
- CECT
  - Simple cysts: No enhancement
  - Neoplastic cystic masses: Enhancing soft tissue component
  - Enhancement post administration of IV contrast
    - Enhanced HU minus unenhanced HU
      - □ < 10 HU: No enhancement
      - □ 10-20 HU: Indeterminate
      - □ ≥ 20 HU: Enhancement
    - "Pseudoenhancement" refers to artifactual increase in cyst content attenuation (by > 10 HU) on CECT

MR Findings

- T1WI
  - Complicated, hemorrhagic cysts: ↑ signal intensity (signal intensity changes according to stage of hemorrhage)
- T2WI
  - Simple cysts: ↑ signal intensity, homogeneous mass with imperceptible wall
- T1WI C+
  - Neoplastic cystic masses: Enhancing soft tissue component

Imaging Recommendations

- Best imaging tool
  - Management of hyperattenuating cystic lesions on NECT
    - > 70 HU on NECT = hyperdense, benign renal cyst requiring no follow-up or treatment
    - 20-70 HU on NECT: Requires contrast administration to exclude enhancing components; alternatively, US or MR imaging (T1WI, T2WI, DWI) can be used if patient cannot tolerate IV contrast administration
      - □ At US, hyperdense lesions on CT may often appear as anechoic, benign cysts

DIFFERENTIAL DIAGNOSIS

Renal Cell Carcinoma

- Some RCCs are cystic from inception

Renal Abscess

- Enhancing capsule, ± perinephric stranding

Autosomal Dominant Polycystic Kidney Disease

- Inherited polycystic kidney disease

Uremic Cystic Disease

- Multiple renal cysts in patients with end-stage renal disease and no history of hereditary cystic disease

CLINICAL ISSUES

Natural History & Prognosis

- Simple cysts grow slowly
- Complications are rare: Hydronephrosis, hemorrhage, infection, rupture
- Risks of renal cell carcinoma
  - Bosniak classes: I, II (0%); IIF (11-25%); III (28-54%); IV (90%)

(Left) Transverse US shows a simple renal cyst ➡ displaying the typical imaging features, including anechoic content, imperceptible wall, and acoustic enhancement ⏩. (Right) Axial T2WI FS MR shows a simple hyperintense cyst ➡ (Bosniak class 1) in the left kidney.

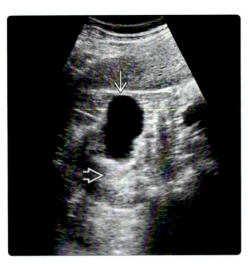 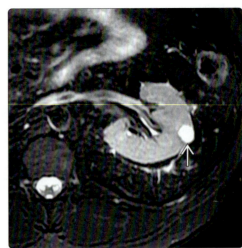

(Left) Axial NECT shows an hyperdense (100-HU) cyst ➡ in the left kidney (Bosniak class 2). (Right) Axial T2WI FS MR shows a lobulated left renal cyst ➡ with multiple internal, thin septations. Though thin, the septations qualitatively enhance on gadolinium-enhanced T1WI MR (not shown). The lesion is a Bosniak class 2F cyst. Class 2F cysts require imaging follow-up with CT or MR imaging.

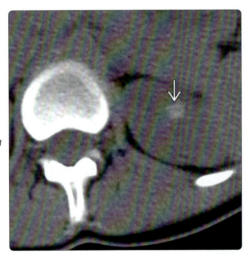 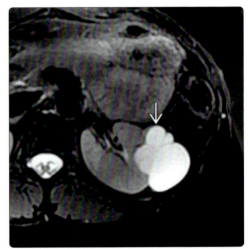

(Left) Axial CECT shows a multiloculated cystic mass ➡ with septa with measurable enhancement (Bosniak class 3). The invagination into the renal sinus ➡ is characteristic of multilocular cystic nephroma. (Right) Axial CECT of the left kidney shows an exophytic complex cystic lesion ➡ with enhancing nodules ➡ and septation ➡ compatible with a Bosniak class 4. At resection, the lesion was proven to be a low-grade oncocytic neoplasm.

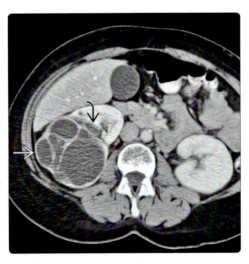 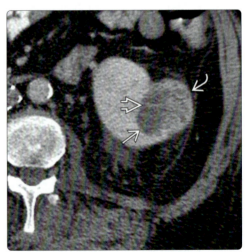

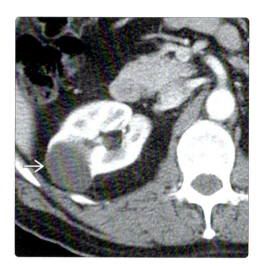
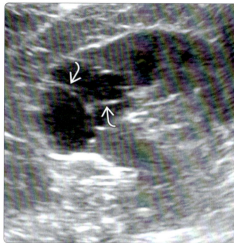

(Left) Axial CECT shows a simple right renal cyst ➡ (Bosniak class 1). (Right) Longitudinal US of the right kidney in the same patient reveals thin septations ➡ within the cyst. Renal cysts may appear more complex on US than on CT.

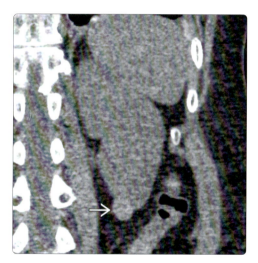
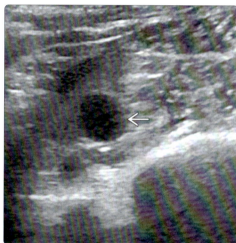

(Left) Coronal NECT shows a small, exophytic, and hyperdense (65-HU) lesion ➡ in the lower pole of the left kidney. (Right) Transverse US of the left kidney in the same patient shows the same lesion as anechoic with imperceptible walls and posterior acoustic enhancement, confirming it as a simple cyst ➡. At US, hyperdense lesions on CT may often appear as anechoic, benign cysts.

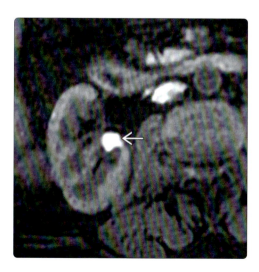
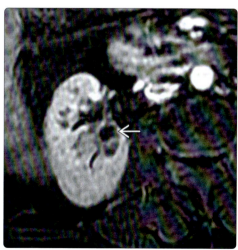

(Left) Axial FS T1WI MR shows a high signal intensity lesion ➡ in the cortex of the right kidney. (Right) Axial T1WI subtraction (postcontrast minus precontrast) MR confirms the lack of enhancement within the lesion ➡. Renal lesions hyperintense on T1WI MR are usually proteinaceous or hemorrhagic lesions; the lack of enhancement confirms the cystic nature.

KEY FACTS

TERMINOLOGY

- Synonym: Renal sinus cysts
- Definitions
  - Parapelvic cyst: Renal cysts extending into renal sinus fat
  - Peripelvic cyst: Originating from renal sinus lymphatics

IMAGING

- Parapelvic cysts
  - Usually single and unilateral
- Peripelvic cysts
  - Usually multiple and bilateral
- IVP
  - Compression and displacement of renal calyces and pelvis
- CECT
  - Excretory phase: Water-attenuation cysts separate from enhanced renal collecting system
- Ultrasound
  - Anechoic lesions in renal sinus

- No connection among cysts
- Best diagnostic clue
  - Contrast-enhanced CT or MR obtained during excretory phase shows enhanced collecting system separate from nonenhancing renal cysts

TOP DIFFERENTIAL DIAGNOSES

- Hydronephrosis
- Renal lipomatosis
- Renal lymphangiomatosis

CLINICAL ISSUES

- Most commonly asymptomatic
- Treatment for symptomatic cysts
  - Laparoscopic, ureteroscopic, or percutaneous ablation

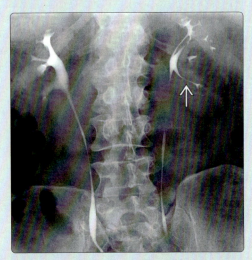
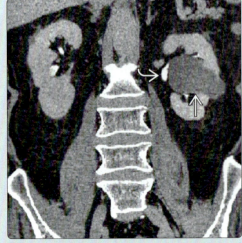

(Left) Retrograde pyelogram shows a displaced and compressed left renal collecting system ➡. (Right) Coronal CECT obtained during the excretory phase in the same patient shows a large nonenhancing left parapelvic cyst ➡ displacing the enhancing renal collecting system ➡.

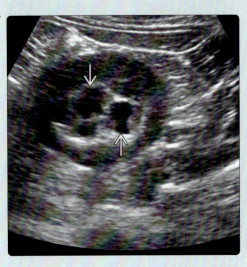
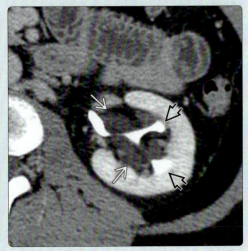

(Left) Transverse ultrasound of the left kidney shows multiple anechoic cysts in the renal pelvis ➡ simulating hydronephrosis. (Right) Axial CECT obtained during the excretory phase in the same patient demonstrates peripelvic cysts ➡ displacing the enhanced renal collecting system ➡. Excretory phase of CECT or MR helps in differentiating cysts from enhancing renal collecting system.

KEY FACTS

TERMINOLOGY

- Inherited polycystic renal disease characterized by progressive cystic growth and multiple systemic manifestations

IMAGING

- Enlarged kidneys replaced by innumerable cysts
  - Simple ± complicated (hemorrhagic, infected) cysts
  - Progressive increase in cyst and renal volume
- Extrarenal manifestations
  - Polycystic liver disease, intracranial arterial aneurysm, cysts in other organs, abdominal hernias

TOP DIFFERENTIAL DIAGNOSES

- Multiple simple cysts
- Acquired (uremic) cystic disease
- von Hippel-Lindau disease
- Medullary cystic kidney disease

PATHOLOGY

- Autosomal dominant inheritance
  - *PKD1* gene mutation (85% of cases)
  - *PKD2* gene mutation (15% of cases)
- Enlarged kidneys (2-4 kg; normal kidney = 150 g), multiple cysts of various size in cortex and medulla

CLINICAL ISSUES

- Incidence in USA: 1:400-1,000
- Asymptomatic, abdominal pain, hematuria, hypertension
- Complications
  - 50% evolve to end-stage renal disease by 6th decade
  - Renal function is related to kidney volume

DIAGNOSTIC CHECKLIST

- Enlarged kidneys with multiple, bilateral cysts
- ± polycystic liver disease and cysts in other organs (e.g., epididymis, pancreas, spleen)

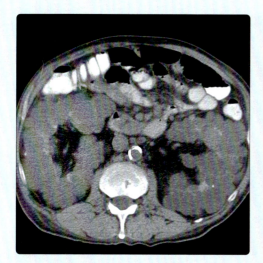

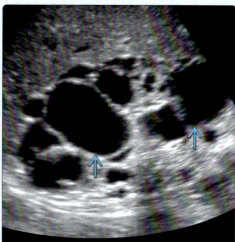

(Left) Axial NECT in patient with autosomal dominant polycystic kidney disease shows massively enlarged kidneys replaced by innumerable simple cysts. (Right) Longitudinal ultrasound of the right kidney in a patient with autosomal dominant polycystic kidney disease shows multiple varying size simple anechoic cysts ➡ that replace and enlarge the kidney.

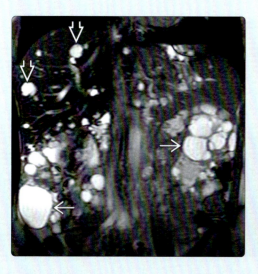

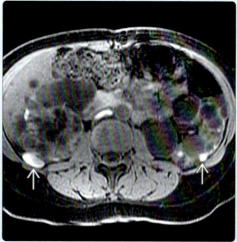

(Left) Coronal T2WI MR shows enlarged kidneys replaced by innumerable T2-hyperintense cysts ➡ and multiple liver cysts ➡. Liver cysts are the most common extrarenal manifestation in patients with autosomal dominant polycystic kidney disease. (Right) Axial T1WI FS MR in the same patient shows multiple renal cysts with varying signal intensity. Complicated, hemorrhagic cysts ➡ appear hyperintense on T1WI.

KEY FACTS

IMAGING

- Radiographs: Bulging, lateral abdominal contours with displaced bowel gas centrally due to large kidneys
  - Bell-shaped thorax ± pneumothorax, pneumomediastinum
- US: Bilaterally enlarged echogenic kidneys with loss of corticomedullary differentiation
  - 2-6 standard deviations above mean size for age
  - Dilated, radially arranged tubules on high-resolution linear transducers ± small cysts (< 1 cm)
  - Tiny, punctate hyperechoic foci (likely calcium deposits) develop with time & correlate with renal failure
- MR: Large kidneys of diffusely high signal intensity on T2
  - Intervening low-signal septa
- Variable degrees of liver disease (congenital hepatic fibrosis)

PATHOLOGY

- Autosomal recessive, due to mutation of polycystic kidney & hepatic disease 1 gene (*PKHD1*) on chromosome 6p12.2
  - Ciliopathy effecting epithelial cells in renal collecting ducts, loops of Henle, & liver bile ducts
  - Bilateral renal enlargement due to dilated distal tubules & collecting ducts; hepatic bile duct dilatation & cysts

CLINICAL ISSUES

- Variable genotype expressivity
- Perinatal form: More severe renal disease with oligohydramnios & pulmonary hypoplasia, less hepatic disease
  - 30% perinatal mortality (respiratory insufficiency)
- Juvenile form: Less renal disease, more severe hepatic disease
  - Portal hypertension & fibrosis develop in 50%
- Survival rate for milder forms up to 82% at age 3 years & 79% at 15 years

(Left) *Coronal SSFSE T2 fetal MR shows marked enlargement and increased signal of both kidneys* ⇒ *without hydronephrosis. Note the lack of amniotic fluid around this fetus, reflecting poor renal function in this case of autosomal recessive polycystic kidney disease (ARPKD).* (Right) *Frontal view of a newborn infant with a history of oligohydramnios shows bowel loops displaced centrally by bilateral flank "masses"* ⇒ *(due to massively enlarged kidneys). Note the bell-shaped thorax and left pneumothorax* ⇒.

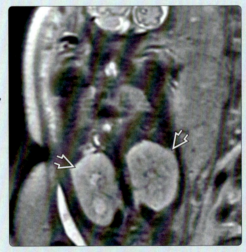
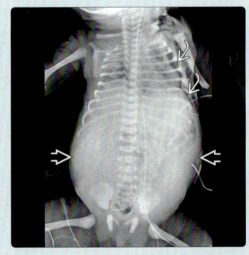

(Left) *Extended field-of-view US shows a large newborn kidney measuring > 10 cm in length* ⇒ *(normal: 4-6 cm) with no corticomedullary differentiation and replacement of renal parenchyma by microscopic cysts and dilated tubules with hyperechoic walls.* (Right) *Sagittal CECT shows innumerable ill-defined hypodensities* ⇒ *throughout the right kidney, a nodular liver contour* ⇒, *and ascites* ⇒ *in this 8-year-old boy with ARPKD and congenital hepatic fibrosis and more severe liver involvement.*

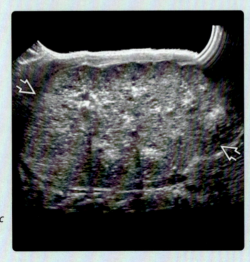
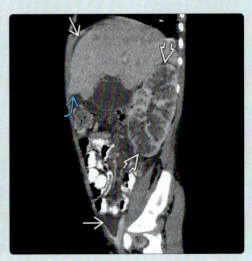

Multicystic Dysplastic Kidney

KEY FACTS

TERMINOLOGY

- Congenital nonfunctional kidney replaced by multiple cysts and dysplastic tissue
- Tend to involve with time: Cysts shrink, and residual tissue may lose reniform shape

IMAGING

- Reniform-shaped multicystic mass occupying renal fossa
  - ± lobulated outer contour (due to cysts of variable size)
  - Wide range of sizes: up to 15 cm in length in newborn period; may be only 1-2 cm after years of involution
- Cysts of varying size do not connect
  - Largest cyst typically peripheral, not central
  - Helpful to distinguish from hydronephrosis
- Poorly defined intervening echogenic parenchyma without normal corticomedullary architecture
- Can be segmental in duplicated kidneys
- Nuclear scintigraphy documents lack of renal function in multicystic dysplastic kidney (MCDK)

PATHOLOGY

- Probably due to atresia of ureter or ureteropelvic junction (UPJ) during fetal metanephric stage

CLINICAL ISSUES

- MCDK 2nd most common abdominal mass in neonate (after hydronephrosis)
- > 50% discovered antenatally or in infancy as palpable mass
- Up to 40% of patients with MCDK have contralateral renal abnormality
  - UPJ obstruction and vesicoureteral reflux most common
- Unilateral MCDK with normal contralateral kidney: Excellent prognosis
  - Vast majority involve with time and remain asymptomatic
  - Rare reports of Wilms tumor developing in MCDK
- Unilateral MCDK with abnormal contralateral kidney: May develop renal insufficiency
- Bilateral MCDK: Incompatible with life

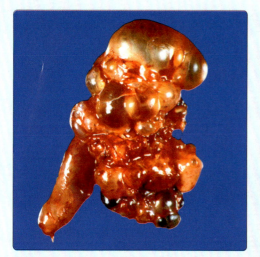
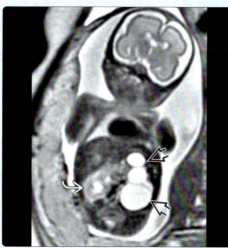

(Left) Gross pathology shows numerous cysts replacing the renal parenchyma and distorting the contour of this multicystic dysplastic kidney (MCDK). Note that the largest cyst in this specimen is in the upper pole, not in the renal hilum. (Right) Coronal SSFSE T2 fetal MR shows a multicystic mass in the left renal fossa ⊟ with no discernible normal left renal tissue, most consistent with a left MCDK. The right kidney ⊞ and volume of amniotic fluid appear normal.

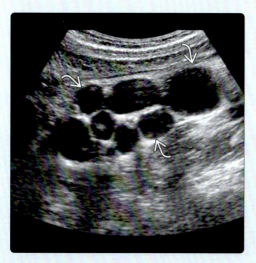
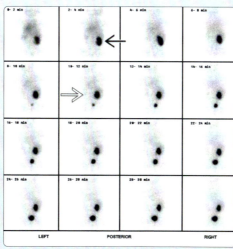

(Left) Prone postnatal US of the left flank in the same patient shows multiple noncommunicating cysts ⊟ of varying size replacing the left kidney. A reniform shape is retained, but no normal left renal parenchyma is seen. (Right) Posterior images of the same infant during a Tc-99m MAG3 renal scan show normal function of the right kidney ⊟ but no function on the left side ⊟, confirming a left MCDK. Early transient activity in MCDK on nuclear scans merely reflects that the tissue is being perfused, but continued images show no function.

Acquired Cystic Renal Disease

KEY FACTS

TERMINOLOGY
- Acquired cystic kidney disease (ACKD)/uremic cystic disease
- ≥ 3 cysts per kidney in patients with end-stage renal disease and no history of hereditary cystic disease

IMAGING
- Imaging findings
  - Atrophic kidneys
  - Multiple cysts
    - Hemorrhagic cysts in 50% of cases
  - Renal cell carcinoma (RCC) in 3-6% of cases
- Best imaging tools
  - Ultrasound: Screening
  - CT or MR: Complications, diagnosis of RCC

PATHOLOGY
- Multiple cysts of various size
  - Single layer of hyperplastic epithelium
- Histological subtypes of RCC

- Papillary (most common among subtypes similar to sporadic RCC), clear cell, chromophobe
- Acquired cystic disease-associated RCC (most common in ACKD), clear cell papillary RCC of end-stage kidney

CLINICAL ISSUES
- Usually asymptomatic
  - Pain, hematuria in case of hemorrhage into cyst or cyst rupture
- Incidence increases with duration of dialysis
  - > 90% of patients will develop ACKD after 5-10 years of hemodialysis
- Complications
  - Hemorrhage into renal cysts
  - RCC
    - Risk factors: Male gender, length of dialysis, kidney weight > 150 g
    - Screening with ultrasound (controversial)

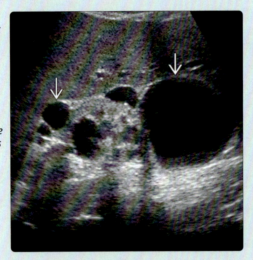
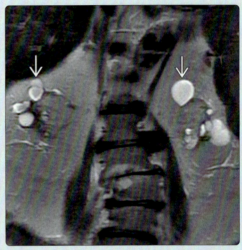

(Left) Longitudinal ultrasound of the right kidney in a patient with end-stage renal disease shows an atrophic echogenic kidney with multiple varying size and anechoic cysts ➡, an appearance compatible with acquired cystic kidney disease (ACKD). (Right) Coronal T2WI MR in a patient with end-stage renal disease and ACKD shows small, atrophic kidneys with multiple simple cysts ➡.

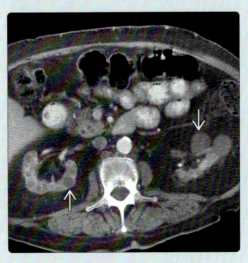
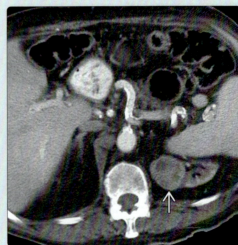

(Left) Axial CECT in a patient with ACKD shows small kidneys replaced by innumerable cysts ➡. (Right) Axial CECT in the same patient shows a heterogeneous enhancing mass ➡ in the upper pole of the left kidney. The lesion is a biopsy-proven chromophobe renal cell carcinoma (RCC). The prevalence of RCC in patients with ACKD is 3-6%.

von Hippel-Lindau Disease

KEY FACTS

TERMINOLOGY

- Hereditary, autosomal dominant disease affecting several organs and associated with multiple neoplasms

IMAGING

- Best imaging tool: Contrast-enhanced CT or MR with renal mass protocol
- Renal manifestations
  - Renal cysts (59-63%)
    - Usually multiple and bilateral
  - Renal cell carcinoma (RCC) (25-45%)
    - Frequently multiple and bilateral
- Extrarenal manifestations
  - Hemangioblastomas in central nervous system (13-72%)
  - Retinal hemangioblastoma (45-59%)
  - Pancreatic lesions (17-56%)
  - Pheochromocytomas (0-60%)

TOP DIFFERENTIAL DIAGNOSES

- Adult polycystic kidney disease
- Acquired cystic kidney disease of uremia

PATHOLOGY

- Mutation of *VHL* tumor-suppressor gene on chromosome 3 (3p25-p26)
- Type 1: Pheocromocytoma absent
- Type 2: Pheochromocytoma present

CLINICAL ISSUES

- Age: Infancy to 7th decade (average age: 26 years)
- Prevalence: 1:30,000 to 1:50,000
- Natural history and prognosis
  - RCC responsible for 50% of deaths in VHL patients
  - Surgery: Nephron-sparing approach
    - Preferred because of high morbidity/mortality associated with dialysis
    - 10-year disease-specific survival = 81-94%

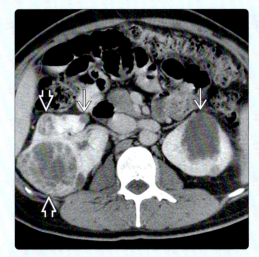
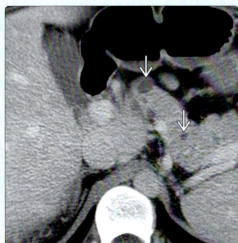

(Left) Axial CECT in a patient with von Hippel-Lindau (VHL) disease shows bilateral renal cysts ➡ and multiple complex cystic masses ⇨ with enhancing nodules and septations that are compatible with cystic renal cell carcinomas (RCC). Renal cysts and RCCs are common visceral manifestations of VHL. (Right) Axial CECT in the same patient shows multiple pancreatic cysts ➡.

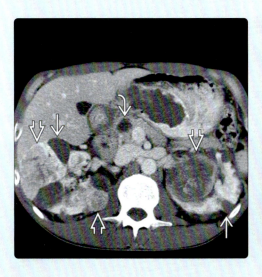
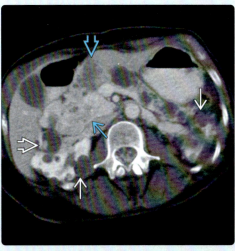

(Left) Axial CECT in a patient with VHL shows multiple and bilateral renal cysts ➡ and RCCs ⇨. A cystic neoplasm is noted in the pancreatic head ➡. Pancreatic manifestations of VHL include cysts, cystic neoplasms (microcystic adenoma), and neuroendocrine tumors. (Right) A 60-year-old man with multiple manifestations of VHL, including renal cysts ➡, cystic RCC ⇨, pancreatic neuroendocrine tumor ⇨, and serous cystic neoplasm ⇨, is shown.

KEY FACTS

TERMINOLOGY

- Spectrum of functional and structural renal damage caused by lithium ingestion
- Nephrogenic diabetes insipidus and chronic renal insufficiency are most common presentations

IMAGING

- Numerous nonenhancing microcysts in patient with history of chronic lithium use
  - Normal-sized kidneys, numerous (few to innumerable) microcysts (1-2 mm in diameter)
- On ultrasound, microcysts can manifest as small anechoic lesions or tiny echogenic foci
- Imaging usually not needed for diagnosis

TOP DIFFERENTIAL DIAGNOSES

- Autosomal dominant polycystic kidney disease
- Medullary cystic disease
- Acquired cystic disease of uremia

PATHOLOGY

- Distal tubular dilatation and microcysts (33-62%)
- Chronic interstitial nephritis, tubular atrophy

CLINICAL ISSUES

- Nephrotoxicity usually occurs within 1 month of onset of drug
- Polyuria, polydipsia, urine osmolarity < 100 mOsm/kg; normal or ↑ serum osmolarity (diabetes insipidus)
- 20-54% of those taking lithium have urine-concentrating defects
- Renal insufficiency is less common
- Structural damage (microcysts) is correlated with degree of renal failure (↓ glomerular filtration rate)
- Diabetes insipidus may be reversible after discontinuing drug
- Acute intoxication requires aggressive correction of fluid and electrolyte abnormalities ± dialysis

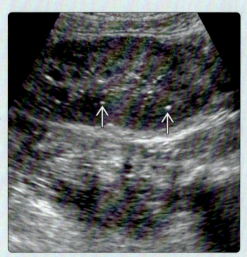
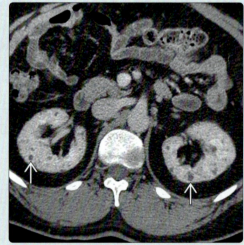

(Left) Longitudinal ultrasound shows the right kidney of a 49-year-old woman with a history of long-term lithium intake. Scattered, tiny echogenic foci ➡ are seen within the right kidney, compatible with lithium nephropathy. The microcysts may be too small to resolve as fluid-containing structures on ultrasound. (Right) Axial CECT in patient with lithium nephropathy shows innumerable, bilateral, tiny renal cysts ➡.

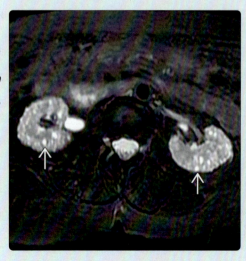
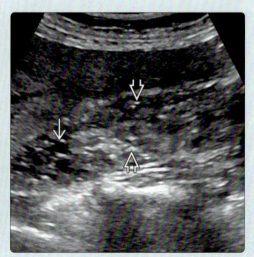

(Left) Axial fat-suppressed T2WI shows innumerable, small renal cysts ➡ in a 69-year-old woman with a history of bipolar disease and lithium intake compatible with lithium nephropathy. (Right) Longitudinal ultrasound of the right kidney in the same patient shows some renal cysts as small anechoic lesions ➡ and multiple other tiny echogenic foci ➡.

Localized Cystic Renal Disease

KEY FACTS

TERMINOLOGY

- Benign nonneoplastic proliferation of cysts, usually within normally functioning kidney

IMAGING

- Nonencapsulated collection of cysts of varying sizes separated by normal (or compressed) renal parenchyma
  - Cyst clustering helps distinguish from hydronephrosis at ultrasound
- Always unilateral
- Usually involves only part of kidney but can affect entire kidney
- Renal tissue in between cysts and in uninvolved portions of kidney functions, enhances normally
- Ipsilateral ureter normal

TOP DIFFERENTIAL DIAGNOSES

- Multilocular cystic nephroma
- Autosomal dominant polycystic disease

- Cystic renal cell carcinoma

PATHOLOGY

- Simple cysts with normal renal tissue in between

CLINICAL ISSUES

- Usually asymptomatic
- Occasionally flank pain or palpable mass, hematuria, hypertension
- Young adults to elderly
- Benign, stable, or slowly progressive
- Conservative management; imaging follow-up

DIAGNOSTIC CHECKLIST

- Important to not label patient as having inherited, progressive, or neoplastic disease
- Key is to distinguish from multilocular cystic nephroma and cystic renal cell carcinoma
  - Both of these have irregular cystic spaces surrounded by thick capsule

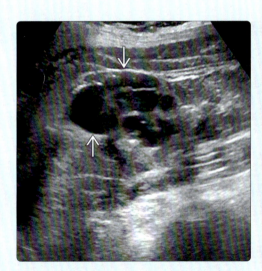

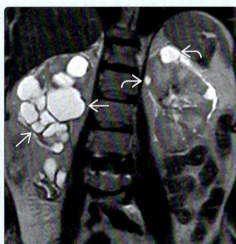

(Left) Longitudinal ultrasound through the right kidney shows a cluster of multiple cysts ➡. Each cyst has a typical benign appearance. (Right) Coronal T2WI MR in the same patient shows a cluster of cysts ➡ in the lower pole of the right kidney. Absence of a capsule is in keeping with localized cystic renal disease. Note scattered left renal cysts ➡.

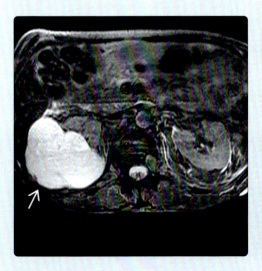

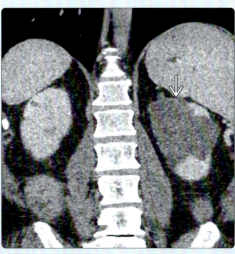

(Left) Axial fat-suppressed T2WI MR shows a cluster of high signal intensity cysts ➡ in the right kidney without a capsule, compatible with localized cystic renal disease. (Right) Coronal CECT demonstrates the lack of a capsule associated to the collection of cysts ➡, consistent with localized cystic renal disease.

KEY FACTS

TERMINOLOGY

- Benign renal tumor composed of abnormal blood vessels, smooth muscle, and adipose components

IMAGING

- Most common benign renal neoplasm
- 90% are unilateral and solitary: Usually not associated with tuberous sclerosis (TSC)
- 10% are multiple and bilateral: Usually due to TSC
  - 80% of TSC patients have renal angiomyolipomas (AMLs)
- Solid, heterogeneous, renal cortical mass in adult with macroscopic fat is reliable sign of AML
  - Variable amounts of fat may be present
  - ~ 5% of AMLs contain minimal fat and cannot be reliably diagnosed by imaging
- Lipid-poor AMLs are often hyperdense on NECT

TOP DIFFERENTIAL DIAGNOSES

- Renal cell carcinoma (RCC)

- Rarely reported to contain fat (engulfed sinus or perirenal fat)
  - Calcification/ossification within tumor is highly suggestive of RCC
- Perirenal liposarcoma
  - Smooth compression of kidney and extension beyond perirenal space favor liposarcoma
  - Renal parenchymal defect and enlarged vessels favor AML
- Wilms tumor
  - If child has TSC, mass more likely to be AML
  - Otherwise suspect Wilms tumor
- Other less common considerations: Metastases, lymphoma, oncocytoma, lipoma, teratoma

CLINICAL ISSUES

- Most common complication: Hemorrhage
- Small subgroup of AMLs can be angioinvasive, affect local lymph nodes, and rarely metastasize

(Left) Graphic shows a vascular renal mass ➡ with prominent fatty and soft tissue components. Note the large "feeding" arteries. This hypervascularity predisposes these tumors to spontaneous hemorrhage. (Right) Sagittal US shows an echogenic lesion ➡ in the superior cortex of the left kidney due to an incidental angiomyolipoma. Color flow was not identified in the lesion.

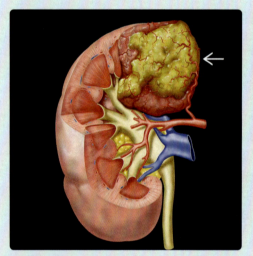
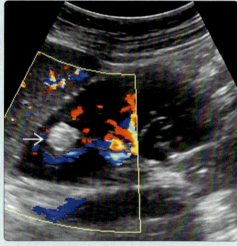

(Left) Axial NECT in the same patient demonstrates a fat attenuation lesion ➡ in the superior cortex of the left kidney, consistent with an incidental angiomyolipoma. (Right) Axial T1 postcontrast MR with fat saturation reveals an angiomyolipoma ➡ that extends into the perinephric space. A cortical defect (notch sign) ➡ identifies the origin of the angiomyolipoma from the kidney. A large vessel ➡ also extends into the neoplasm from the kidney.

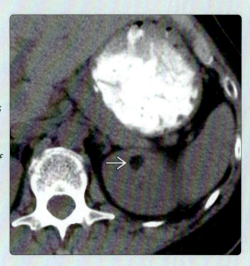
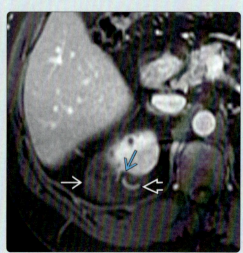

Renal Angiomyolipoma (AML)

TERMINOLOGY

Definitions

- Benign renal neoplasm composed of abnormal blood vessels, smooth muscle, and adipose components

IMAGING

General Features

- Best diagnostic clue
  - Solid, heterogeneous, renal cortical mass containing macroscopic fat in adult

CT Findings

- NECT
  - Well-marginated, heterogeneous mass with macroscopic fat arising from renal cortex
    - Notch sign: Angiomyolipoma (AML) originates from triangular or rectangular notch-like defect in cortex
  - Solid renal mass with predominance of macroscopic fat is reliable sign of AML
    - Tissue attenuation of -10 HU or lower is reliable indicator of fat
      □ Specificity of fat detection increases with use of lower attenuation values
    - However, amount of fat is variable
    - ~ 5% of AMLs contain minimal fat and cannot be reliably diagnosed by CT, pixel analysis, or MR
  - Minimal fat AMLs are often hyperattenuating relative to normal renal parenchyma on NECT
    - Not sufficient to allow diagnosis due to overlap with renal cell carcinomas (RCCs)
    - CT histogram analysis and pixel mapping have not reliably been able to differentiate minimal fat AMLs from RCCs
  - Hemorrhage more likely in large (≥ 4 cm) AMLs
    - AML size > 4.0-4.5 cm considered relative indication for partial nephrectomy or embolization in past
  - Rare calcification; if present, suspect RCC
- CECT
  - Varied enhancement pattern based on tumor composition
  - Without macroscopic fat, enhancement alone does not differentiate AML from renal tumors
    - Minimal fat AMLs typically show more homogeneous and prolonged enhancement than RCCs during nephrographic phase
    - However, differentiation remains difficult and biopsy of small, solid minimal fat lesions should be considered
  - Invasion of renal vein/inferior vena cava by AML is extremely rare
  - Hemorrhage from ruptured AML can extend into perinephric space and renal hilum
- CTA
  - Disorganized tumoral vessels, aneurysms, and pseudoaneurysms may be seen within and around tumor

MR Findings

- AML typically heterogeneous signal intensity
  - Variable proportion of vessels, muscle, and fat
  - Macroscopic fat: High signal intensity on T1WI and T2WI

- MR techniques for localization of fat
  - Fat suppression (frequency selective): Loss of signal
  - Opposed-phase imaging
    - Signal loss on out-of-phase images
      □ Not specific; can occur in various types of renal neoplasms
- Caveat: Clear cell RCC also loses signal on out-of-phase sequence
- T1 C+
  - Variable enhancement due to tumor composition
    - Hypointense compared to renal parenchyma
    - Signal intensity similar to hypovascular RCCs
  - In cases without macroscopic fat, enhancement cannot reliably differentiate AML from malignant and other benign renal lesions
- DWI
  - Not useful for differentiating AML from other renal lesions
- Minimal fat AMLs (~ 5% of all AMLs)
  - Often indistinguishable from RCC
  - Signal decrease with opposed-phase imaging for tissues containing intracellular lipid
    - Nonspecific: Opposed-phase signal decrease also observed in various benign and malignant renal cortical tumors
  - Smaller size and low T2 signal intensity compared to clear cell RCC

Ultrasonographic Findings

- Grayscale ultrasound
  - Classic appearance: Well-defined, markedly hyperechoic mass relative to normal renal parenchyma with acoustic shadowing
    - However, subset of minimal fat AMLs are isoechoic to slightly hypoechoic and lack shadowing
    - Minimal fat AMLs are typically homogeneously isoechoic
  - Small RCC may also be hyperechoic
    - AML and RCC can be difficult to distinguish on US
- Color Doppler
  - Pseudoaneurysm detection
    - Color-filled ovoid or round structures within or adjacent to AML
    - Color flow appears as swirling or yin and yang sign
- Power Doppler
  - Most AMLs show intratumoral focal pattern
    - Central, internal flow that does not extend to margins of tumor
  - Conversely, most small RCCs have mixed peripheral and penetrating pattern
    - Flow present in center and extends to margins/periphery of tumor

Angiographic Findings

- Tumor with increased vascular component
  - Highly vascular mass with disorganized, long, and tortuous vessels
  - Sacculated pseudoaneurysms

(Left) *Axial T2 MR shows a lesion ⇨ with signal intensity similar to fat arising from the posterior renal cortex via a small defect ⇨.* **(Right)** *Axial postcontrast T1 MR with fat suppression in the same patient shows that the lesion ⇨ loses signal intensity with application of fat saturation. A cortical defect (notch sign) and a feeding vessel ⇨ are shown.*

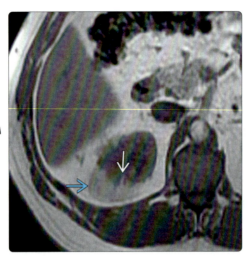 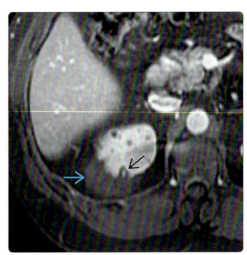

(Left) *Sagittal US of the right kidney shows a round, echogenic lesion ⇨ within the posterior cortex.* **(Right)** *Axial CECT in the same patient shows the cortical defect ⇨ from which the angiomyolipoma ⇨ originates and extends into the perinephric space.*

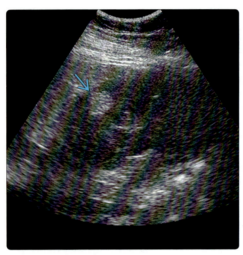 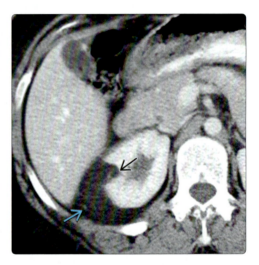

(Left) *Axial CECT in a 61-year-old woman with tuberous sclerosis shows bilateral renal masses, some of which contain obvious fat ⇨ (due to angiomyolipoma), while others represent cysts ⇨.* **(Right)** *Coronal CECT reformation in the same patient shows multiple bilateral cysts ⇨ and solid masses (angiomyolipomas) with both fatty ⇨ and soft tissue density ⇨ components. The presence of multiple and bilateral angiomyolipomas is strong evidence for tuberous sclerosis.*

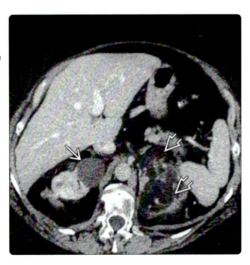 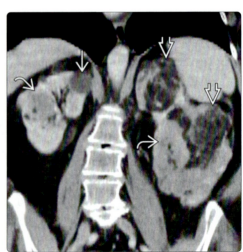

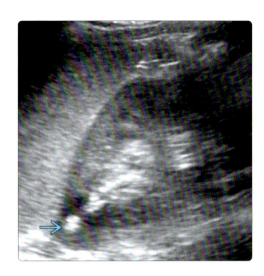
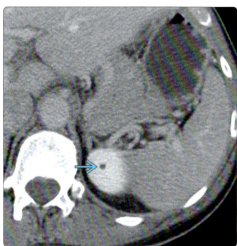

(Left) *Sagittal US shows an echogenic lesion* ⮕ *at the superior pole of the kidney, consistent with an angiomyolipoma.* (Right) *Axial postcontrast CT shows a fat attenuation lesion* ⮕ *in the superior pole of the left kidney that corresponds to the echogenic lesion noted on prior US, consistent with angiomyolipoma.*

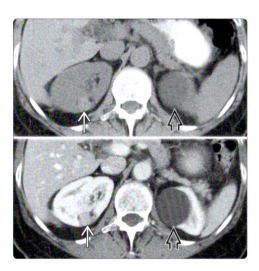
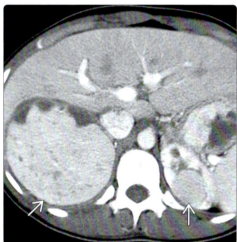

(Left) *Axial NECT and CECT show subtle foci of fat within multiple angiomyolipomas in the right kidney* ⮕*. Note the simple cyst in the left kidney* ⮕*.* (Right) *Axial CECT shows bilateral enhancing renal masses* ⮕ *in a patient with tuberous sclerosis, angiomyolipomas without an obvious fat component.*

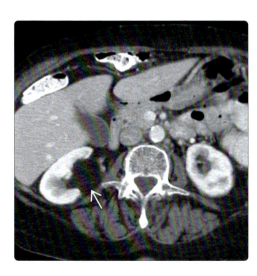
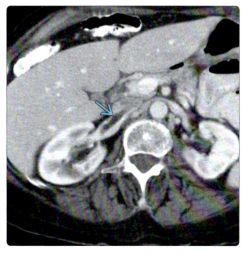

(Left) *Axial contrast-enhanced CT shows an angiomyolipoma* ⮕ *in the right renal hilum.* (Right) *Axial contrast-enhanced CT in the same patient reveals fat attenuation in the lumen of the right renal vein* ⮕*, consistent with renal vein invasion by angiomyolipoma.*

KEY FACTS

TERMINOLOGY

- Benign renal tumor composed of eosinophilic epithelial cells, arising from collecting ducts

IMAGING

- Solid renal cortical mass lesion ± central stellate scar
- Dynamic postcontrast imaging is highly variable and depends on degree of cellularity and stroma
- Absence of malignant features
  - No invasion of vessels, perinephric fat, or collecting system
  - No adenopathy or metastases
- Other general features
  - 2nd most common benign renal tumor after angiomyolipoma
  - Accounts for 3-7% of all renal cortical neoplasms
  - ~ 3-16% are multifocal and 4-14% are bilateral

TOP DIFFERENTIAL DIAGNOSES

- Renal cell carcinoma (RCC)
  - Necrotic, calcific, hemorrhagic, cystic components often seen in RCC but rare or absent in oncocytoma
  - Central necrosis of RCC may mimic central scar of oncocytoma
- Renal angiomyolipoma
  - Well-defined cortical heterogeneous tumor with foci of fat density (-30 to -100 HU)
  - CTA: Aneurysmal renal vessels may be seen
- Renal metastases and lymphoma
  - Solid, hypoattenuating masses showing moderate enhancement
  - Usually known primary tumor and metastases in other sites strongly suggest renal metastases

DIAGNOSTIC CHECKLIST

- Not possible to distinguish from RCC on imaging alone
- May suggest diagnosis → nephron-sparing surgery

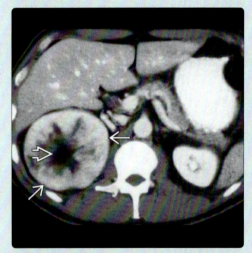

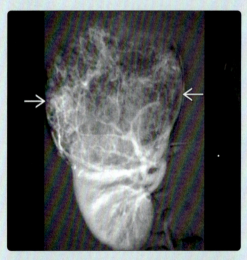

(Left) *Axial CECT shows an exophytic, solid, enhancing mass ⟹ extending from the superior pole of the right kidney. Note the large central scar ⟹. Oncocytomas appear as encapsulated, well-marginated masses with smooth contour.* (Right) *Digital subtraction angiography in the same patient shows hypervascularity of the large mass ⟹. Note the absence of bizarre tumor neovascularity that is often seen with renal cell carcinoma (RCC).*

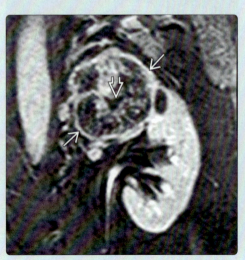

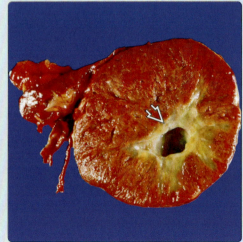

(Left) *Coronal T1WI C+ MR demonstrates a well-defined, spherical renal mass ⟹ with a pseudocapsule and a central scar ⟹, findings that are characteristic, but not diagnostic, of an oncocytoma. Some variants of RCC share many imaging features and some histologic features with oncocytomas.* (Right) *Surgical photograph shows a resected oncocytoma with a central scar ⟹ and thin septa within a homogeneous, sharply marginated, solid mass.*

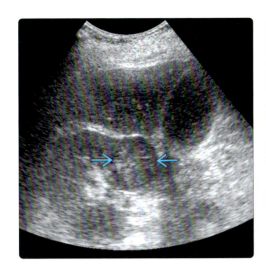 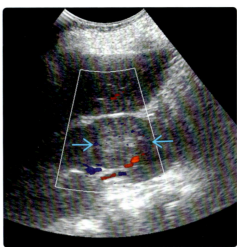

(Left) *Transverse US of the right upper quadrant reveals an incidental solid right renal mass ⇨ with heterogeneous echotexture.* (Right) *Longitudinal color Doppler US in the same patient shows minimal, peripheral, low-level color flow within the right renal mass ⇨. These findings are consistent with a renal neoplasm, but further characterization is not possible by US alone. Flow may be better assessed with contrast-enhanced US, CT, or MR. Surgical resection was consistent with oncocytoma.*

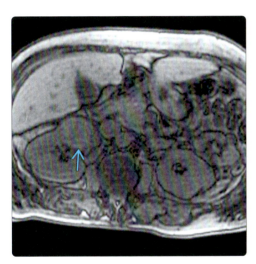 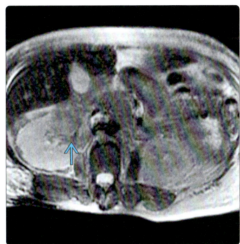

(Left) *Axial T1WI out-phase MR shows a solid mass ⇨ in the anterior cortex of the right kidney with mildly increased signal intensity compared to the renal parenchyma. Compared to the in-phase image, there was no loss of signal.* (Right) *Axial T2WI MR in the same patient shows heterogeneous, intermediate signal intensity of the right renal mass ⇨. The intermediate T2 signal intensity is due to the highly cellular components of the tumor.*

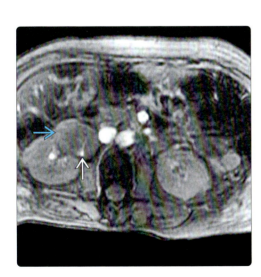 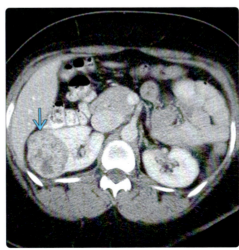

(Left) *Axial T2WI MR in the same patient shows the presence of vessels ⇨ within the mass ⇨ that is isointense to the renal parenchyma on this sequence. Although these findings suggest that the mass is due to renal neoplasm, the MR findings of oncocytoma do not allow definitive characterization or differentiation from RCC. Surgical resection was consistent with oncocytoma.* (Right) *Axial CECT during the nephrographic phase shows heterogeneous enhancement of a partially exophytic renal mass ⇨ due to oncocytoma.*

KEY FACTS

IMAGING

- Encapsulated, multilocular cystic mass herniating into renal hilum
  - Typically solitary and unilateral
- Ultrasound
  - Anechoic cystic components: Thin, echogenic capsule and septa
- CT
  - Low-attenuation cystic components without enhancement; fibrous septa and capsule enhance
- MR
  - T1WI: Typically low signal intensity of cystic components (occasional ↑ T1 signal due to protein)
  - T2WI: High signal intensity of cystic components
  - Capsule and septa: Low signal intensity on T1WI and T2WI

TOP DIFFERENTIAL DIAGNOSES

- Cystic renal cell carcinoma

- Cystic Wilms tumor
- Localized cystic renal disease
- Multicystic dysplastic kidney
- Cortical (simple) cysts
- Mixed embryonal and stromal tumor of kidney

CLINICAL ISSUES

- Biphasic age distribution
  - Males: 3 months to 2 years; females: < 5 years and 40-60 years

DIAGNOSTIC CHECKLIST

- Multilocular cystic nephroma (MLCN) qualifies as Bosniak class 3 or 4 cystic mass
- Difficult to distinguish from multilocular cystic renal cell carcinoma
- Imaging features suggestive of MLCN
  - Cystic spaces in MLCN are enclosed within capsule
  - Herniation of cystic spaces into renal hilum

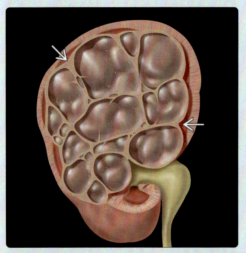
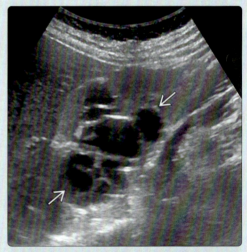

(Left) Graphic shows an encapsulated ➡, multilocular cystic mass that herniates into the renal hilum. (Right) Sagittal US in a 48-year-old woman shows a multiloculated cystic mass ➡ invaginating into the renal hilum. The mass consists of numerous, well-marginated cystic spaces separated by thin, echogenic septa. Occasionally, a cluster of small cysts, or low-level echoes within larger cysts, may mimic a solid component. Although the septa can enhance at CT or MR, detection of color Doppler flow is often difficult.

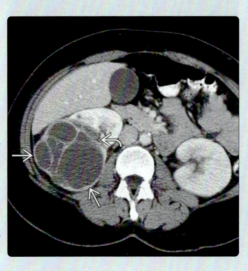
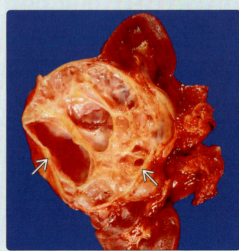

(Left) Axial CECT in a middle-aged woman with flank discomfort shows an encapsulated, multiloculated mass ➡ with septa that enhances after contrast administration. Note the invagination of the mass into the renal hilum ➡, a characteristic feature of this tumor. (Right) Coronal surgical cross section photograph of an excised kidney in the same patient shows a multiloculated cystic mass extending into the renal hilum. Note the presence of a capsule ➡ completely surrounding the cystic mass.

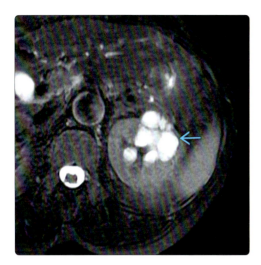

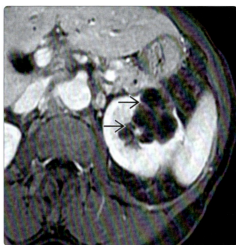

(Left) *Axial T2WI MR with fat saturation shows high signal intensity in a multiloculated cystic lesion ➡ that arises from the superior pole of the left kidney and extends toward the renal sinus. Note that the high signal intensity in the cystic portion is homogeneous.* (Right) *Axial postcontrast T1WI MR with fat saturation in the same patient shows enhancement within the thin septa ➡ of the multiloculated cystic mass. There is also enhancement of the thin fibrous capsule but none within the cystic components.*

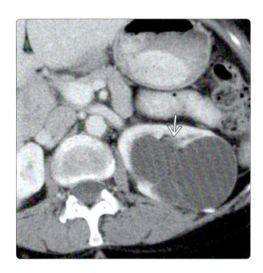

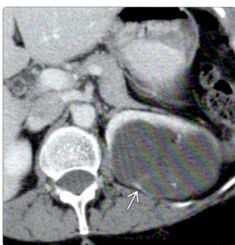

(Left) *Axial CECT shows a classic multilocular cystic nephroma as a multiseptated cystic mass that herniates into the renal sinus ➡. The kidney functions normally, and there is no evidence of vascular invasion, lymphadenopathy, or other signs of malignancy.* (Right) *Axial CECT in the same patient shows a classic, multilocular cystic nephroma as an encapsulated ➡ multicystic mass with herniation into the renal sinus. Note that while there is no enhancement of the cystic portion, there is enhancement of the thin septa.*

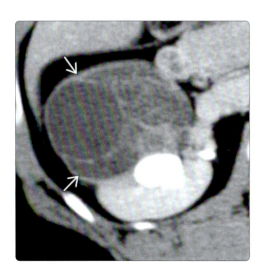

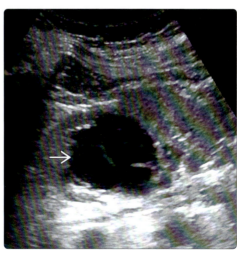

(Left) *Axial CECT shows an encapsulated ➡, multiloculated cystic mass with enhancing septa herniating into the renal hilum. The presence of the capsule encircling the cysts is a key feature that distinguishes multilocular cystic nephroma from other multicystic renal masses.* (Right) *Sagittal US demonstrates an encapsulated, multiloculated cystic mass ➡ in the superior pole of the kidney that herniates toward the renal sinus. Note the thin septa are without nodularity.*

KEY FACTS

TERMINOLOGY

- Rare, benign epithelial renal neoplasm

IMAGING

- Best imaging tool
  - CECT or MR
- Ultrasound
  - Solid expansile mass without specific features
  - May range from hypoechoic to echogenic mass
  - Color Doppler: Variable degree of internal flow
- NECT
  - Soft tissue attenuation mass
    - Frequently hyperattenuating
  - Calcification in ~ 20%
- CECT
  - Well-circumscribed mass
  - Mild, delayed enhancement
  - Large tumors: Heterogeneity due to areas of necrosis and hemorrhage

- MR
  - T1WI: Low signal intensity
  - T2WI: Isointense to slightly hyperintense signal intensity
  - Enhancement is similar to CT

TOP DIFFERENTIAL DIAGNOSES

- Renal cell carcinoma (RCC)
- Oncocytoma
- Wilms tumor (nephroblastoma)

PATHOLOGY

- Epithelial cells with tubulopapillary architecture
- Foci of hemorrhage and necrosis are common
- Immunohistochemical staining facilitates differentiation from papillary RCC

DIAGNOSTIC CHECKLIST

- Consider in middle-aged patient with solitary renal mass that is sightly hyperattenuating on NECT
- Excellent prognosis

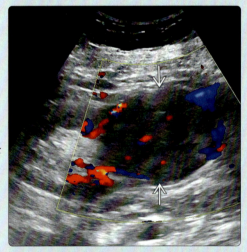
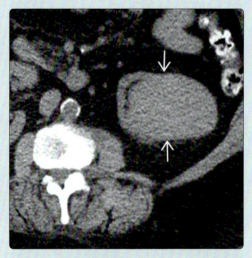

(Left) Longitudinal US shows a solid, exophytic mass ➡ extending from the inferior pole of the left kidney. The mass is isoechoic to renal cortex and has internal color flow. (Right) Axial NECT in the same patient shows that the mass ➡ is slightly hyperattenuating to the renal parenchyma. Although pathology proved metanephric adenoma, these imaging features are nonspecific and differential considerations can include various other renal neoplasms, such as renal cell carcinoma and oncocytoma.

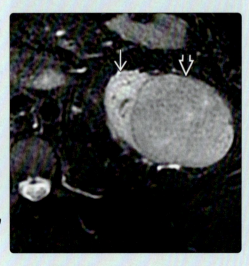
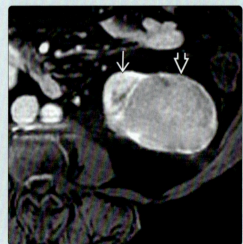

(Left) Axial T2WI MR with fat saturation in the same patient demonstrates that the exophytic left renal mass ➡ has mildly heterogeneous signal intensity that is slightly less than the adjacent renal parenchyma ➡. (Right) Axial postcontrast T1WI MR with fat saturation in the same patient reveals that the mass ➡ is hypovascular compared to the adjacent normal renal parenchyma ➡. There was no vascular invasion, metastases, or regional adenopathy. Pathology was consistent with metanephric adenoma.

Mixed Epithelial and Stromal Tumor

KEY FACTS

TERMINOLOGY

- Rare, benign cystic renal neoplasm that contains stromal and epithelial components

IMAGING

- Well-marginated, multiseptate cystic and solid mass with delayed contrast enhancement
  - Septa are typically ≥ 5 mm in thickness
- Variable appearances due to differential components of cystic and solid components
- Very rare calcification or fatty component

TOP DIFFERENTIAL DIAGNOSES

- Cystic renal cell carcinoma
- Complex renal cyst
- Renal abscess
- Adult cystic nephroma
- Multicystic dysplastic kidney

PATHOLOGY

- Stromal elements: Spindle cells that mimic ovarian stroma
- Epithelial elements: Epithelial-lined cysts and microcysts

CLINICAL ISSUES

- Almost exclusively found in perimenopausal women
- Common symptoms: Hematuria, flank pain, palpable mass, urinary tract infection
  - ~ 25% are asymptomatic
- ~ 70% of mixed epithelial and stromal tumors (MESTs) are Bosniak 4 lesions and resected

DIAGNOSTIC CHECKLIST

- Consider diagnosis of MEST in
  - Perimenopausal women
  - Patients with chronic estrogen use
  - Cystic tumors with delayed enhancement
  - Renal pelvis tumors with negative urine cytology
  - Obstructed duplicated collecting system

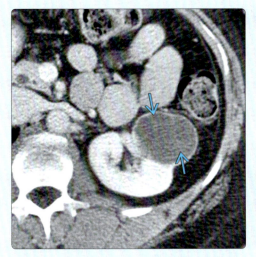
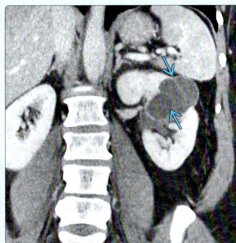

(Left) Axial CECT shows an ovoid, well-circumscribed mass that is partially exophytic from the left kidney. Note several thin, mildly enhancing septa ⊒. Pathology revealed mixed epithelial and stromal tumor (MEST). (Right) Coronal CECT in the same patient shows the multiple, enhancing thin septa ⊒ in the MEST to better advantage. Multiplanar reformatted images are often useful for detecting and assessing the thickness of intratumoral septa and preoperative planning.

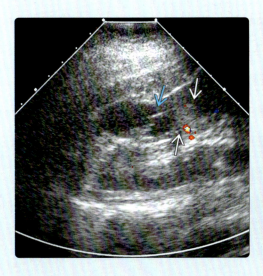
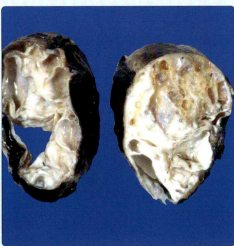

(Left) Longitudinal color Doppler US of the right kidney in a different patient shows an ovoid, predominantly cystic mass with internal septum ⊒ and a small solid component ➡ that shows color flow. The patient underwent partial nephrectomy. Cystic renal cell carcinoma was suspected at imaging. The pathology revealed MEST. (Right) Longitudinal bisected gross surgical specimen of MEST demonstrates numerous cysts and microcysts of variable size interspersed between septa and solid components.

IMAGING

- 2% of sporadic renal cell carcinomas (RCCs) are bilateral, and 16-25% of sporadic RCCs are multicentric in same kidney
- Exophytic: Projects from cortical surface, distinct from parenchyma
- Most are hypervascular (not papillary RCC)
- Rarely, small areas of fat attenuation (-80 to -120 HU)
  - Combination of fat and calcification suggests RCC, not renal angiomyolipoma (AML)
- Renal venous (23%) and inferior vena cava (IVC) tumor extension (7%)
- Metastases (most to least common): Lung, liver, bone, adrenal, opposite kidney, and brain
- Cystic RCC: Enhancing, smooth or nodular septa
- Multiphase CT
  - Mandatory: Nonenhanced and parenchymal phase
  - Optional: Corticomedullary, excretory phases

- Multiphase MR
  - T1WI: Typically low signal intensity (SI)
  - T2WI: High to heterogeneous SI due to necrosis
  - Post contrast: Heterogeneous due to areas of viable, hypervascular tumor and necrosis

TOP DIFFERENTIAL DIAGNOSES

- Renal oncocytoma
- Renal AML
- Renal transitional cell carcinoma
- Renal metastases and lymphoma
- Renal abscess
- Complex renal cysts (Bosniak classification types II and III)

PATHOLOGY

- Clear cell (70%), papillary (10-15%), granular cell (7%), chromophobe cell (5%), sarcomatoid (1.5%), collecting duct (< 1%)

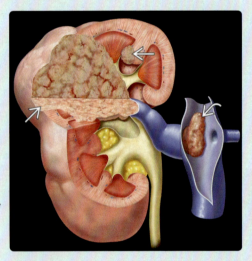
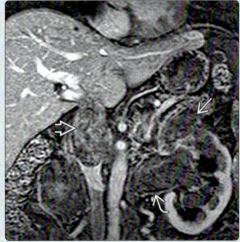

(Left) Graphic shows a heterogeneous, vascular, expansile mass arising from the renal cortex, invading the renal vein and inferior vena cava (IVC) ➡. The tumor is multicentric ➡, as is the case in 16-25% of sporadic RCCs and in a higher percentage of syndromal or inherited cases. (Right) Coronal T1WI MR with contrast enhancement shows an expansile mass ➡ in the upper pole of the left kidney, extending into the renal vein ➡ and IVC ➡. The propensity for venous invasion leads to a high prevalence of pulmonary metastases.

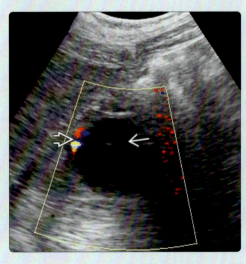
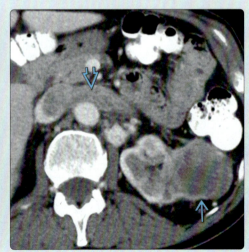

(Left) Sagittal color Doppler US shows a cystic lesion in the superior pole of the right kidney. The lesion has a thick septum ➡ and mural nodule with internal color flow ➡. Partial nephrectomy was performed, confirming cystic RCC. (Right) Axial CECT demonstrates a heterogeneously enhancing, solid mass ➡ with central necrosis that is exophytic from the lateral cortex of the left kidney. There is enhancing tumor thrombus ➡ in the left renal vein and IVC. The tumor was confirmed to be clear cell RCC.

IMAGING

CT Findings

- NECT
  - Heterogeneous mass ± cystic components
    - High attenuation (hemorrhage)
    - Low attenuation (≤ 20 HU) due to necrosis or cystic component
  - Rare calcifications (< 10% of cases)
  - Rare, small areas of fat attenuation (-80 to -120 HU)
    - Usually due to enveloping perirenal or sinus fat
    - Dedifferentiated renal cell carcinoma (RCC) → fat and calcification
    - Fat + calcification suggests RCC > angiomyolipoma (AML)
  - Cystic RCC
    - Uni- or multilocular cystic mass with thick wall
    - Calcification of septa or tumor capsule
- CECT
  - Enhancement (attenuation value ↑ by ≥ 20 HU compared to NECT)
    - < renal parenchyma on nephrographic and pyelographic phases
  - Heterogeneous enhancement (necrosis)
  - ± infiltrating mass may simulate urothelial carcinoma
  - ± subcapsular or perinephric hemorrhage
  - ± invasion of renal veins or inferior vena cava (IVC)
  - Metastases to local lymph nodes (≥ 1 cm) or viscera
  - Cystic RCC: Enhancing, smooth or nodular septa

MR Findings

- T1WI
  - Typically isointense (~ 60%) to hypointense
  - ↑ signal intensity (SI) if internal hemorrhage (methemoglobin)
- T2WI
  - Clear cell RCC: Typically ↑ SI
  - Papillary RCC: Typically ↓ SI
    - Appears same as AML with minimal fat
- T1WI C+ FS
  - Enhancement is usually < normal renal tissue
- In/out of phase
  - Clear cell RCC can lose SI on out-of-phase images
  - Loss of signal on out-of-phase sequence cannot be reliably used to differentiate RCC from AML

Ultrasonographic Findings

- Grayscale ultrasound
  - Detect 85% of masses > 3 cm; ≤ 60% < 2 cm
  - Hyperechoic (48%), isoechoic (42%), or hypoechoic (10%) renal mass
  - Cystic RCC
    - Septa, nodules, necrosis
- Color Doppler
  - Most prominent color flow around periphery of mass

PATHOLOGY

Staging, Grading, & Classification

- TNM staging (7th edition)
  - T (tumor size)
    - T1: Limited to kidney but ≤ 7 cm
      - T1a: ≤ 4 cm
      - T1b: > 4 cm but ≤ 7 cm
    - T2: Limited to kidney but > 7 cm
      - T2a: > 7 cm but ≤ 10 cm
      - T2b: > 10 cm
    - T3: Extension into major veins or perinephric fat or renal sinus but not into ipsilateral adrenal or beyond Gerota fascia
      - T3a: Spread to renal vein
      - T3b: Spread to infradiaphragmatic IVC
      - T3c: Spread to supradiaphragmatic IVC or invades wall of IVC
    - T4: Into ipsilateral adrenal gland or beyond Gerota fascia
  - N (lymph nodes)
    - N0: No nodal involvement
    - N1: Regional nodal involvement
  - M (metastases)
    - M0: No metastases
    - M1: Distant metastases
- Bosniak classification for management of cystic renal lesions
  - Bosniak 1 cystic lesion
    - Simple cyst: Water attenuation; round; well marginated; hairline-thin wall; no septa, calcification, solid components, or enhancement
    - Malignant: 0%
  - Bosniak 2 cystic lesion (minimally complex)
    - Few hairline-thin septa ± perceived enhancement (not measurable)
    - Fine calcifications or short segment of slightly thickened calcification in wall or septa
    - Homogeneously high-attenuation masses (≤ 3 cm) that are sharply marginated and do not enhance
    - Malignant: 0%
  - Bosniak 2F cystic lesion (minimally complex but require follow-up)
    - Multiple hairline-thin septa ± perceived enhancement (not measurable)
    - Thick or nodular calcifications; minimal smooth thickening of wall or septa that may show perceived (not measurable) enhancement
    - Intrarenal, nonenhancing, high-attenuation masses (> 3 cm); no enhancing soft tissue components
    - Work-up: Follow-up imaging (US, CT, MR); typically performed at 6 and 12 months, then annually for 5 years
    - Malignant: ~ 5%
  - Bosniak 3 cystic lesion
    - Indeterminate cystic renal lesions: Thickened, irregular or smooth walls or septa with measurable enhancement
    - Work-up: Partial nephrectomy; radiofrequency ablation in elderly or poor surgical candidates
    - Percentage malignant: ~ 54%
  - Bosniak 4 cystic lesion
    - Clearly malignant: Criteria of category 3 but also containing enhancing soft tissue components
    - Work-up: Partial or complete nephrectomy
    - Malignant: 100%

(Left) Coronal CECT reformation shows a large mass ⮞ replacing all but the superior pole of the left kidney. The mass is heterogeneous due to areas of viable, enhancing tumor and necrosis. (Right) Coronal CECT of a different plane in the same patient shows invasion of the left renal vein and IVC ⮞. Even patients with invasion of the IVC are often candidates for surgical resection. It is important to determine the complete extent of the venous invasion and whether the wall of the vein is involved.

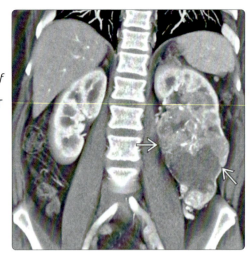
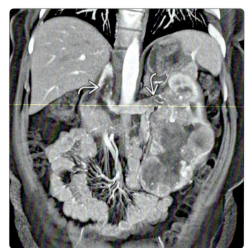

(Left) Sagittal color Doppler US shows a solid, heterogeneous, and slightly hyperechoic mass ⮞ within the posterior aspect of the interpolar cortex. The mass results in a mild contour deformity of the posterior renal cortex. Several areas ⮞ of color flow are present within the mass due to tumor neovascularity. (Right) Axial CECT in the same patient shows a heterogeneously enhancing mass ⮞ in the lateral cortex of the right kidney that corresponds to the abnormality found on prior US.

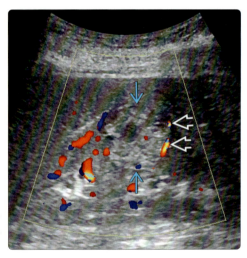
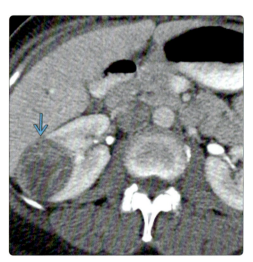

(Left) Coronal T2WI MR in the same patient shows that the mass ⮞ has heterogeneous signal intensity and is partially exophytic along the posteroinferior border of the right renal cortex. (Right) Coronal T1WI MR with fat saturation demonstrates heterogeneous enhancement of the right renal mass ⮞ due to small areas of central necrosis. There was no vascular invasion, adenopathy, or metastatic disease. Due to these factors and the size and location of the tumor, the patient was cured by partial nephrectomy.

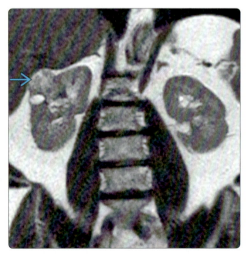
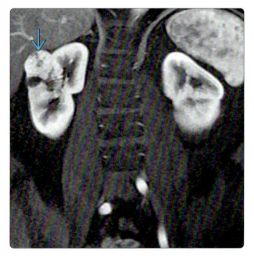

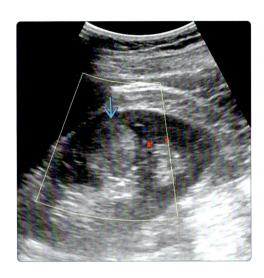

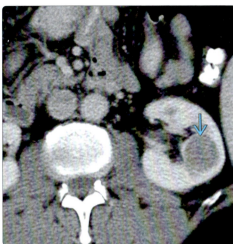

(Left) Sagittal color Doppler US of the left kidney reveals an incidental round, echogenic mass ➡ in the interpolar cortex. No demonstrable color Doppler flow was shown within the mass. (Right) Axial CECT during the nephrographic phase in the same patient shows a solid, round mass ➡ that has minimal enhancement (30 HU above NECT). The nephrectomy specimen was consistent with a papillary RCC. Papillary RCCs are hypovascular compared to clear cell RCCs.

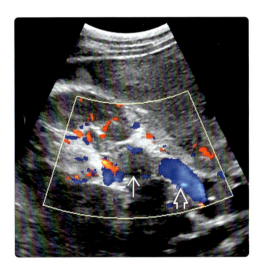

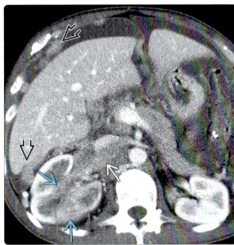

(Left) Axial color Doppler US reveals echogenic thrombus ➡ in a segment of the left renal vein near the renal hilum. Flow is preserved in the segment of renal vein ➡ closest to the IVC. (Right) Subsequent follow-up axial CECT in the same patient demonstrates tumor thrombus in the right renal vein ➡, peritoneal carcinomatosis ➡, and ill-defined tumor ➡ in the right kidney due to infiltrative papillary RCC. Type 2 papillary RCCs typically present at a more advanced stage compared to type 1 tumors.

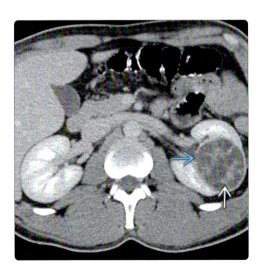

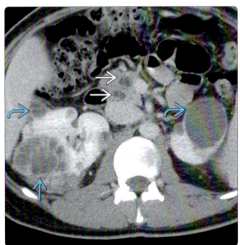

(Left) Axial CECT reveals an incidental heterogeneous, cystic mass ➡ in the left kidney. This is a Bosniak 4 cystic lesion due to the numerous thick, enhancing septa and enhancing nodular components ➡. The surgical resection specimen was consistent with a clear cell RCC. (Right) Axial CECT in a patient with von Hippel Lindau disease demonstrates renal cysts ➡, pancreatic cysts ➡, and a RCC ➡ in the right kidney. The patient also had hemangioblastomas in the brain and spinal cord.

T | Definition of Primary Tumor (T)

T Category	T Criteria
TX	Primary tumor cannot be assessed
T0	No evidence of primary tumor
T1	Tumor ≤ 7 cm in greatest dimension, limited to kidney
T1a	Tumor ≤ 4 cm in greatest dimension, limited to kidney
T1b	Tumor > 4 cm but ≤ 7 cm in greatest dimension, limited to kidney
T2	Tumor > 7 cm in greatest dimension, limited to kidney
T2a	Tumor > 7 cm but ≤ 10 cm in greatest dimension, limited to kidney
T2b	Tumor > 10 cm, limited to kidney
T3	Tumor extends into major veins or perinephric tissues, but not into the ipsilateral adrenal gland and not beyond Gerota's fascia
T3a	Tumor extends into the renal vein or its segmental branches, or invades the pelvicalyceal system, or invades perirenal &/or renal sinus fat but not beyond Gerota's fascia
T3b	Tumor extends into the vena cava below the diaphragm
T3c	Tumor extends into the vena cava above the diaphragm or invades the wall of the vena cava
T4	Tumor invades beyond Gerota's fascia (including contiguous extension into the ipsilateral adrenal gland)

Adapted with permission from AJCC Cancer Staging Manual 8th ed., 2017.

N | Definition of Regional Lymph Node (N)

N Category	N Criteria
NX	Regional lymph nodes cannot be assessed
N0	No regional lymph node metastasis
N1	Metastasis in regional lymph node(s)

Adapted with permission from AJCC Cancer Staging Manual 8th ed., 2017.

M | Definition of Distant Metastasis (M)

M Category	M Criteria
M0	No distant metastasis
M1	Distant metastasis

Adapted with permission from AJCC Cancer Staging Manual 8th ed., 2017.

AJCC | Prognostic Stage Groups

When T is...	And N is...	And M is...	Then the stage group is...
T1	N0	M0	I
T1	N1	M0	III
T2	N0	M0	II
T2	N1	M0	III
T3	N0	M0	III
T3	N1	M0	III
T4	Any N	M0	IV
Any T	Any N	M1	IV

Adapted with permission from AJCC Cancer Staging Manual 8th ed., 2017.

Comparison of Robson and TNM Staging

Robson Stage	Definitions	TNM
I	Tumor ≤ 2.5 cm and confined to kidney	T1
	Tumor > 2.5 cm and confined to kidney	T1-T2
II	Tumor extends into perinephric fat or adrenal	T3a if involves perinephric fat, T4 if involves ipsilateral adrenal
IIIA	Tumor invades renal vein	T3a
	Tumor extends into inferior vena cava	T3b below diaphragm
IIIB	Lymph node involvement	N0-N1, M0
IIIC	Involvement of local vasculature and lymph nodes	T3a-c, N0-N1
IVA	Involvement of adjacent organs (except ipsilateral adrenal)	T4
IVB	Distant metastases	M1

T1a

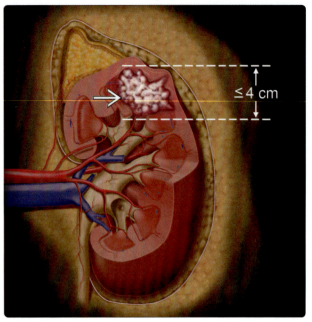

Coronal graphic shows a typical T1a lesion ➡, defined as ≤ 4 cm and confined to the kidney.

T1a

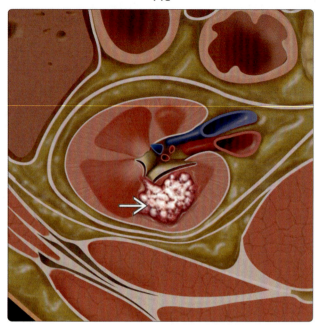

Axial graphic shows a T1a renal cell carcinoma ➡, defined as ≤ 4 cm and confined to the kidney. Lesions may be exophytic or more centrally located, as is the T1a depicted here.

T1b

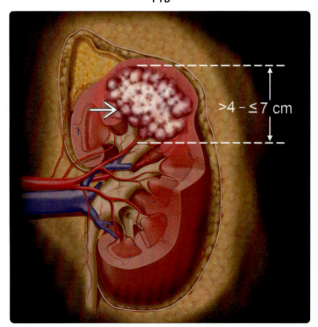

Coronal graphic shows a typical T1b lesion ➡, defined as > 4 cm but ≤ 7 cm and confined to the kidney.

T1b

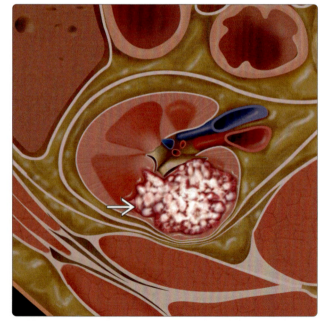

Axial graphic shows a T1b renal cell carcinoma ➡, defined as > 4 cm but ≤ 7 cm and confined to the kidney. These lesions may be exophytic but will still be categorized as T1 as long as there is no extension outside of the kidney.

T2a

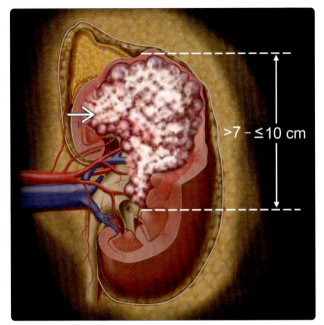

Coronal graphic shows a T2a renal cell carcinoma ➡, defined as > 7 cm but ≤ 10 cm and confined to the kidney. These lesions may also be described as exophytic but do not invade outside of the kidney.

T2b

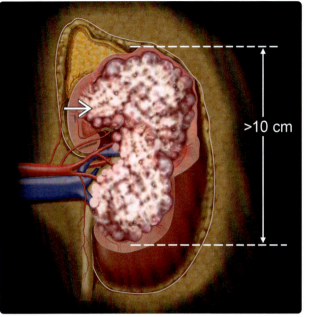

Coronal graphic shows a typical T2b renal cell carcinoma ➡, defined as > 10 cm but confined to the kidney.

T3a

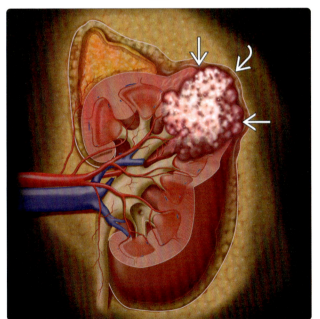

Coronal graphic shows a T3a renal cell carcinoma with tumor extension ➡ into the perirenal fat but not beyond the confines of the Gerota fascia ➡.

T3a

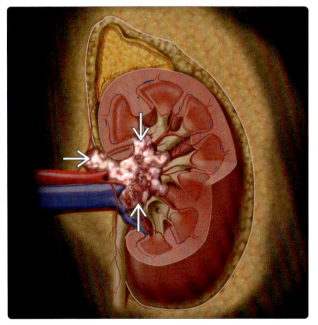

Coronal graphic shows another example of a T3a lesion with extension into the perirenal or renal sinus fat ➡. Again, the tumor is limited by the confines of the Gerota fascia.

T3a

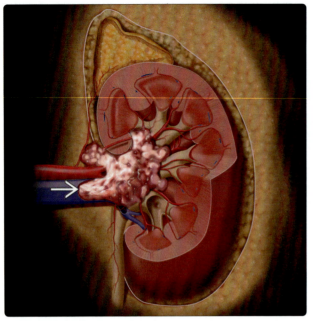

Coronal graphic shows a T3a renal cell carcinoma with extension of tumor into the renal vein ➡. Extension beyond the renal vein into the inferior vena cava would be defined as a T3b lesion.

T3b

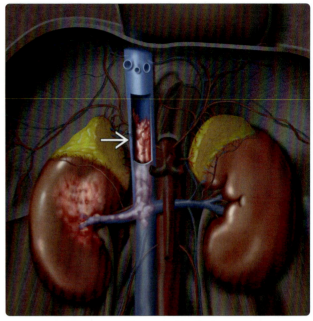

Coronal graphic shows a T3b renal cell carcinoma with extension of tumor not only into the renal vein but also into the inferior vena cava ➡. T3b lesions do not extend above the diaphragm.

T3c

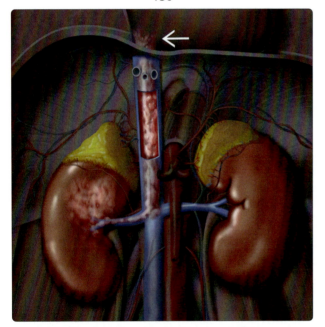

Coronal graphic shows a T3c renal cell carcinoma with involvement of tumor in the renal vein and inferior vena cava, as well as extension of tumor within the inferior vena cava above the diaphragm ➡.

T4

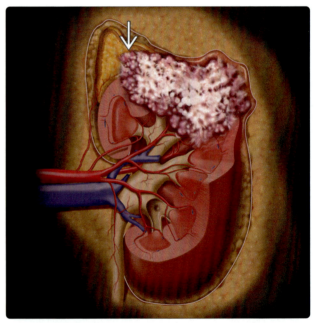

Coronal graphic shows a T4 renal cell carcinoma with extension into the ipsilateral adrenal gland ➡.

T4

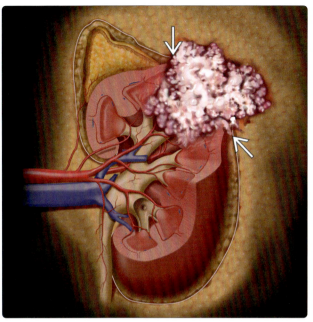

Coronal graphic shows another example of a T4 lesion with invasion into not only the perirenal fat but also with extension beyond the Gerota fascia ➡.

N1 Disease (Stage III or IV)

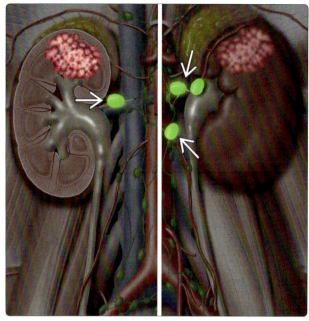

Coronal graphic shows retroperitoneal adenopathy on both sides of the midline ➡. N0 disease is classified as no regional lymph node metastasis, while N1 disease is classified as metastatic disease in regional lymph nodes.

Metastases, Organ Frequency

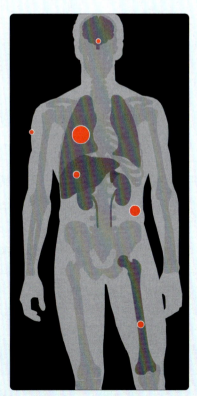

Lung	75%
Soft tissue	35%
Bone	20%
Liver	20%
Adrenal gland	19%
Cutaneous tissues	8%
Central nervous system	8%

25-40% of patients present with metastatic disease.

TERMINOLOGY

- Highly aggressive, infiltrative malignancy arising in collecting duct

IMAGING

- CECT
  - Ill-defined, infiltrative central renal mass
  - Hypovascular; heterogeneous enhancement
  - Caliectasis without pelviectasis
  - Necrosis and hemorrhage are common
- MR
  - T1WI: Low signal intensity
  - T2WI: Low to intermediate signal intensity
  - DWI: Restricted diffusion in areas of viable tumor
- Ultrasound
  - Mixed echogenicity central mass
  - Loss of normal renal architecture
  - Hypovascular: Color Doppler flow typically absent

TOP DIFFERENTIAL DIAGNOSES

- Transitional cell carcinoma
- Lymphoma
- Renal cell carcinoma
- Pyelonephritis

PATHOLOGY

- Central location in kidney; ± satellite lesions in cortex
- Sheets of poorly differentiated, eosinophilic cells
- Inflammatory, edematous stroma; mucin production

CLINICAL ISSUES

- Common symptoms: Flank pain, hematuria, weight loss
- Poor prognosis: Mean survival: ~ 15 months

DIAGNOSTIC CHECKLIST

- Suspect in young African American with sickle cell trait
- Adenopathy and metastases are common at presentation

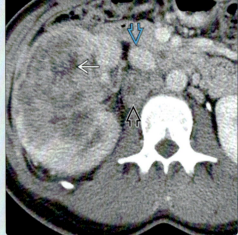
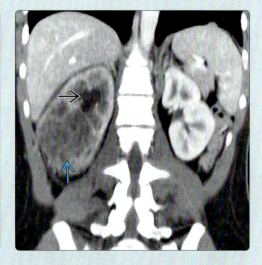

(Left) Axial CECT in a patient with sickle cell trait who presented with right flank pain and hematuria shows an ill-defined, infiltrative mass in the right kidney. The mass enhances heterogeneously due to areas of necrosis ➡. Note the retrocaval adenopathy ➡ resulting in anterior displacement of the inferior vena cava ➡. (Right) Coronal CECT in the same patient reveals that the ill-defined mass ➡ results in caliectasis ➡ in the superior collecting system but no pelviectasis. Pathology was consistent with medullary carcinoma.

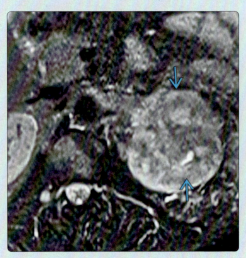
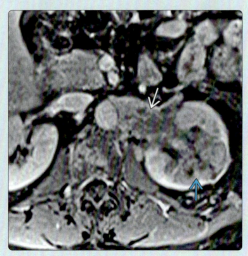

(Left) Axial T2WI MR with fat saturation shows an ill-defined mass ➡ that infiltrates the renal cortex, medulla, and collecting system. The mass has heterogeneous low to intermediate signal intensity. (Right) Axial T1WI C+ MR with fat saturation slightly more inferiorly in the same patient shows heterogeneous enhancement of the infiltrative, hypovascular mass ➡. The tumor also extends into the expanded left renal vein ➡. Heterogeneity within the vein reflects hypovascular tumor and contrast material within the lumen.

Collecting Duct Carcinoma

KEY FACTS

TERMINOLOGY

- Rare, aggressive neoplasm arising in renal medulla
- Synonym: Duct of Bellini carcinoma

IMAGING

- US
  - Ill-defined, hyperechoic mass
  - Obscuration of normal renal architecture
- CT
  - Infiltrative, solid mass centered in renal medulla
    - Invasion of renal sinus ~ 90-95%
  - Hypovascular to heterogeneous enhancement
  - Vascular invasion in ~ 25%
  - Cystic component: ~ 50%
  - Preservation of renal contour > expansile appearance
- MR
  - T1WI: Hypo- to isointense relative to renal parenchyma
  - T2WI: Hypointense relative to renal parenchyma

TOP DIFFERENTIAL DIAGNOSES

- Urothelial carcinoma
- Renal cell carcinoma
- Lymphoma
- Renal medullary carcinoma
- Pyelonephritis

PATHOLOGY

- Arises from collecting ducts in renal medulla
- Columnar cells with variable pleomorphism

CLINICAL ISSUES

- ~ 40% of patients present with metastasis at diagnosis
- Poor prognosis: 2-year survival rate is only ~ 33%
- Presentation: Hematuria, flank pain, palpable mass

DIAGNOSTIC CHECKLIST

- Consider collecting duct carcinoma in middle-aged patient with infiltrative renal mass centered in renal medulla

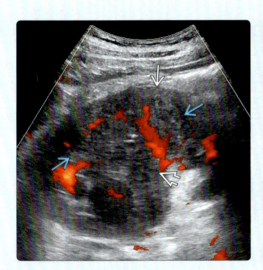

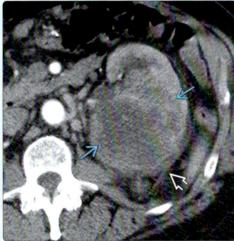

(Left) Longitudinal power Doppler US demonstrates poor definition of the central kidney with obscuration of the normal anatomic landmarks due to an infiltrating mass ➡, which invades the renal sinus ➡, medulla, and cortex ➡. Flow is evident throughout the abnormal soft tissue. (Right) Axial CECT in the same patient confirms an infiltrating, hypovascular mass ➡. The mass originates in the medulla but extends through the cortex into the perinephric fat ➡. Pathology proved collecting duct carcinoma.

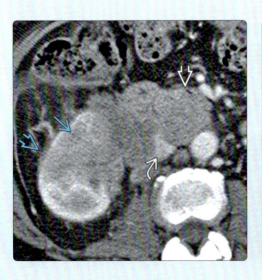

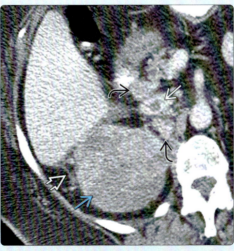

(Left) Axial CECT during the corticomedullary phase shows an ill-defined, hypovascular mass ➡ that infiltrates from the collecting system into the perinephric fat ➡. Tumor also extends medially to surround and compress the IVC ➡ and fills the aortocaval space ➡. Pathology revealed collecting duct carcinoma. (Right) Axial CECT shows a hypovascular mass ➡ replacing the entire superior pole of the right kidney. The mass infiltrates into the perinephric fat ➡. Note metastatic pericaval adenopathy ➡ and tumor thrombus in the IVC ➡.

KEY FACTS

IMAGING

- Bladder: Site of 90% of all cases of urothelial carcinoma
  - Kidney (8%): Extrarenal part of renal pelvis more common than infundibulocalyceal
  - Ureter and proximal 2/3 of urethra (2%)
- Most are low-grade, superficial, papillary masses within renal collecting system
  - Sessile, flat, or polypoid solid mass
- ~ 15% are aggressive and invade renal parenchyma, renal sinus, etc.
  - Maintains bean-shaped renal contour
- Best clue: Irregular filling defect in renal pelvis with tumor infiltration of parenchyma
- CT urography
  - Axial NECT through abdomen and pelvis; CECT (nephrographic, 80- to 140-second delay) through kidneys
  - Excretory phase (5- to 10-minute delay) through abdomen and pelvis
  - Provides "IVP"-type image plus conventional CT views
- Ultrasound
  - Solid mass in collecting system that may efface renal sinus fat and invade into renal parenchyma
- MR
  - Iso- to slightly ↓ signal intensity (SI) on T1WI; iso- to mildly ↑ SI on T2WI

TOP DIFFERENTIAL DIAGNOSES

- Urolithiasis (renal calculi)
- Blood clot
- Infection (e.g., tuberculosis)
- Papillary necrosis
- Renal cell carcinoma
- Xanthogranulomatous pyelonephritis

DIAGNOSTIC CHECKLIST

- Synchronous or metachronous tumors
- Cystoscopy still necessary to diagnose bladder cancer

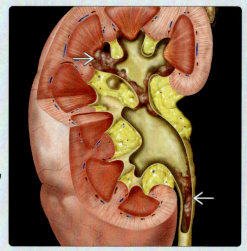
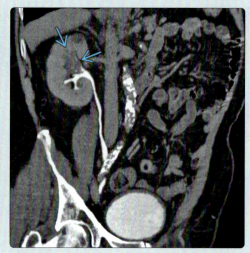

(Left) Graphic shows multifocal urothelial carcinoma ➡ involving the proximal ureter and superior pole calyces. Partial obstruction of the upper pole infundibulum can result in hydronephrosis of a superior calyx with filling defects ("oncocalyces"). (Right) Coronal CECT during the excretory phase shows a soft tissue mass ➡ filling the superior pole collecting system due to urothelial carcinoma.

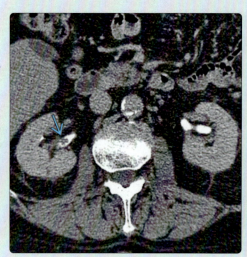
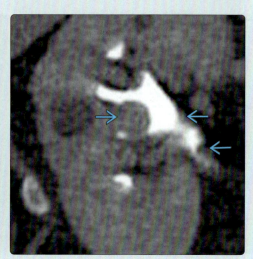

(Left) Axial CECT during the excretory phase in the same patient shows the urothelial carcinoma as a filling defect ➡ in the right renal collecting system. (Right) Coronal CECT in a different patient shows papillary projections of the tumor ➡ at multiple sites along the renal pelvis and proximal ureter. There was no infiltration of the renal parenchyma (best evaluated on nephrographic-phase images, not shown).

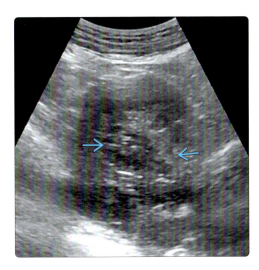

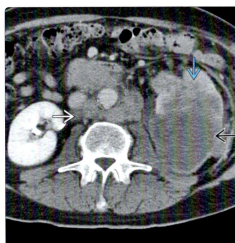

(Left) Transverse ultrasound of the left kidney shows replacement of the normal sinus fat with an ill-defined soft tissue mass ➡ due to urothelial carcinoma. (Right) Axial CECT during the nephrographic phase in the same patient reveals a heterogeneously enhancing mass ➡ effacing the renal sinus and extending posteriorly into the renal parenchyma ➡. Note metastatic retroperitoneal adenopathy ➡.

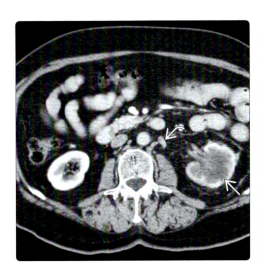

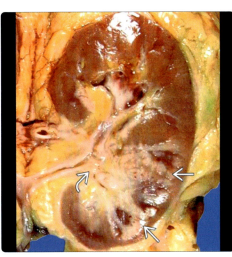

(Left) Axial CECT shows infiltration of the renal parenchyma ➡ by urothelial carcinoma from an inferior pole calyx that was "amputated" on pyelographic-phase images. Renal contour is preserved. Nodal metastases ➡ were better shown on adjacent images. (Right) Gross pathology of the bivalved resected kidney (coronal plane) in the same patient shows a tumor along the surface of the inferior pole collecting system ➡ and invading into the parenchyma ➡ with preservation of the normal renal contour.

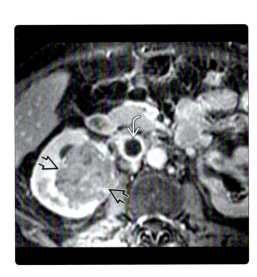

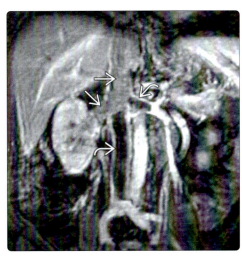

(Left) Axial T1WI C+ FS MR shows a tumor arising from the renal pelvis ➡ and infiltrating the renal parenchyma without altering the renal contour. Note the thrombus in the inferior vena cava (IVC) ➡. (Right) Coronal T1 C+ FS MR shows an enhancing tumor thrombus ➡ within the right renal vein and suprarenal IVC, along with diffuse infiltration of the kidney but preservation of the renal contour. Thrombus is present in the infrarenal IVC and left renal vein ➡.

T | Definition of Primary Tumor (T)

T Category	T Criteria
TX	Primary tumor cannot be assessed
T0	No evidence of primary tumor
Ta	Papillary noninvasive carcinoma
Tis	Carcinoma in situ
T1	Tumor invades subepithelial connective tissue
T2	Tumor invades muscularis
T3	
Renal Pelvis only	Tumor invades beyond muscularis into peripelvic fat or the renal parenchyma
Ureter only	Tumor invades beyond muscularis into periureteric fat
T4	Tumor invades adjacent organs or through kidney into perinephric fat

Adapted with permission from AJCC Cancer Staging Manual 8th ed., 2017.

N | Definition of Regional Lymph Node (N)

N Category	N Criteria
NX	Regional lymph nodes cannot be assessed
N0	No regional lymph node metastasis
N1	Metastasis in a single lymph node, ≤ cm in greatest dimension
N2	Metastasis in a single lymph node, > 2 cm; or multiple lymph nodes

Adapted with permission from AJCC Cancer Staging Manual 8th ed., 2017.

M | Definition of Distant Metastasis (M)

M Category	M Criteria
M0	No distant metastasis
M1	Distant metastasis

Adapted with permission from AJCC Cancer Staging Manual 8th ed., 2017.

AJCC | Prognostic Stage Groups

When T is...	And N is...	And M is...	Then the stage group is...
Ta	N0	M0	0a
Tis	N0	M0	0is
T1	N0	M0	I
T2	N0	M0	II
T3	N0	M0	III
T4	N0	M0	IV
Any T	N1	M0	IV
Any T	N2	M0	IV
Any T	Any N	M1	IV

Adapted with permission from AJCC Cancer Staging Manual 8th ed., 2017.

Ta

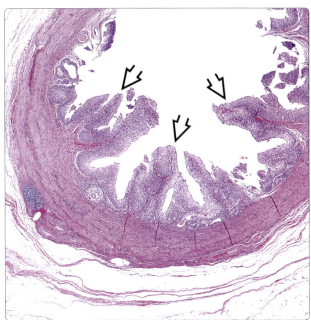

Low-power magnification (H&E stain) shows a cross section of proximal ureter with papillary noninvasive urothelial carcinoma. Note the multiple papillary fronds ➯ lined by variably thickened epithelium extending into the lumen.

Ta

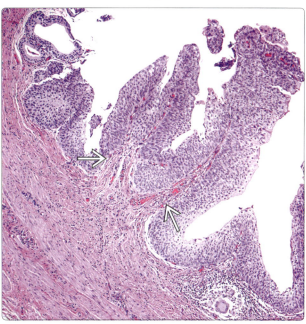

Higher power magnification of the previous image shows fibrovascular cores ➡ surrounded by an increased number of cells compared to normal urothelium. Cells are oriented perpendicular to basement membrane and lack cytologic atypia and pleomorphism.

Tis

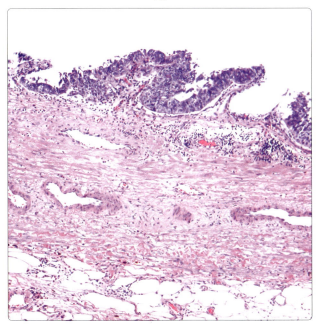

H&E shows that, in contrast to cells in the previous images, the neoplastic cells are markedly pleomorphic and hyperchromatic. The nuclei lack polarity to basement membrane. Note also the propensity of these cells to become detached from basement membrane focally.

T1

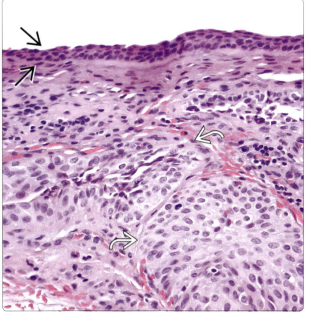

H&E stain demonstrates uninvolved superficial urothelium ➯ with underlying nests of neoplastic urothelium ➡ that invade the subepithelial connective tissue.

T2

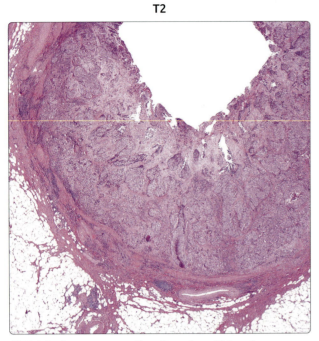

H&E stain shows a cross section of a ureter with invasive urothelial carcinoma. Tumor nests invade almost the entire thickness of the muscularis propria but do not extend into the periureteric fat.

T2

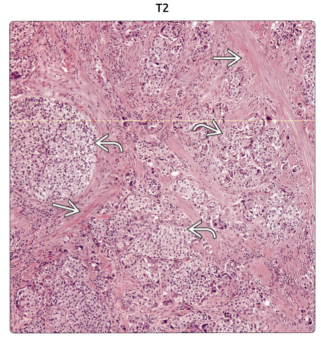

High-power magnification of the previous image shows nests of urothelial carcinoma ⮞ invading and disrupting the muscularis propria (pink bundles of smooth muscles) ⮞.

T3

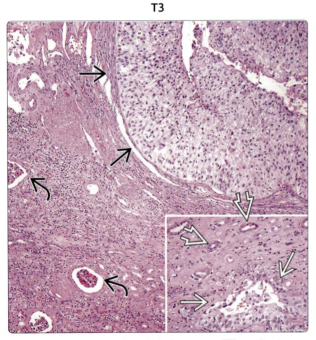

H&E stain shows a nest of urothelial carcinoma ⮞ invading into renal parenchyma; note the renal glomeruli ⮞. The inset shows a nest of urothelial carcinoma ⮞ invading renal parenchyma in proximity to renal tubules ⮞.

T4

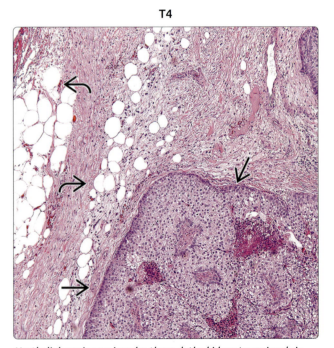

Urothelial carcinoma invades through the kidney to perinephric fat. The large nests of urothelial carcinoma ⮞ infiltrate the perinephric fat (white round cells) ⮞ with prominent pink desmoplastic reaction.

Ta, T1, and T2

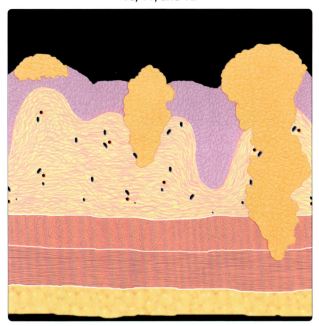

Graphic shows local extent of early stages of ureteric carcinoma: Ta is papillary noninvasive carcinoma, T1 is tumor invading subepithelial connective tissue, and T2 is tumor invading the muscularis.

T3: Renal Pelvis and Calyceal Carcinoma

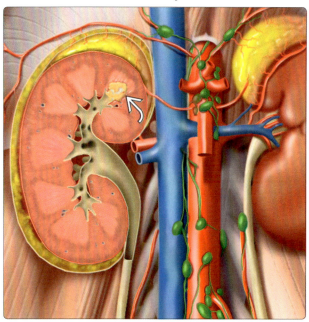

Graphic shows T3 tumor of the upper calyx ➡ with extension through the muscularis layer into the peripelvic fat or renal parenchyma.

T3: Ureteral Carcinoma

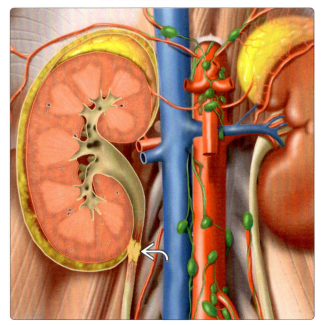

Graphic shows T3 tumor of the ureter ➡ with extension through the muscularis layer into the periureteric fat without invasion of surrounding organs or structures.

T4: Renal Pelvis and Calyceal Carcinoma

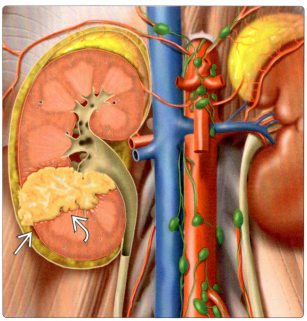

Graphic shows T4 tumor of the lower calyx ➡ with invasion through the renal parenchyma into the perinephric fat ➡.

T4: Ureteral Carcinoma

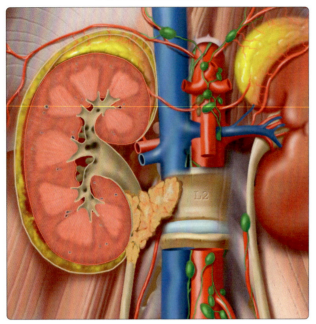

T4 ureteric tumors invade through the surrounding organs and structures. Graphic shows a T4 tumor of the upper ureter invading L2 vertebral body.

T4: Ureteral Carcinoma

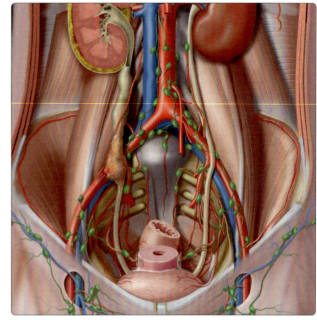

T4 ureteric tumors invade through the surrounding organs and structures. Graphic shows a T4 tumor of the middle ureter invading the right iliac vessels.

T4: Ureteral Carcinoma

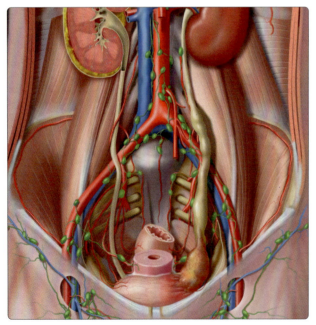

T4 ureteric tumors invade through the surrounding organs and structures. Graphic shows a T4 tumor of the lower ureter invading the urinary bladder.

Nodal Drainage of Renal Pelvis and Calyces

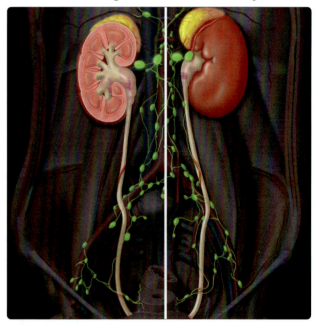

Right renal pelvis tumors spread to renal hilar, paracaval, and retrocaval nodes, whereas left renal pelvic tumors spread to renal hilar and paraaortic nodes.

Nodal Drainage of Upper 2/3 of Ureters

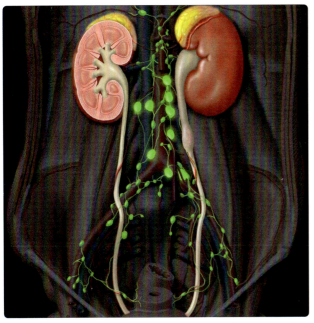

Tumors of the upper 2/3 of the right ureter spread to retrocaval and aortocaval nodes, and tumors of the upper 2/3 of the left ureter spread to paraaortic nodes, nodes at the origin of the inferior mesenteric artery, and common iliac nodes.

Nodal Drainage of Lower 1/3 of Ureters

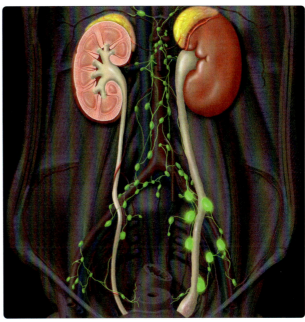

Tumors of the distal 1/3 of either ureter spread to common iliac, internal iliac, external iliac, obturator, and presacral nodes.

Metastases, Organ Frequency

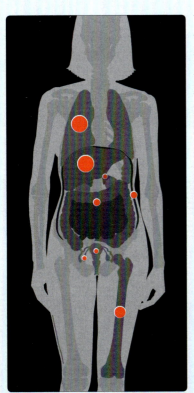

Liver	63%
Lung	58%
Bone	43%
Gastrointestinal tract	20%
Peritoneum	18%
Adrenal gland	15%
Ovary	13%
Uterus	10%

Data from Batata MA et al: Primary carcinoma of the ureter: a prognostic study. Cancer. 35:1626-32, 1975.

KEY FACTS

IMAGING

- CECT
  - Multiple bilateral renal masses (40-60%)
  - Homogeneous, mild enhancement (10-20 HU)
  - Retroperitoneal adenopathy (25%), splenomegaly, or lymphadenopathy at other sites
  - Infiltration of renal parenchyma or sinus with maintenance of reniform shape; may simulate transitional cell carcinoma
  - Extranodal sites: Bowel, brain, liver, bone marrow
- MR
  - T1: Iso- to slightly hypointense
  - T2: Typically hypointense
  - T1WI C+ FS: Mild enhancement
- US
  - Solid, hypoechoic lesions relative to renal parenchyma
  - ± internal flow; power Doppler improves sensitivity

TOP DIFFERENTIAL DIAGNOSES

- Renal cell carcinoma
- Transitional cell carcinoma
- Infection

PATHOLOGY

- Renal involvement of non-Hodgkin lymphoma to Hodgkin lymphoma ratio = 10:1

CLINICAL ISSUES

- Usually asymptomatic
- ± flank pain, fever, weight loss

DIAGNOSTIC CHECKLIST

- CECT or MR is best for evaluation of indeterminate renal masses
- Consider renal lymphoma when there are discreet or infiltrative renal masses in setting of systemic adenopathy
- Biopsy often required for diagnosis

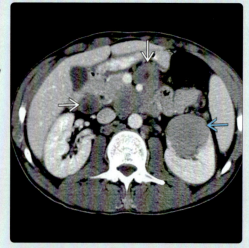
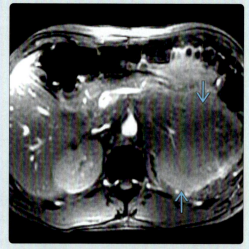

(Left) Axial CECT in a 34-year-old man with AIDS shows a well-circumscribed, mildly enhancing mass ➡ in the left kidney. There are also several enlarged lymph nodes ➡ with hypoattenuating areas of necrosis due to non-Hodgkin lymphoma. (Right) Axial T2* GRE MR shows an ill-defined tumor ➡ infiltrating the left kidney and perirenal space. The patient also had systemic adenopathy that is not shown on this image. Biopsy of the mass revealed B-cell non-Hodgkin lymphoma, the most common type of lymphoma involving the kidney.

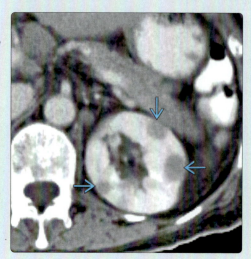
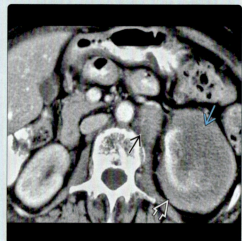

(Left) Axial CECT shows multiple small, homogeneous, hypoattenuating masses ➡ in a patient with systemic non-Hodgkin lymphoma. Renal lymphoma may present as numerous hypoattenuating lesions or as an infiltrating mass that invades the kidney and perinephric space. (Right) Axial CECT shows ill-defined tumor ➡ infiltrating the left kidney and extending into the perirenal space ➡. An adjacent retroperitoneal node ➡ is enlarged. Pathology revealed non-Hodgkin lymphoma.

KEY FACTS

IMAGING

- Renal metastases often found in setting of other visceral and nodal metastases
- CT
  - Multiple solid, hypoattenuating renal masses
  - Typically located in renal cortex or at corticomedullary junction
  - Variable enhancement (depending on primary tumor type)
    - Hypervascular: Melanoma, breast, neuroendocrine
- MR
  - T1WI: Typically iso- to hypointense
  - T2WI: Typically hyperintense
- Best advice for evaluation of indeterminate renal lesions
  - Contrast-enhanced CT or MR
  - PET/CT for staging of malignancy
- US
  - Multiple solid, hypoechoic masses at grayscale
  - Variable color Doppler flow (depending on tumor type)

TOP DIFFERENTIAL DIAGNOSES

- Renal cell carcinoma
- Transitional cell carcinoma
- Lymphoma
- Infection (pyelonephritis, abscess)

PATHOLOGY

- Common etiologies for renal metastases
  - Bronchogenic carcinoma
  - Breast carcinoma
  - Melanoma
  - Gastric carcinoma
  - Contralateral renal cell carcinoma

DIAGNOSTIC CHECKLIST

- Imaging features of renal metastases often nonspecific
- Percutaneous biopsy may be required for definitive diagnosis

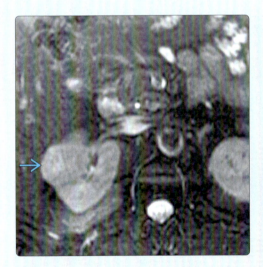
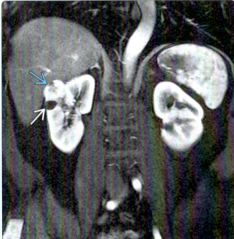

(Left) Axial T2WI MR with fat suppression reveals a solid mass ➡ centered in the lateral cortex of the right kidney that has intermediate to slightly increased signal intensity relative to the normal adjacent renal parenchyma. (Right) Postcontrast coronal T1WI MR with fat suppression in the same patient shows a hypervascular mass ➡ with central necrosis in the right kidney. Pathology was consistent with metastatic breast carcinoma. An incidental cyst ➡ is inferior to the metastasis.

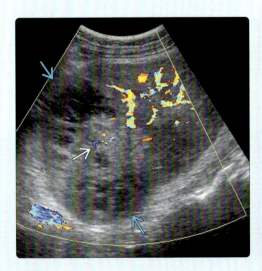
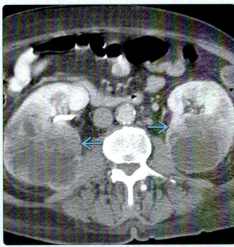

(Left) Sagittal color Doppler ultrasound shows a large, heterogeneous mass ➡ replacing the superior pole of the right kidney due to metastatic non-small cell lung carcinoma. Note internal color flow ➡ within the metastasis. There was a similar-appearing mass in the contralateral kidney (not shown). (Right) Subsequent axial CECT in the same patient demonstrates bilateral, heterogeneously enhancing renal masses ➡ with areas of necrosis due to metastatic non-small cell lung carcinoma.

KEY FACTS

TERMINOLOGY

- Malignant tumor of primitive metanephric blastema
- Accounts for 90% of pediatric renal tumors
- 80% of cases in children < 5 years old

IMAGING

- Ultrasound frequently 1st study performed; CT and MR better characterize tumor and stage
  - Large, heterogeneous but predominantly solid hypoechoic (ultrasound), hypoenhancing renal mass
  - Careful evaluation of
    - Adjacent soft tissues for tumor rupture, adenopathy
    - Renal vein and inferior vena cava for tumor thrombus
    - Contralateral kidney for synchronous tumor or nephrogenic rests
- Chest CT: Lung metastases in 10-20%

TOP DIFFERENTIAL DIAGNOSES

- Neuroblastoma: Extrarenal, more often calcified

- Congenital mesoblastic nephroma: < 3-12 months
- Renal cell carcinoma: Equal incidence to Wilms after age 12

PATHOLOGY

- Arises from primitive metanephric blastemal tissue
  - Persistence after 36 weeks gestation termed nephroblastomatosis → found in 40% of kidneys resected for Wilms tumor
- Associated predisposing syndromes in 10%, including Beckwith-Wiedemann, WAGR syndromes
  - Quarterly screening renal ultrasounds until age 8

CLINICAL ISSUES

- Biopsy increases stage (considered tumor spill)
- Treatment: Radical nephrectomy + chemotherapy, ± radiation
  - Neoadjuvant chemotherapy if unresectable or tumor thrombus above hepatic veins; consider if background nephroblastomatosis or bilateral tumors
- > 90% 5-year survival for localized abdominal disease

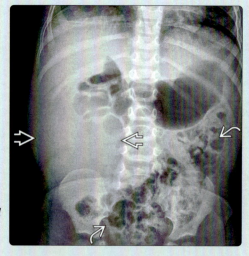
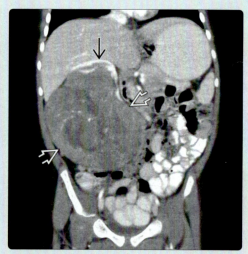

(Left) AP abdominal radiograph of a 3-year-old child with a firm, palpable mass shows leftward displacement of bowel loops ⇒ by a right-sided soft tissue mass ⇒. CT was performed next in this child due to suspicion for a Wilms tumor. (Right) Coronal CECT in the same patient confirms a large, heterogeneous, solid mass ⇒ arising from the right kidney. A residual "claw" of normal renal tissue ⇒ is splayed along the upper pole of this Wilms tumor. No contralateral lesions or venous invasion were identified.

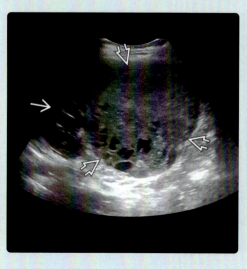
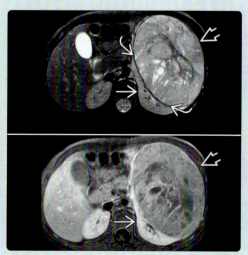

(Left) Longitudinal ultrasound in a 5 year old with hypertension and abdominal fullness shows a round heterogeneous mass ⇒ extending out of the lower pole of the left kidney ⇒. Wilms tumor was confirmed after resection. (Right) Axial T2 (top) and T1 C+ (bottom) MR images show a large, well-defined, heterogeneous mass ⇒ arising from a splayed "claw" of the left kidney ⇒ in a 6 year old with a Wilms tumor. Note the presence of a T2-hypointense pseudocapsule ⇒ around the tumor.

Nephroblastomatosis

TERMINOLOGY

- Nephrogenic rests (NR): Persistent metanephric blastema; precursor to Wilms tumor
  - Perilobar NR: At periphery of kidney
  - Intralobar NR: Within central kidney
- Nephroblastomatosis: Multiple or diffuse NR

IMAGING

- Homogeneous, multifocal, ovoid or subcapsular, rind-like renal masses that enhance < normal kidney on CT/MR
  - Diffuse disease: Thick, uniform, homogeneous peripheral rind of hypoenhancing abnormal tissue
  - Multifocal disease: Scattered nodules resembling normal renal cortex on precontrast imaging
- Differentiating NR from Wilms tumor
  - NR: Diffusely homogeneous appearance; Wilms tumor: Heterogeneous
  - NR: Usually < 2 cm; Wilms tumor: Usually > 3 cm

- NR: Usually oval or lenticular in shape; Wilms tumor: Usually spherical
- Imaging findings suggesting conversion of NR to Wilms
  - Rapid ↑ in size
  - Stable or ↑ size while on chemotherapy
  - Nodule within initial lesions
  - New heterogeneous appearance of mass

PATHOLOGY

- Biopsy often not helpful as microscopic patterns of NR and Wilms tumor can appear similar

CLINICAL ISSUES

- Most NR spontaneously regress; treatment controversial
- Common associated syndromes
  - Perilobar NR: Beckwith-Wiedemann syndrome, hemihypertrophy, Perlman syndrome, trisomy 18
  - Intralobar NR: Drash syndrome, sporadic aniridia, WAGR syndrome

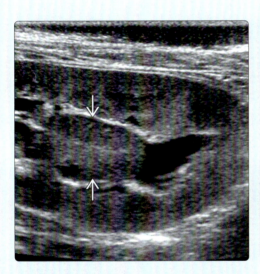

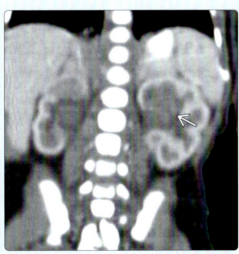

(Left) Longitudinal ultrasound of the left kidney in a 4 day old shows a centrally located, ovoid, isoechoic nephrogenic rest ➡. Intralobar nephrogenic rests are less common than the perilobar form but have a higher risk of malignant transformation to Wilms tumor. (Right) Coronal CECT of the abdomen in the same patient shows a homogeneously hypodense, intralobar nephrogenic rest ➡. Intralobar rests are associated with the WT1 gene, sporadic aniridia, and Drash syndrome.

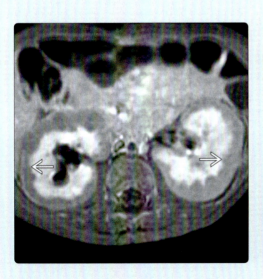

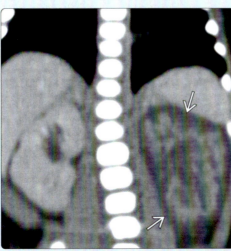

(Left) Axial T1WI C+ MR in a young patient shows diffuse enlargement of the kidneys and a homogeneous lobulated rim of decreased enhancement ➡ surrounding both kidneys, consistent with perilobar nephrogenic rests. (Right) Coronal CECT in a neonate shows the unilateral, diffuse perilobar nephrogenic rests ➡ of the left kidney. Perilobar nephrogenic rests are more common than the intralobar form and are associated with the WT2 gene, Beckwith-Wiedemann syndrome, and hemihypertrophy.

KEY FACTS

TERMINOLOGY

- Hamartomatous renal tumor of young infants
- Classic benign vs. more aggressive cellular variants
  - Studies vary on which type more common

IMAGING

- Solitary renal mass in fetus or infant
- Well-defined oval/round mass
  - Classic benign type usually solid, smaller
  - Cellular type usually larger with cystic/necrotic/hemorrhagic foci

PATHOLOGY

- Classic type similar to infantile fibromatosis
- Cellular type thought to be visceral form of infantile fibrosarcoma
  - Local recurrence, metastases
  - Polysomies of chromosome 11, *ETV6-NTRK3* gene fusion
- Composed predominantly of elongated spindle cells

CLINICAL ISSUES

- Most common renal tumor < 5 months of age
- 3-6% of childhood renal tumors
- Presentations include
  - Palpable abdominal mass in young infant
  - Hypertension, hypercalcemia, hematuria
  - Prenatally detected renal mass with polyhydramnios (70%), preterm labor
- Most mesoblastic nephroma (MN) diagnosed before 3 months of age (90% by 1 year)
  - Classic type more common < 3 months
- After age 3 months
  - Wilms tumor becomes more common
  - Remaining MN more likely to be cellular
- Nephrectomy usually curative

DIAGNOSTIC CHECKLIST

- Preoperative feature for best differentiating solid renal masses in children: Age

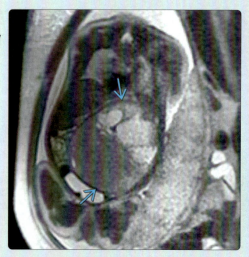
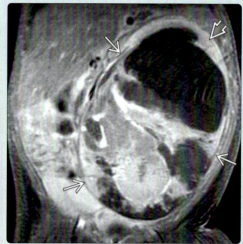

(Left) Coronal T2 fetal MR in a 37-week gestation fetus shows a large mixed cystic and solid mass ⇨ in the left abdomen. (Right) Coronal T1 C+ MR in a 5 day old with abdominal fullness shows a heterogeneously enhancing tumor ⇨ with large foci of nonenhancement. A "claw" of residual renal parenchyma is seen superiorly ⇨. Resection of this cellular mesoblastic nephroma was complicated by intraoperative rupture/spill.

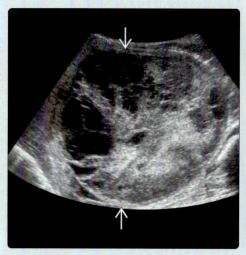
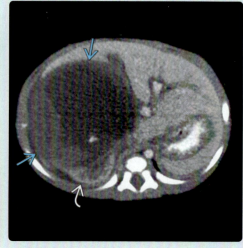

(Left) Longitudinal oblique ultrasound in a 1-month-old infant with a palpable mass shows a heterogeneous, mixed solid and cystic lesion almost completely replacing the right kidney ⇨. Given the patient's age, mesoblastic nephroma is the most likely diagnosis. (Right) Axial CECT in a patient with cellular mesoblastic nephroma shows a claw of residual right kidney ⇨ splayed along the posterior margin of the heterogeneous mass ⇨. This claw sign helps to identify the kidney as the organ of origin for the tumor.

Rhabdoid Tumor

KEY FACTS

TERMINOLOGY

- Rare, highly aggressive neoplasm in young children
- ~ 2% of pediatric renal tumors
- Extrarenal sites include CNS, soft tissues > liver, lung

IMAGING

- Contrast-enhanced CT or MR most useful
  - Large, heterogeneous renal mass
    - Foci of hemorrhage, necrosis, &/or Ca²⁺ separating tumor lobules
      - □ Ca²⁺ more common than Wilms
  - Crescentic subcapsular fluid collection common
  - Sinus/hilar, local, and vascular invasion common
  - Metastasizes most frequently to lungs

PATHOLOGY

- Likely arises from primitive cells in renal medulla
- Associated with inactivation or deletion of *SMARCB1* (hSNFS/INI1) gene on chromosome 22q11

CLINICAL ISSUES

- Mean age of presentation: ~ 11 months
  - Younger than mean age for Wilms tumor
- Signs/symptoms
  - Most common: Palpable abdominal mass, hematuria (gross or microscopic)
  - Others include fever, anemia, hypercalcemia
- Aggressive neoplasm with poor prognosis
  - Patients often present with advanced disease
    - Stages 3-4 in ~ 70% at presentation
  - Overall 5-year survival around 20%
  - Prognosis worse in younger patients (< 6 months of age)

DIAGNOSTIC CHECKLIST

- If neurologic symptoms, consider brain MR to evaluate for synchronous or metachronous CNS neoplasm (present in 15%)

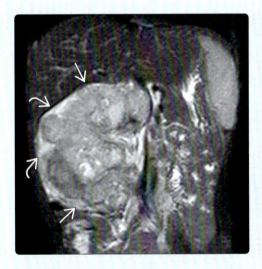
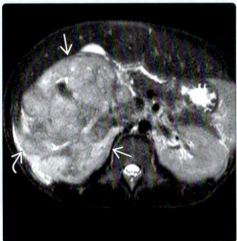

(Left) *Coronal T2 MR with fat saturation in an 11-month-old boy ultimately diagnosed with a rhabdoid tumor shows a large, heterogeneous, lobulated mass ➡ replacing the right kidney. A thin subcapsular fluid collection ➡ is noted at the periphery of the mass.* (Right) *Axial T2 MR with fat saturation in the same patient with a right renal rhabdoid tumor shows a crescentic focus of subcapsular fluid ➡ at the periphery of the heterogeneous tumor ➡.*

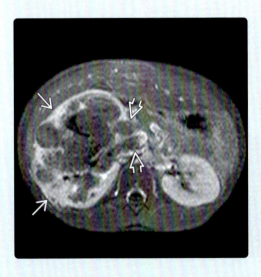
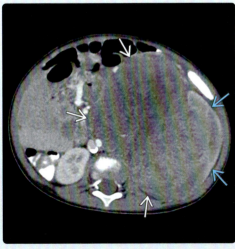

(Left) *Postcontrast T1 C+ MR with fat saturation in the same patient demonstrates heterogeneous enhancement of the large right renal mass ➡. Note the hilar invasion by the tumor lobules ➡.* (Right) *Axial CECT in a 14-month-old patient with a renal rhabdoid tumor demonstrates a very large heterogeneously enhancing central mass ➡ in the left kidney ➡.*

TERMINOLOGY

- Rare malignant renal neoplasm in children < 4 years
  - 2nd most common malignant childhood renal tumor after Wilms
  - 3-5% of pediatric renal tumors
  - Metastasizes to bone, brain

IMAGING

- CECT or MR best for characterizing tumor and evaluating local extension
  - Large, heterogeneous, circumscribed, unilateral renal mass + osseous metastases in young child
    - Cystic and necrotic foci common
    - Calcification: 25%
    - Vascular invasion: 5%
    - Regional lymph node involvement: up to 30%
  - Staging similar to Wilms tumor
- Metastasis evaluation
  - Chest CT, nuclear medicine bone scan

CLINICAL ISSUES

- Most common presentation: Palpable abdominal mass
  - ± hematuria
  - ± hypertension
  - Rarely presents with pain from osseous metastases
- Mean age at presentation: 36 months
- M > F (2:1)
- 5-year survival: ~ 70%
  - Up to 98% for stage I disease
  - ~ 50% for stage IV disease
- Treatment: Combination chemotherapy (including doxorubicin), radiation, resection (depending on stage)
- Delayed recurrence in bones, lungs

DIAGNOSTIC CHECKLIST

- Pediatric solid renal masses are rarely distinguishable by imaging alone
  - Age, clinical history, pattern of spread helpful

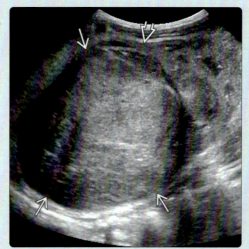
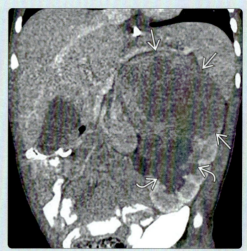

(Left) *Sagittal ultrasound in a 2-year-old boy with a palpable mass shows a circumscribed solid mass ➡ arising from the upper pole of the left kidney. Note the splayed adjacent renal parenchyma ➡, the so-called "claw" sign, which is helpful for determining the organ of origin.* (Right) *Coronal CECT in the same patient shows a large, hypoenhancing mass ➡ arising from the upper pole of the left kidney. The mass obstructs the collecting system of the lower pole ➡. Clear cell sarcoma was confirmed at resection.*

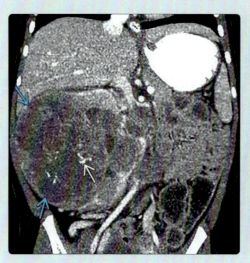
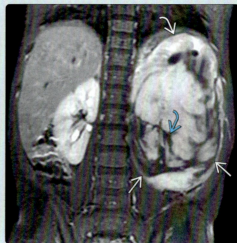

(Left) *Coronal CECT in a 3-year-old girl with clear cell sarcoma shows a heterogeneous mass ➡ arising from the right kidney. Note the calcification ➡ within the mass.* (Right) *Coronal T1 C+ MR in an 18-month-old boy with clear cell sarcoma shows a large, heterogeneous mass ➡ arising from the left kidney with areas of nonenhancement corresponding to necrosis ➡. Some preserved renal parenchyma is seen in the upper pole ➡.*

Ossifying Renal Tumor of Infancy

KEY FACTS

IMAGING

- Small renal pelvis mass with calcification
- Ultrasound
  - Echogenic mass within renal collecting system
    - ± collecting system dilatation due to partial obstruction
  - Posterior acoustic shadowing due to calcification
  - True internal Doppler flow helps distinguish from nonneoplastic material in collecting system
- CECT
  - Polypoid or lobulated mass within pelvicalyceal system
  - Calcification typically present
    - If only microcalcifications, may appear as vague hyperdensity
  - Variable enhancement
- MR
  - May be low in signal intensity on T2 due to calcification

TOP DIFFERENTIAL DIAGNOSES

- Mesoblastic nephroma
  - Most common renal neoplasm < 3 months old
  - Solid or mixed solid and cystic; calcification uncommon
- Wilms tumor
  - Most common pediatric renal neoplasm > 3 months old
  - Typically solid; calcification uncommon
- Staghorn calculus
  - Large calcification filling variable degrees of collecting system
  - No true internal Doppler flow
  - Extremely rare in young children

CLINICAL ISSUES

- Extremely rare benign tumor presenting with gross hematuria in infants age 6 days to 2.5 years
- M > F
- Surgical resection curative, nephron sparing if possible
  - No reports of metastasis or recurrence after resection

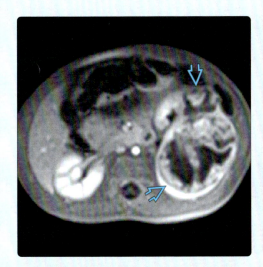
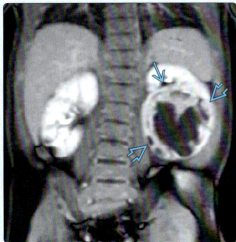

(Left) *Axial T1 C+ FS MR in a 5-month-old boy with hematuria shows a lobulated, heterogeneously enhancing mass ➡ in the left kidney.* (Right) *Coronal T1 C+ FS MR in the same patient shows that the heterogeneously enhancing mass is centered in the left lower pole kidney ➡ but protrudes into the collecting system centrally ➡. The mass is larger than typically seen with an ossifying renal tumor of infancy.*

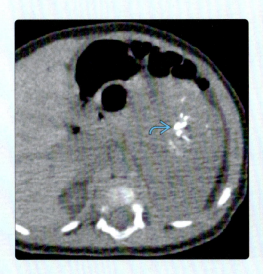
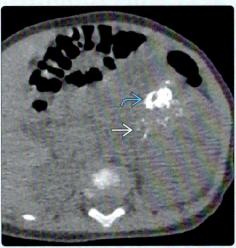

(Left) *Axial NECT of the upper abdomen (done as part of a metastatic work-up chest CT in the same 5-month-old patient) shows coarse calcification ➡ within the left renal mass, typical of an ossifying renal tumor of infancy.* (Right) *Slightly inferior axial NECT of the upper abdomen in the same patient shows the calcification within the left renal mass ➡ extends into the region of the central collecting system ➡, typical of an ossifying renal tumor of infancy.*

Nephrocalcinosis

IMAGING

- Renal parenchymal sites of calcinosis
  - Medullary nephrocalcinosis (95%)
  - Cortical nephrocalcinosis (5%)
- Scattered punctate calcifications in renal medulla
  - Common in medullary sponge kidney
- Dense, confluent medullary calcification
  - Renal tubular acidosis > hyperparathyroidism
- Tram line calcification in renal cortex
  - Especially in acute cortical necrosis

TOP DIFFERENTIAL DIAGNOSES

- Renal papillary necrosis
- Renal tuberculosis
- Extrapulmonary *Pneumocystis carinii* or *Mycobacterium avium-intracellulare* infection in AIDS patients

PATHOLOGY

- Medullary nephrocalcinosis
  - Hyperparathyroidism > renal tubular acidosis > medullary sponge kidney
- Cortical nephrocalcinosis
  - Chronic glomerulonephritis > cortical necrosis > rejected renal allograft
- 3 primary mechanisms for calcium deposition
  - Metastatic: Metabolic abnormality leads to calcium deposition in normal kidneys
  - Dystrophic: Calcium deposition in damaged renal parenchyma
  - Urinary stasis: Calcium salts precipitate in dilated tubules (medullary sponge kidney)

CLINICAL ISSUES

- Nephrocalcinosis is most often asymptomatic
- Increased intestinal absorption of calcium
  - Sarcoidosis and milk-alkali syndrome
- Best imaging tool: Noncontrast CT

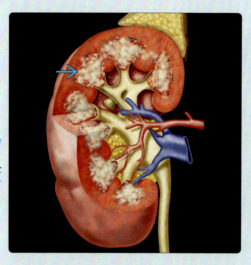
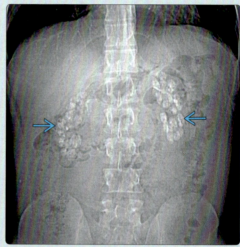

(Left) Graphic shows calcification ➡ in the renal pyramids, representing nephrocalcinosis. Severe, diffuse calcification of this type would be typical of renal tubular acidosis. (Right) AP radiograph shows extensive, dense calcifications in the renal medulla due to medullary nephrocalcinosis ➡ in a patient with hyperparathyroidism, the most common etiology of medullary nephrocalcinosis.

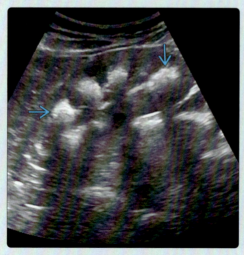
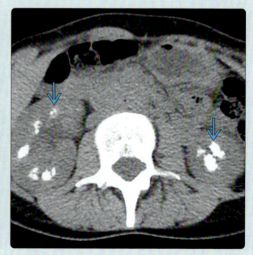

(Left) Sagittal US in a patient with renal tubular acidosis shows increased echogenicity ➡ of the renal pyramids due to extensive nephrocalcinosis. Note that there is shadowing posterior to the annotated pyramids, while others do not show shadowing. Medullary nephrocalcinosis can also produce ring-like echogenicity on US. (Right) Axial NECT in the same patient demonstrates the calcifications ➡ in the renal medullae bilaterally. The calcifications can erode through the renal papillae and enter the collecting system.

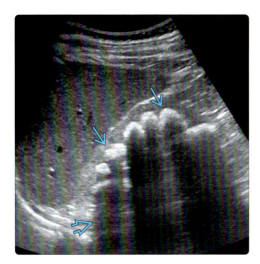
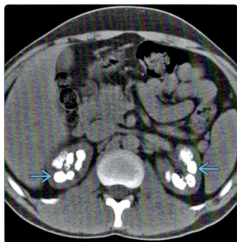

(Left) Sagittal US demonstrates dense calcification ⇨ in the renal medulla due to extensive medullary nephrocalcinosis in a patient with renal tubular acidosis. Note the extensive posterior shadowing ⇨ that obscures the posterior aspect of the kidney. (Right) Axial NECT in the same patient reveals the extensive, dense calcifications ⇨ in the renal medulla bilaterally. Unlike medullary sponge kidney, medullary nephrocalcinosis due to hyperparathyroidism and renal tubular acidosis is usually very dense.

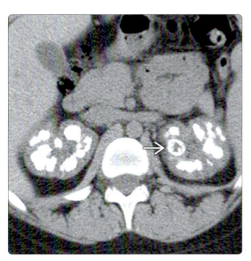
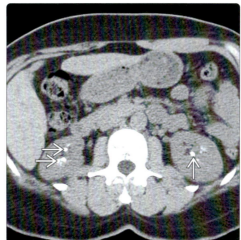

(Left) Axial NECT in a patient with medullary nephrocalcinosis due to sarcoidosis shows densely calcified renal pyramids. Note the ring-like pattern ⇨ at the corticomedullary junction. (Right) Axial NECT in a patient with medullary sponge kidney disease shows multiple discrete calcifications ⇨ in the medulla of both kidneys. Medullary sponge kidney usually results in multifocal, but not diffuse, calcification in the medullae near the tips of the renal pyramids.

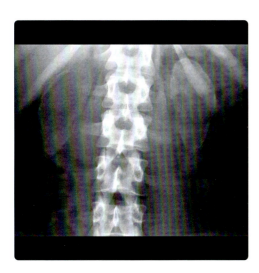
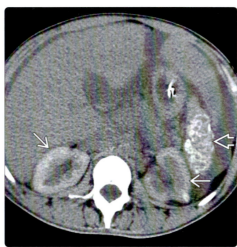

(Left) AP radiograph demonstrates cortical nephrocalcinosis in a patient with chronic glomerulonephritis. Note that the patient has not received any intravenous contrast material. The cortical calcification is dystrophic due to longstanding inflammation. (Right) Axial NECT in a young woman with sickle cell anemia and cortical nephrocalcinosis shows diffuse calcification in both renal cortices ⇨ and diffuse calcification of a chronically infarcted and atrophic spleen ⇨.

IMAGING

- Calculi are uniformly dense, except matrix and indinavir stones
- Indinavir calculi: Soft tissue density; deduced from secondary findings (obstruction)
  - Imaging pearl: In AIDS patient with flank pain and obstructed ureter without visible calculi, consider indinavir calculus
- CT findings
  - Dense (several hundred Hounsfield units) foci in calyces, renal pelvis, ureter, or bladder
  - Soft tissue rim sign: Ureteral wall edema surrounds stone
  - Perinephric stranding: Inflammation/fluid in perinephric space
  - Hydroureteronephrosis if full or partial obstruction
- US findings
  - Round or ovoid echogenic foci
  - Posterior shadowing: Hypoechoic posterior band

- "Twinkle" artifact: Disorganized, alternating color band posterior to calculus

TOP DIFFERENTIAL DIAGNOSES

- Renal artery calcification
  - Radiography: Curvilinear parallel lines of calcification in extrarenal, intrarenal, or pelvic arteries
- Nephrocalcinosis
  - Parenchymal calcification: Medulla > cortex
  - May erode and cause nephrolithiasis
- Phlebolith
  - Pelvic phleboliths usually caudal to ureterovesical junction (level of cervix or seminal vesicles)
  - May require excretory phase imaging to differentiate
- Congenital megacalyces and megaureter

CLINICAL ISSUES

- Small, "nonobstructing" renal calculi can be symptomatic

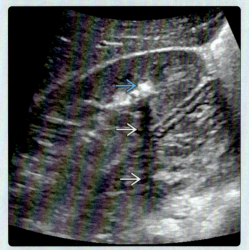
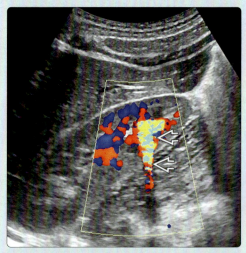

(Left) Sagittal US shows an echogenic calculus ➡ within a superior pole calyx and posterior shadowing shown by a linear hypoechoic band ➡. In the absence of the shadowing artifact, it may be difficult to differentiate this calculus from sinus fat. (Right) Sagittal color Doppler US in the same patient reveals "twinkle" artifact ➡ due to the highly refractive calculus; the "twinkle" artifact appears as a linear band or tail of disorganized, rapidly changing color posterior to the calculus. Other areas of color flow are due to blood vessels.

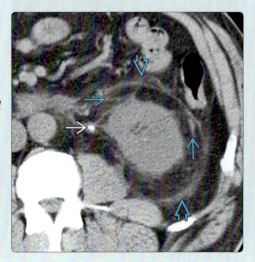
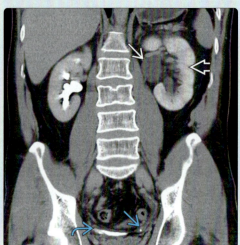

(Left) Axial NECT shows a proximal ureteral stone ➡ with a "rim" of soft tissue, which represents the ureteral wall. Note the moderate degree of perinephric stranding ➡ and fascial thickening ➡. (Right) Coronal CECT during the excretory phase shows moderate left hydronephrosis ➡ and delayed nephrogram ➡ due to a 3-mm calculus ➡ in the distal left ureter. Note the small volume of contrast in the urinary bladder ➡ due to excretion from the right kidney.

Urolithiasis

IMAGING

General Features

- Best diagnostic clue
  - Small dense focus in ureter with proximal hydronephrosis and perinephric stranding
- Location
  - Upper urinary tract (UT): Calyceal, renal pelvis, or ureteropelvic junction (UPJ)
  - Ureteral calculi: Ureter or ureterovesical junction (UVJ)
  - Lower UT: Bladder, urethral
- Other general features
  - Types of calculi
    - Calcium stones (75-80%): Oxalate &/or phosphate
    - Struvite calculi (15-20%): Magnesium ammonium phosphate (struvite), magnesium ammonium phosphate, and calcium phosphate (triple phosphate)
    - Uric acid calculi (5-10%)
    - Cystine calculi (1-3%)
    - Matrix calculi (rare): Mucoproteins
    - Xanthine calculi (extremely rare)
    - Protease inhibitor calculi: Indinavir induced
    - Milk of calcium: Calcium carbonate & calcium phosphate (carbonate apatite)

Radiographic Findings

- Radiography
  - Based on CT correlation, radiography misses majority of calculi
    - Due to small size, insufficient radiopacity, overlying bones, bowel, etc.
  - Calcium oxalate or phosphate calculi
    - Usually very opaque; variable shape
  - Struvite and cystine calculi
    - Staghorn calculi: Conform to pelvocalyceal system
    - Usually opaque
  - Uric acid and xanthine calculi
    - Usually small, smooth, disc-shaped
    - Rarely opaque or detectable on radiograph
  - Milk of calcium
    - Liquid suspension of calcium salts that are "trapped" in calyceal diverticulum or ureterocele
  - Protease inhibitor calculi
    - Nonopaque on radiography (and sometimes CT)
- IVP
  - Ureteral calculi
    - Enlarged, hydronephrotic kidney
    - Delayed ("obstructive," peak at 6 hours); prolonged (> 24 hours) nephrogram
    - Dense, striated, or absent nephrogram
    - Contrast extravasation; ± forniceal rupture

CT Findings

- NECT
  - Calculi are all uniformly dense except matrix and indinavir stones
  - Radiopacity: Calcium oxalate &/or phosphate > cystine > struvite > uric acid
  - Calcium calculi: 400-600 HU
  - Uric acid and cystine calculi: 100-300 HU
  - Matrix calculi
    - Soft tissue attenuation (pure, rare)
    - Laminated peripheral calcification, diffuse ↑ density or round, faintly opaque nodules with densely calcified center (when mixed with calcium salts)
  - Milk of calcium: Layered opaque suspension; stone movement in calyceal diverticulum
  - Indinavir calculi: Not or faintly opaque; deduced from secondary findings (obstruction)
  - Ureteral calculi
    - **Soft tissue rim sign**: Ureteral wall edema at calculus
    - Pseudoureterocele: UVJ edema around calculus
    - Hydroureteronephrosis: Perinephric stranding
- CECT
  - Lucent filling defects (matrix and indinavir stones) during excretory phase
  - Delayed nephrogram during excretory phase
- Dual-energy CT (DECT)
  - Calculi have different attenuation values when imaged at low and high energies
  - Analysis of energy-dependent changes in attenuation allow determination of chemical composition
    - Stone analysis is compared to referenced material-specific attenuation curves
  - Specificity of chemical composition decreases with
    - Small (< 3 mm) calculi
    - Large patient body habitus

MR Findings

- Calculi appear as signal voids (due to lack of mobile protons)
- Secondary signs
  - Renal edema: ↑ T2 signal intensity (SI), ↓ T1 SI of parenchyma
  - Perinephric stranding: ↑ T2 SI of perinephric fat
- Pregnant patients: Use noncontrast T2WI MR
  - Calculus shows ↓ T2 SI while surrounding urine shows ↑ T2 SI

Ultrasonographic Findings

- Grayscale ultrasound
  - Focal echogenic foci
    - Not dependent on chemical consistency
  - Posterior shadowing: Linear hypoechoic artifact
- Color Doppler
  - "Twinkle" artifact: Linear band of disorganized, rapidly changing color deep to highly refractive surface
  - Lack of urine jet from UVJ into bladder is associated with obstructing ureteral calculus

DIAGNOSTIC CHECKLIST

Consider

- Avoid repeat CT in young patients with known or clinically evident calculi (excessive radiation)
- In pregnant patients with renal colic symptoms, begin imaging work-up with US
  - If US is inconclusive, consider MR before CT

Image Interpretation Pearls

- Small dense focus in course of ureter with perinephric stranding ± hydronephrosis

(Left) *Axial CECT obtained during the corticomedullary phase reveals moderate left hydronephrosis ➡. On the excretory phase (not shown), the left nephrogram was delayed.* **(Right)** *Axial CECT more inferiorly in the same patient during the corticomedullary phase reveals a calculus ➡ in the lumen of the midleft ureter. Note the "soft tissue rim" sign ➡ due to the edematous ureteral wall surrounding the calculus. Recognition of this sign allows differentiation of ureteral calculi from phleboliths.*

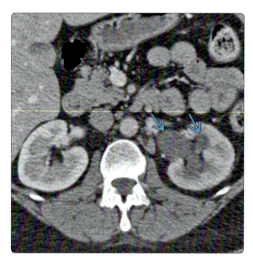 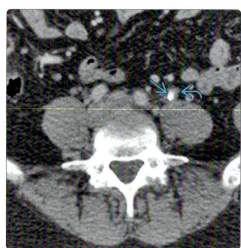

(Left) *Sagittal color Doppler US in the same patient shows the echogenic calculus ➡ in the ureteral lumen; its location can be aided by shadowing ➡ & "twinkle" artifact ➡, shown by the focus of disorganized color Doppler signal posterior to the calculus.* **(Right)** *Axial CECT using dual-energy technique shows a nonobstructing calculus ➡ in a right inferior calyx. Dual-energy CT can be used to characterize the composition of renal calculi by exploiting the change in attenuation when images are acquired at different energies.*

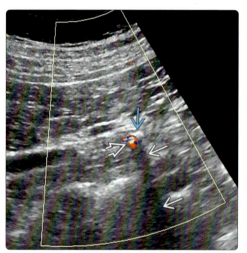 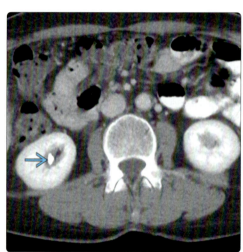

(Left) *Axial virtual noncontrast dual-energy CT shows a region of interest (ROI) ➡ drawn over the right renal calculus.* **(Right)** *Spectral attenuation curve from dual-energy CT shows a plot of attenuation in Hounsfield units (HU, y-axis) vs. energy level (keV, x-axis) that has been generated from the ROI. The curve of the calculus ➡ most closely approximates the curve of calcium oxalate dihydrate ➡, 1 of several included attenuation profiles for calculi of known composition. The effective Z value was also consistent with the above.*

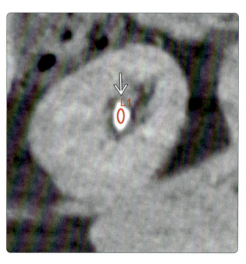 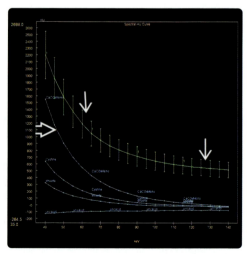

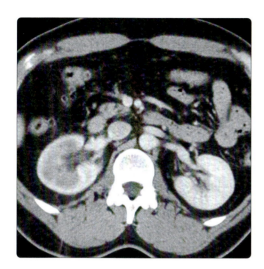

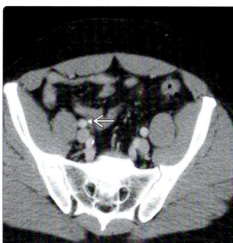

(Left) Axial CECT shows a delayed nephrogram and mild caliectasis of the right kidney. (Right) Axial CECT more inferiorly in the same patient shows a small ureteral calculus ➡ as the cause of the ureteral obstruction and delayed nephrogram. The dilated ureter could be followed directly to this stone on sequential axial images.

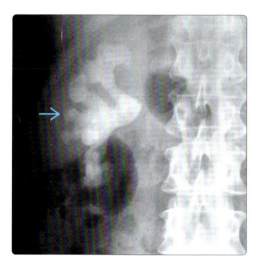

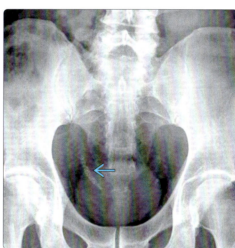

(Left) Anteroposterior radiograph shows a large staghorn calculus ➡ that could be concealed by dense urine on a contrast-enhanced, delayed-phase CT or IVU. (Right) Anteroposterior radiograph in the same patient shows multiple stone fragments ➡ filling the distal ureter (a.k.a. steinstrasse) after the large staghorn calculus has fragmented into smaller components.

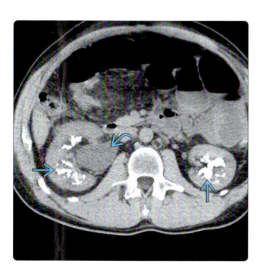

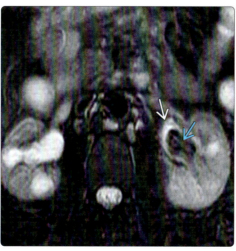

(Left) Axial NECT shows severe medullary nephrocalcinosis in both kidneys ➡. As small calculi erode through the papillae and enter the calyceal system, they can give rise to obstructing ureteral calculi. Note the right-side hydronephrosis ➡ due to a ureteral calculus (not shown). (Right) Axial T2 MR with fat saturation shows a low signal intensity stone ➡ in the left renal pelvis; the high signal intensity of urine ➡ in the renal pelvis outlines the stone. (Courtesy R. Cohan, MD.)

TERMINOLOGY

- Rare, acquired stem cell disorder that results in predisposition to complement-mediated hemolysis
  - Commonly abbreviated as PNH

IMAGING

- CT
  - No specific CT findings
  - ± ↑ attenuation of renal cortices on NECT
- MR
  - Low signal intensity (SI) in renal cortices is characteristic but not pathognomonic
  - T1W: Reverse of normal pattern of corticomedullary SI
    - ↓ SI in renal cortices; medulla not affected, so appears as relatively ↑ SI
  - T2W: ↓ SI in renal cortices
    - Medulla is not affected so appears relatively ↑ SI
  - Liver, spleen, and bone marrow usually have normal SI

TOP DIFFERENTIAL DIAGNOSES

- Low MR signal intensity in renal cortices
  - Malfunctioning prosthetic heart valves
  - Sickle cell anemia
  - Diffuse renal cortical calcification

PATHOLOGY

- Characterized by acute and chronic intravascular hemolysis
- Hemosiderin deposition in epithelial cells of proximal convoluted tubules in renal cortex

CLINICAL ISSUES

- Venous thrombosis (hepatic, sagittal sinus, mesenteric)

DIAGNOSTIC CHECKLIST

- Important to consider PNH in patients with Budd-Chiari, as treatment is systemic (bone marrow transplant) rather than hepatic (surgical decompression vs. transjugular intrahepatic portosystemic shunt creation)

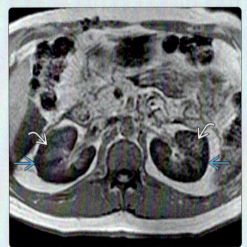
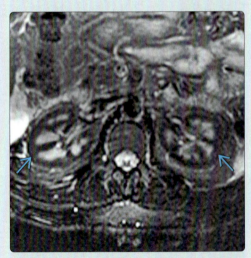

(Left) Axial T1W in-phase MR shows low signal intensity ⇨ in the renal cortices due to hemosiderin deposition from PNH. Note that the medulla ⇨ is not affected by PNH and has a relatively higher signal intensity relative to the cortices. This is the reverse of the normal corticomedullary signal intensity. (Right) Axial T2W MR with fat saturation in the same patient shows low signal intensity ⇨ in the renal cortices. The more profoundly low signal intensity on the T2W sequence occurs because there is more susceptibility of ferric iron with a longer TE.

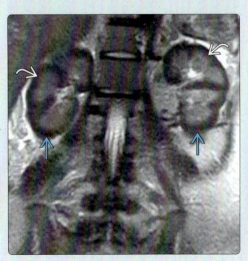
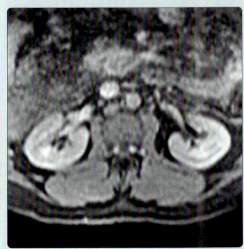

(Left) Coronal T2 MR in the same patient demonstrates low signal intensity ⇨ in the renal cortices and normal signal intensity in the medulla ⇨. PNH is due to acute on chronic intravascular hemolysis, direct release of hemoglobin into the plasma and resorption by the proximal convoluted tubule. (Right) Post-contrast T1W MR with fat saturation in the same patient shows normal size morphology and enhancement of the kidneys. PNH does not affect these qualities unless sequelae of chronic renal failure develop.

Hydronephrosis

TERMINOLOGY

- Dilatation of collecting system

IMAGING

- Best diagnostic clue
  - Pyelocalyceal ± ureteral dilatation
- Best imaging tool
  - US for initial diagnosis
    - In acute kidney injury, US is preferred imaging modality to exclude postrenal causes
  - CECT
    - Problem solving; e.g., distinguishing hydronephrosis from renal sinus cysts
    - Identification of cause of hydronephrosis

TOP DIFFERENTIAL DIAGNOSES

- Congenital megacalyces and megaureter
- Parapelvic (peripelvic) cyst
- Pyonephrosis

PATHOLOGY

- Etiology
  - Obstructive: Partial or complete obstruction anywhere from proximal ureter to urethral meatus
    - Young adults: Calculi
    - Children: Ureteropelvic junction (UPJ) obstruction
    - Adults: Gynecological cancers and pregnancy (female); benign prostatic hyperplasia (male)
  - Nonobstructive
    - Vesicoureteral reflux

CLINICAL ISSUES

- Acute obstruction: Flank pain, nausea, vomiting
  - ↑ pain with acute UPJ obstruction: Dietl crisis
- Obstruction represents 10-15% of acute kidney injury cases
- Treatment
  - Correct underlying cause (obstruction)
  - If complicated by pyonephrosis (infected collecting system with sepsis), must be treated emergently

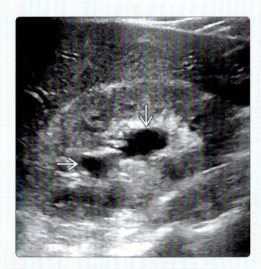

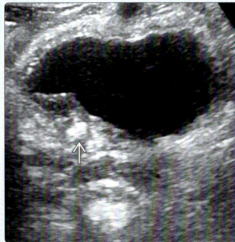

(Left) Longitudinal ultrasound of the right kidney shows mild hydronephrosis ➡ in a patient presenting with right flank pain. (Right) Transverse ultrasound of the pelvis in the same patient shows an echogenic stone ➡ impacted at the right ureterovesical junction causing obstructive hydronephrosis. Ureteral calculi are the most common cause of obstructive hydronephrosis in the young adult population.

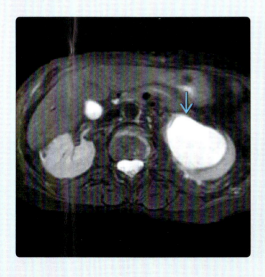

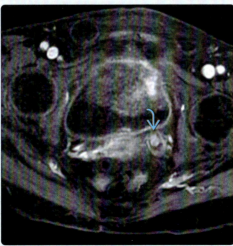

(Left) Axial T2WI MR shows severe left hydronephrosis ➡ in this 80-year old man presenting with hematuria. (Right) Axial postcontrast T1WI MR through the pelvis in the same patient reveals an obstructing polypoid mass in the distal left ureter ➡ causing severe dilatation of the ureter and renal collecting system.

Glomerulonephritis

TERMINOLOGY

- Inflammation and proliferation of glomerular tissue

IMAGING

- Nonspecific imaging findings
  - Enlarged, diffusely echogenic kidneys: Acute glomerulonephritis (GN)
  - Small kidneys: Chronic GN
- US useful to rule out hydronephrosis and to document signs of chronic vs. acute renal failure
- Color Doppler: Apply to exclude renal vein thrombosis

TOP DIFFERENTIAL DIAGNOSES

- Bilateral smooth renal enlargement
  - Amyloidosis, multiple myeloma
  - Acute tubular necrosis
  - Acute interstitial nephritis
- Bilateral small kidneys with smooth contour
  - Arteriosclerosis, nephrosclerosis

PATHOLOGY

- Primary GN: Confined to kidney
  - Systemic features secondary to renal dysfunction
  - Most are immune mediated (post *Streptococcus* infection)
- Secondary: Part of multisystem disorder
  - Many autoimmune disorders (e.g., systemic lupus)
- Associated abnormalities
  - Renal vein thrombosis
  - Hemolytic uremic syndrome

CLINICAL ISSUES

- Major presentations of glomerular disease
  - Acute nephritic or nephrotic syndrome
  - Asymptomatic urinalysis abnormalities

DIAGNOSTIC CHECKLIST

- US to exclude renal vein thrombosis and hydronephrosis

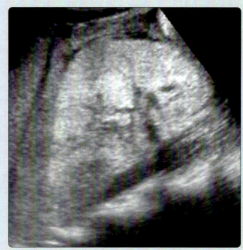
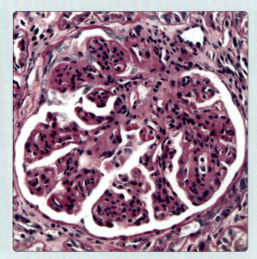

(Left) *Coronal oblique US shows a markedly echogenic kidney in a patient with acute renal failure due to glomerulosclerosis. There is nothing specific about the US appearance of the kidney to suggest a diagnosis other than general renal parenchymal disease. (Courtesy H. Harvin, MD.)* **(Right)** *Micropathology shows a diffusely enlarged glomerulus with increased cellularity and thickening of the glomerular capillary walls in membranoproliferative glomerulonephritis associated with hepatitis C virus.*

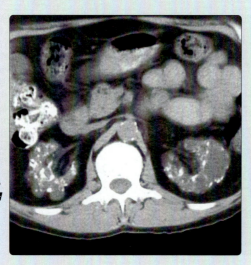
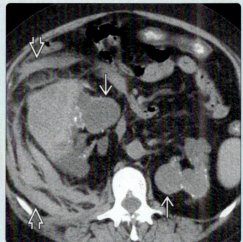

(Left) *Axial NECT shows punctate parenchymal calcification in a patient on dialysis with chronic glomerulonephritis and secondary hyperparathyroidism. Also note the acquired cystic renal disease.* **(Right)** *Axial CECT shows kidneys that are small and nonfunctional with innumerable cysts ➡, characteristic of acquired cystic disease of uremia. There is an extensive hemorrhage ⇨ into the right perirenal and other retroperitoneal spaces. The cause of renal failure was chronic glomerulonephritis.*

KEY FACTS

TERMINOLOGY

- Renal cause of acute kidney injury (AKI) characterized by tubular epithelial cell damage from toxins or ischemia

IMAGING

- Ultrasound
  - To assess renal morphology and echogenicity
  - Exclude other causes of AKI (i.e., obstruction)
  - Renal length: Normal or ↑
  - Renal echogenicity: Normal or ↑
- NECT
  - Persistent patchy nephrogram (following prior contrast administration)

TOP DIFFERENTIAL DIAGNOSES

- Acute glomerulonephritis
- HIV nephropathy
- Acute interstitial nephritis

PATHOLOGY

- Ischemia: Hypotension (most common cause)
- Toxins
  - Exogenous: Iodinated contrast media, antibiotics, chemotherapeutic drugs, organic solvents, heavy metals
  - Endogenous: Hemolysis, rhabdomyolysis, uric acid, oxalate

CLINICAL ISSUES

- Most common form of reversible AKI
- Renal failure develops quickly and lasts 10-20 days
- Mortality rates ↑ in intensive care unit patients (50-80%)
- Presentation
  - Oliguria/anuria, water/salt overload, azotemia, ↑ serum potassium, metabolic acidosis
- Treatment
  - Correction of volume depletion or overload, electrolyte imbalance, metabolic acidosis
  - Dialysis

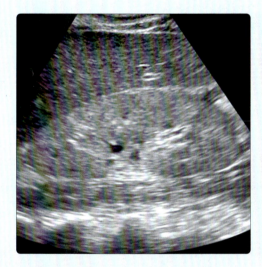
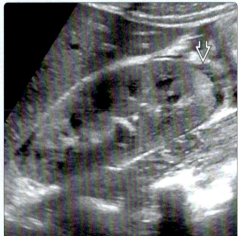

(Left) Ultrasound of a patient with acute kidney injury shows an enlarged, echogenic right kidney, findings commonly seen in the setting of medical renal disease. Note the absence of collecting system dilatation. (Right) Ultrasound of a patient with acute tubular necrosis following cardiac arrest shows an enlarged and echogenic right kidney. Note a small amount of perinephric fluid ("kidney sweat") ➡, a sign often seen in patients with renal failure.

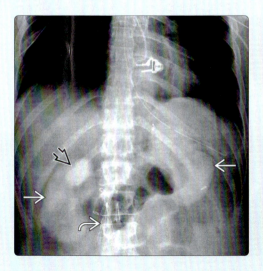
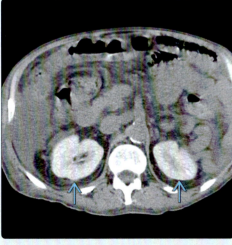

(Left) Abdominal film shows dense bilateral nephrograms ➡ and vicarious (biliary) excretion of contrast medium causing dense opacification of the gallbladder ➡, a sign of shock and acute tubular necrosis. This followed a diagnostic angiogram and placement of an IVC filter ➡ for pulmonary embolism. (Right) Axial NECT shows dense persistent nephrograms ➡ 24 hours following coronary angiography. Acute kidney injury in this case is likely due to hypotension, heart failure, and contrast-induced nephropathy.

TERMINOLOGY

- Rare form of acute renal injury characterized by necrosis of renal cortex

IMAGING

- Best imaging tools: Ultrasound and CT
- Ultrasound
  - Hypoechoic cortical rim
- CT
  - Acute
    - ↓ enhancement of renal cortex
    - Preserved enhancement of thin rim of subcapsular cortical tissue
    - ↓ excretion of contrast media into collecting system
  - Chronic
    - Calcifications in renal cortex and columns of Bertin
- MR: ↓ signal intensity inner cortex and columns of Bertin

TOP DIFFERENTIAL DIAGNOSES

- Acute tubular necrosis
- Renal infarction

CLINICAL ISSUES

- Rare cause of acute kidney injury in developed countries; more common in infants and young women
- Neonates
  - Severe perinatal conditions: e.g., abruptio placentae, congenital heart disease, sepsis, dehydration
- Adults
  - Obstetrical complications (> 50% of cases)
  - Other causes: e.g., hemolytic uremic syndrome, disseminated intravascular coagulopathy, shock
- Poor prognosis
  - Evolution toward chronic renal failure and end-stage renal disease
- Treatment
  - Dialysis; transplantation

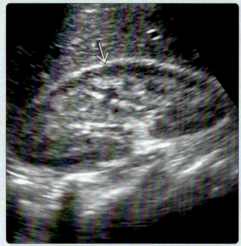
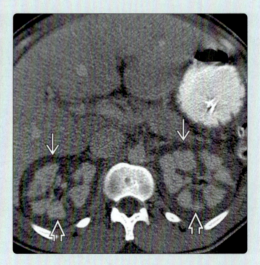

(Left) Longitudinal ultrasound of the right kidney in a patient with sickle cell anemia developing renal cortical necrosis shows decreased renal cortical echogenicity ➡ compared to the medulla. (Right) Axial CECT in the same patient shows bilateral lack of renal cortical enhancement ➡ and preserved medullary enhancement ➡, compatible with bilateral renal cortical necrosis.

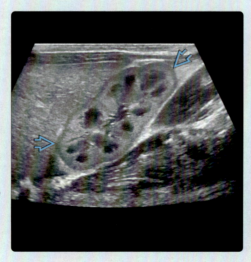
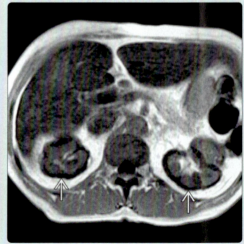

(Left) Sagittal ultrasound in a 12-day-old term infant with congenital heart disease, severely decreased left ventricle function, and persistently elevated creatinine shows decreased echogenicity of the renal cortex ➡ compared to the parenchyma, suspicious for cortical necrosis. (Right) Axial T1WI GRE in a patient with sickle cell anemia shows reversal of the usual corticomedullary pattern with the cortex ➡ being hypointense to the medulla from hemosiderin deposition or cortical necrosis.

Renal Papillary Necrosis

KEY FACTS

TERMINOLOGY

- Necrosis of renal papilla within medulla secondary to interstitial nephritis or ischemia

IMAGING

- Bilateral disease: Analgesics, diabetes, sickle cell disease
- Unilateral disease: Obstruction, infection, venous thrombus
- Triangular or bulbous cavitation adjacent to calyx on IVP, CT urogram, or retrograde pyelogram
- Subtle streak of contrast extending from fornix parallel to long axis of papilla
- Calyx
  - Club-shaped or saccular (sloughed papilla)
  - Widened fornix (necrotic shrinkage of papilla)
- Sloughed papilla
  - Triangular filling defect within calyx, pelvis, ureter
  - May have ring calcification

TOP DIFFERENTIAL DIAGNOSES

- Hydronephrosis
- Medullary sponge kidney
- Congenital megacalyces and megaureter

PATHOLOGY

- Analgesic nephropathy, diabetes, sickle cell
- Urinary tract infection and obstruction, tuberculosis, kidney transplantation, alcoholism

CLINICAL ISSUES

- Complications
  - Obstruction, infection, renal failure, transitional cell carcinoma
- Prognosis
  - Early stage (good), advanced stage (poor)

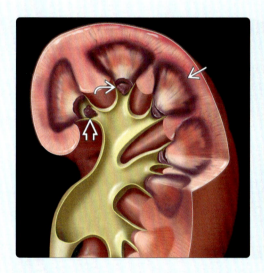

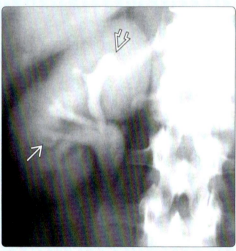

(Left) Graphic shows ischemic injury of some of the renal pyramids ➡ with sloughing of several papillae ➡, 1 of which lies free within the collecting system ➡. (Right) Nephrotomogram of a patient with papillary necrosis obtained 5 minutes after contrast administration shows a sloughed papilla ➡ as a filling defect in the calyx. Deformity ("clubbing") of an upper pole calyx ➡ is due to prior papillary tip necrosis and communication with an adjacent necrotic cavity.

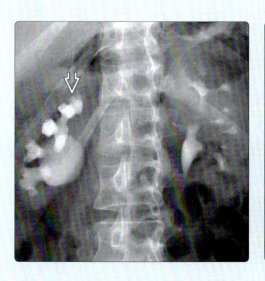

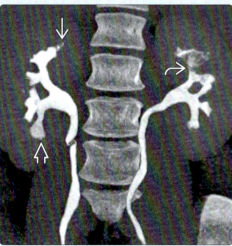

(Left) Excretory urogram of a patient with hematuria shows marked clubbing of right renal calyces ➡, a later manifestation of papillary necrosis. These patients may present with acute episodes (colic, hematuria) or, rarely, renal insufficiency/failure. (Right) Coronal CTU of a patient with sickle cell disease shows clubbing of the calyces ➡, contrast pooling into the site of sloughed papillae ➡, and debris within left upper pole calyces ➡. CTU has replaced IV urography in the imaging evaluation of upper tract disease.

Kidney and Renal Pelvis

TERMINOLOGY

- Multisystem thrombotic microangiopathy typically occurring after diarrheal illness from Shiga toxin-producing bacteria (classically *Escherichia coli* O157:H7)
- Clinical triad of hemolytic anemia, thrombocytopenia, and acute renal failure
  - Affected organ systems: Kidneys > CNS (20-50%) > gastrointestinal tract, heart
- Atypical hemolytic uremic syndrome (HUS) often due to dysregulation in alternative complement pathway

IMAGING

- Kidneys: ↑ renal cortical echogenicity, ↓ vascular perfusion of parenchyma early; perfusion improves in 2nd-4th weeks
  - Resistive index (RI) (peak systolic velocity - end diastolic velocity/peak systolic velocity) most abnormal during oliguric/anuric phase of disease
    - Increased RI with low or absent diastolic flow
  - Improved diastolic flow precedes urine production

- Bowel: Fluid-filled loops with wall thickening
- Brain: Potentially reversible, frequently symmetric lesions

CLINICAL ISSUES

- 1 in 100,000 children affected annually
- Most patients < 5 years of age
- Gastrointestinal illness (hemorrhagic colitis) precedes renal failure by 3-14 days
- Symptoms: Fatigue, pallor, ↓ urine output, anasarca, bruising, ± seizures, altered mental status, visual disturbances
- Full recovery in 70%; 1-4% mortality
- Long-term sequelae: Renal, neurologic
  - Rarely, delayed development of hypertension and proteinuria 1-2 years after full recovery
- Typical HUS treatment: Supportive therapy (including dialysis); ± plasma exchange; no direct treatments
- Atypical HUS treatment: As above + anti-C5 antibody eculizumab for terminal complement blockade

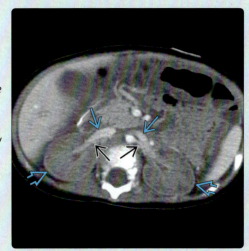

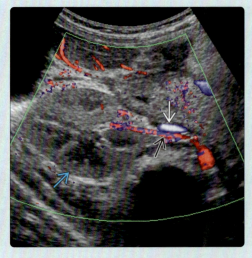

(Left) Axial CECT in a 15 month old with vomiting and altered mental status shows globally decreased enhancement of the bilateral kidneys, though capsular enhancement is intact ➡. The main renal veins ➡ and arteries ➡ appear patent. (Right) Transverse color Doppler US of the right kidney in the same patient shows turbulent flow in the main renal artery ➡. The main renal vein is patent ➡. However, no vascular flow is seen in the renal parenchyma ➡. The renal cortex was mildly echogenic bilaterally.

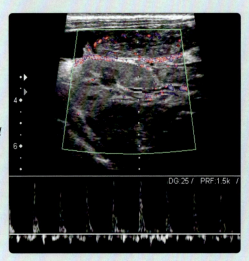

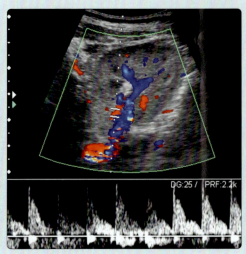

(Left) Transverse pulsed Doppler US in the same patient shows a high-resistance waveform in the right main renal artery with complete reversal of diastolic flow. The left kidney and left main renal artery showed similar findings. However, the aortic waveforms were normal (not shown). (Right) Transverse pulsed Doppler US in the same patient 9 days later shows improved flow in the right renal parenchyma with return of diastolic flow in the main renal artery. The patient began producing urine the following day.

KEY FACTS

TERMINOLOGY

- HIV-associated nephropathy (HIVAN)
- Progressive chronic renal disease in patients with HIV infection histologically, characterized by focal and segmental glomerulosclerosis (collapsing glomerulopathy)

IMAGING

- Symmetric enlargement of kidneys
- Ultrasound
  - Increased renal echogenicity
  - Decreased corticomedullary differentiation
  - Urothelial thickening
  - Decreased renal sinus fat

TOP DIFFERENTIAL DIAGNOSES

- Glomerulonephritis (GN)
- Acute tubular necrosis (ATN)
- Opportunistic renal infections

PATHOLOGY

- Focal and segmental glomerulosclerosis (collapsing glomerulopathy)

CLINICAL ISSUES

- Proteinuria; progressive renal failure
- Higher incidence in African Americans (> 90% of reported cases)
- ↓ incidence after introduction of combination antiretroviral therapy (cART)

DIAGNOSTIC CHECKLIST

- Final diagnosis is made at histology
- Consider other causes of renal disease in HIV-infected patients, including
  - Antiretroviral nephrotoxicity
  - Opportunistic infections
  - Urolithiasis
  - Neoplasms

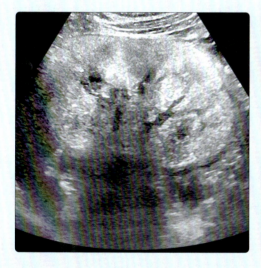

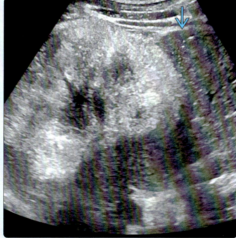

(Left) Longitudinal ultrasound of the left kidney in patient with biopsy-proven HIV-associated nephropathy (HIVAN) shows an enlarged, echogenic kidney. (Right) Transverse olblique ultrasound of the right kidney in the same patient reveals symmetric enlargement of the right kidney. HIVAN typically affects both kidneys. Note the increased echogenicity of the renal parenchyma compared with the adjacent liver ⇒ and the decreased corticomedullary differentiation.

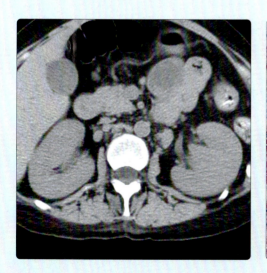

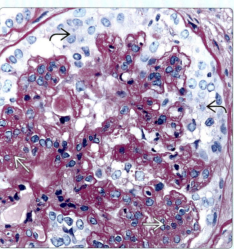

(Left) Axial NECT of the abdomen in an HIV-positive patient shows enlarged kidneys with loss of corticomedullary differentiation and decreased pelvic sinus fat suggesting HIVAN. (Right) Classic appearance of HIV-associated nephropathy (HIVAN) with glomerular collapse ⇒ and proliferation of overlying podocytes ⇒ is well demonstrated by periodic acid-shift (PAS) stain in this HIV-positive man. (From DP: Kidney.)

TERMINOLOGY

- Chronic kidney disease
- Kidney damage or decreased renal function for ≥ 3 months

IMAGING

- Ultrasound
  - ↓ renal length
  - ↓ cortical thickness
  - ↑ echogenicity
  - Multiple cysts (uremic cystic disease)
- NECT
  - Small kidneys; cortical thinning
  - Dilatation of collecting system if cause is obstruction

TOP DIFFERENTIAL DIAGNOSES

- Acute tubular necrosis
- Renal cortical necrosis

PATHOLOGY

- Etiology
  - Diabetic nephropathy, chronic glomerulonephritis, hypertensive nephropathy, polycystic renal disease, chronic pyelonephritis, renal calculi
- Severity stratified by glomerular filtration rate
  - Stage 1: GFR ≥ 90 mL/minute/1.73 m²
  - Stage 2: GFR 60-89 mL/minute/1.73 m²
  - Stage 3: GFR 30-59 mL/minute/1.73 m²
  - Stage 4: GFR 15-29 mL/minute/1.73 m²
  - Stage 5: GFR < 15 mL/minute/1.73 m²

CLINICAL ISSUES

- Symptoms and signs
  - Hypertension, fluid overload, malaise, pericarditis, encephalopathy
- Treatment of underlying etiologies, dialysis, transplantation

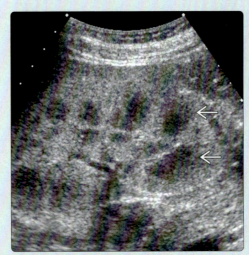
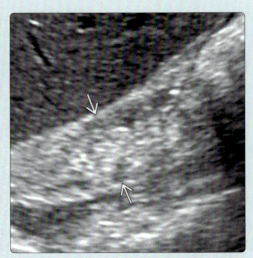

(Left) Longitudinal grayscale ultrasound of end-stage diabetic nephropathy in a 74-year-old man presenting with type 2 diabetes and uremia demonstrates echogenic kidneys with prominent hypoechoic pyramids ➡. (Right) Longitudinal ultrasound of the right kidney shows a small kidney ➡ with decreased cortical thickness and increased echogenicity compatible with a chronic kidney injury.

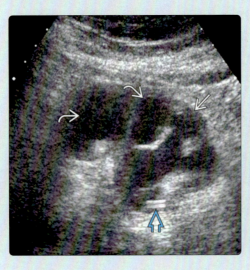
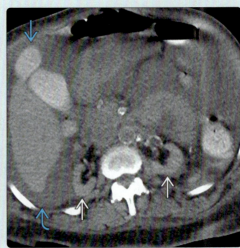

(Left) Longitudinal grayscale ultrasound of end-stage hydronephrosis in an 82-year-old man with prostate cancer and longstanding ureteral obstruction shows marked cortical thinning ➡ and hydronephrosis ➡. Note the ureteral stent ➡ in the proximal renal pelvis. (Right) Axial noncontrast CT in a patient with end-stage renal disease obtained 12 hours after angiography reveals atrophic kidneys with delayed nephrogram ➡ and vicarious excretion of contrast into the gallbladder ➡ and ascites ➡.

Renal Lipomatosis

TERMINOLOGY

- Fatty tissue proliferation in renal sinus (renal sinus lipomatosis) that in extreme cases can replace renal parenchyma (renal replacement lipomatosis)

IMAGING

- Best imaging tool
  - CECT
- Renal sinus lipomatosis
  - Bilateral process, mild associated atrophy
  - Enlarged sinus with fat density (-30 to -90 HU)
- Replacement lipomatosis
  - Unilateral process
  - Enlarged kidney with reniform shape
  - Focal or diffuse renal parenchymal atrophy
  - Fibrofatty proliferation in renal sinus and perirenal space
  - Centrally located calculus in 70%
  - ± hydronephrosis

TOP DIFFERENTIAL DIAGNOSES

- Xanthogranulomatous pyelonephritis
- Renal angiomyolipoma

PATHOLOGY

- Renal sinus lipomatosis
  - Gradual loss of parenchyma replaced by fat
- Renal replacement lipomatosis
  - Sequela of severe renal atrophy or inflammation, usually due to chronic calculous disease

CLINICAL ISSUES

- Renal sinus lipomatosis
  - Normal finding in elderly and obese patients with good prognosis
- Renal replacement lipomatosis
  - Worse prognosis as it is associated with underlying chronic inflammation
  - May require nephrectomy

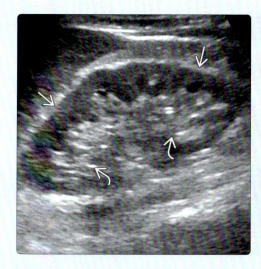

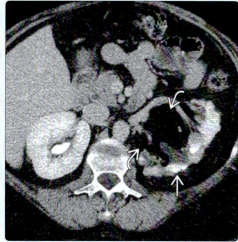

(Left) Longitudinal ultrasound of the right kidney shows mild cortical thinning ➡ and proliferation of sinus fat ➡ compatible with renal sinus lipomatosis. (Right) Axial CECT in a patient with renal replacement lipomatosis shows left side renal cortical atrophy, dilated calyces ➡, and markedly proliferated renal sinus fat ➡. The caliectasis, renal scarring, and lipomatosis were the result of multiple chronic episodes of renal and ureteral calculi and infection.

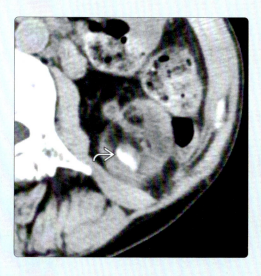

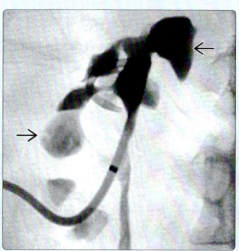

(Left) Axial NECT in a patient with replacement lipomatosis shows a small left kidney, a large renal stone ➡, and dilated calyces with marked cortical thinning and fibrofatty proliferation in the renal sinus and perirenal space. (Right) Percutaneous nephrostogram in the same patient shows dilated calyces ➡. Renal replacement lipomatosis was the result of chronic partial obstruction by the large stone and chronic infection and inflammation of the kidney.

KEY FACTS

IMAGING

- Best diagnostic clue: Focal or segmental luminal narrowing of renal artery (RA)
- Atherosclerotic RA stenosis (RAS): Involves ostium or proximal 2 cm
- Fibromuscular dysplasia (FMD): Involves mid and distal segments of RA ± intrarenal arteries; right > left
- Affected kidney can be normal sized or atrophic
- Doppler findings
  - Direct signs (proximal criteria)
    - ↑ peak systolic velocity **> 200 cm/sec** (> 60% stenosis)
    - ↑ renal:aortic peak velocity ratio **> 3.0-3.5** (> 60% stenosis)
    - ↑ velocity gradient across RA: > 2.7
    - Poststenotic turbulent flow with spectral broadening and color aliasing
  - Indirect signs (distal criteria): Much less reliable and shouldn't be used as sole criteria for diagnosing RAS

- Pulsus tardus-parvus, ↑ acceleration time, ↓ resistive index

PATHOLOGY

- **Atherosclerosis**
  - Most common cause of RAS (60-90%); more common in elderly
- **FMD**
  - 2nd most common cause of RAS (10-30%); more common in young and middle-aged women
  - 2/3 of cases are bilateral

CLINICAL ISSUES

- Majority of cases can be controlled with antihypertensive drugs
- Large randomized clinical trial (ASTRAL) comparing medical therapy alone with revascularization plus medical therapy in patients with atherosclerotic RAS did not show any benefit for revascularization

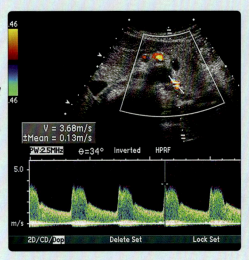

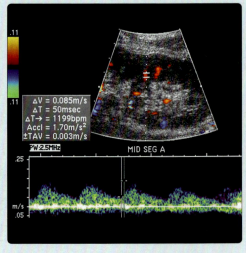

(Left) Spectral Doppler sampling of the proximal left renal artery in a 48-year-old man with a history of intractable hypertension shows high-velocity flow (368 cm/sec) indicating severe renal artery stenosis. The renal:aortic peak velocity ratio was also elevated (~ 4). (Right) Spectral Doppler tracing of the left interpolar segmental artery in the same patient shows parvus tardus waveform with increased acceleration time and borderline low resistive index (0.55).

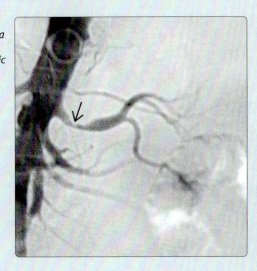

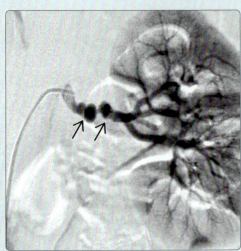

(Left) Anteroposterior catheter angiography shows a variant appearance of renal artery stenosis, as the stenotic region ⊡ is distal to the ostium. Note the focal narrowing of the left renal artery ~ 2 cm from the origin of the renal artery. (Right) Coronal projection from selective catheterization of the renal artery in a young woman with hypertension shows a beaded appearance and stenoses ⊡ of the mid segment of the renal artery, suggestive of fibromuscular dysplasia.

Renal Infarction

KEY FACTS

TERMINOLOGY

- Localized or global area of ischemic necrosis in kidney secondary to interrupted vascular supply

IMAGING

- Best diagnostic clue: Nonenhancing, peripheral, wedge-shaped area with enhancing cortical rim
- Imaging manifestations are variable based on etiology and chronicity
  - Thromboembolic: Usually multifocal and bilateral
  - In situ thrombotic: Unilateral (segmental or global)

TOP DIFFERENTIAL DIAGNOSES

- Pyelonephritis
- Renal mass
- Multiple cortical scars
- Renal laceration or hematoma
- Vasculitis

PATHOLOGY

- Majority of cases are due to sudden occlusion of main renal artery or segmental branch artery
  - Venous infarction is seen in pediatric population (secondary to venous thrombosis); extremely rare in adults
- No causes can be found (idiopathic) in up to 1/3 of patients
- **Arterial infarction**
  - Thromboembolism: From cardiac or aortic source
  - In situ thrombosis: Secondary to trauma, vasculitis, hypercoagulable states, and iatrogenic injury
  - Dissection
- **Venous infarction (rare in adults)**
  - Dehydration is most common risk factor in children
  - Other causes include: Nephrotic syndrome, hypercoagulable states, and renal cell carcinoma
- Torsion (rare)

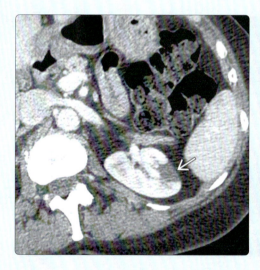

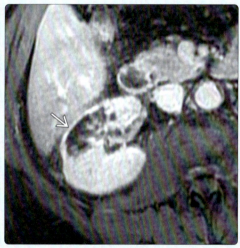

(Left) Axial CECT in a 57-year-old woman with a history of antiphospholipid syndrome presenting with acute onset left flank pain and hematuria illustrates a wedge-shaped area of nonenhancement ➡. (Right) Axial postcontrast T1WI MR in a 55-year-old woman with a history of atrial fibrillation who was being imaged to evaluate a "renal mass" shows a wedge-shaped area of nonenhancement in the right kidney. A rim of cortical enhancement ➡ and preserved renal contour suggest that infarction is acute to subacute.

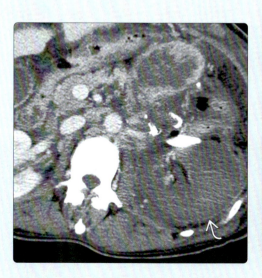

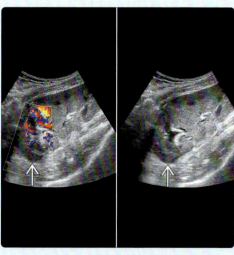

(Left) Axial CECT in a 38-year-old man who sustained a blunt abdominal trauma following a motor vehicle crash demonstrates an extensive renal infarct with lack of enhancement. Note the faint cortical rim enhancement ➡. (Right) Composite grayscale and duplex US images in a female patient post renal transplantation show an area of decreased echogenicity and absent vascularity ➡ in the superior pole of the allograft, corresponding to infarction secondary to injury to a polar artery.

KEY FACTS

IMAGING

- Renal artery aneurysm: Saccular or fusiform dilatation of extrarenal renal artery, typically at branch point
  - CTA/MRA: Focally dilated renal artery segment, enhances similar to adjacent artery unless thrombosed
  - Doppler ultrasound: Turbulent color Doppler flow within dilated arterial segment
- Renal artery pseudoaneurysm (PA): Contained, extraluminal contrast adjacent to injured artery
  - CECT/CTA: Focal eccentric contrast collection adjacent to renal artery
  - Doppler: Yin-yang flow within extrarenal "cyst"; to-and-fro flow within PA neck
- Arteriovenous fistula: Direct communication between renal artery branch and draining vein
  - CECT/CTA/MRA: Arterial enhancement of feeding, tortuous vessels, and early venous drainage (delayed nephrogram due to shunting)
  - Doppler ultrasound: Color flow within vascular tangle, high-velocity, "low-resistance" flow within feeding artery

PATHOLOGY

- Renal artery aneurysms typically idiopathic but may be associated with vasculitides (fibromuscular dysplasia, Ehlers-Danlos)
- False (pseudo-) aneurysms occur with wall injury after trauma (e.g., biopsy), rarely mycotic
- Arteriovenous fistula (AVF) divided into acquired (post trauma, biopsy, malignancy) and rarer congenital types

CLINICAL ISSUES

- Renal artery aneurysms typically incidental, though may present with flank pain, hematuria: Endovascular repair if > 2-3 cm, pregnancy
- High incidence of small AVF post biopsy, usually resolve spontaneously; endovascular therapy of renal PAs and symptomatic AVFs is standard of care

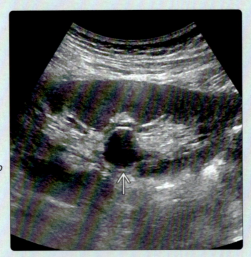
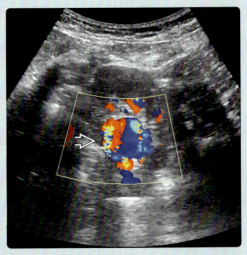

(Left) Sagittal ultrasound of a 32-year-old woman with vague flank pain shows an anechoic renal pelvic "cyst" ⬆. (Right) Renal color Doppler ultrasound of the same patient shows turbulent, swirling flow within the "cyst" ➡. Lack of a history of prior trauma or systemic infection suggests a true rather than a pseudo- (false) renal artery aneurysm. A vasculitis work-up was negative. Endovascular therapy is typically performed for larger (> 2-3 cm) renal artery aneurysms, particularly in females considering pregnancy.

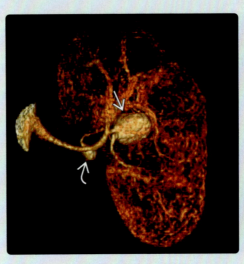
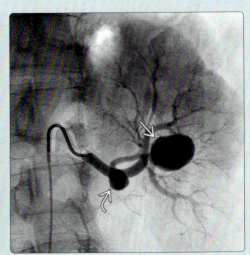

(Left) Coronal volume-rendered CTA of the same patient confirms a sizable main renal artery branch point aneurysm ➡. A smaller polar renal artery aneurysm is also shown ➡. CTA is helpful for endovascular planning and follow-up. (Right) Arteriography performed prior to embolization shows the main renal artery bifurcation aneurysm ➡ and the small polar artery aneurysm ➡. (Courtesy J. Pinter, MD.)

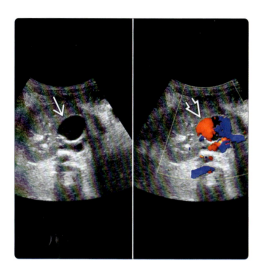

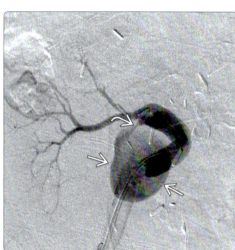

(Left) *Grayscale and corresponding color Doppler ultrasound of a 61-year-old man with renal insufficiency months following angioplasty of a renal artery graft anastomotic stenosis shows an anechoic extrarenal "collection"* ➡. *Color Doppler interrogation confirms turbulent flow* ➡ *within the collection, thus confirming an extrarenal pseudoaneurysm.* **(Right)** *Angiography performed prestent placement in the same patient shows a large perianastamotic pseudoaneurysm (PA)* ➡. *Note the feeding neck* ➡.

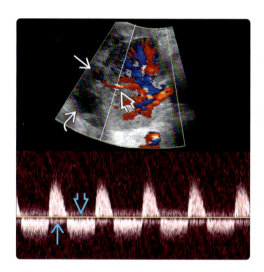

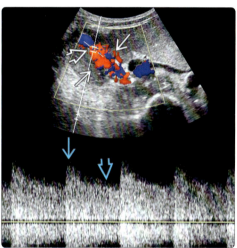

(Left) *Color Doppler ultrasound shows a renal transplant with a small capsular PA* ➡ *and perinephric hematoma* ➡. *With the Doppler gate over the neck* ➡, *a characteristic to-and-fro spectra consisting of forward flow in systole* ➡ *and reversed flow in diastole* ➡ *is shown.* **(Right)** *Color Doppler ultrasound of a post renal transplant biopsy shows a color flurry* ➡. *Pulse wave Doppler of the feeding artery* ➡ *shows high-velocity, "low-resistance" flow. Note high-velocity systolic* ➡ *and diastolic* ➡ *flow.*

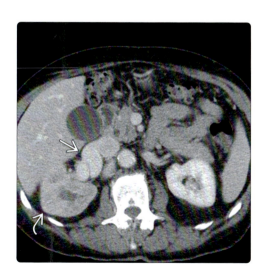

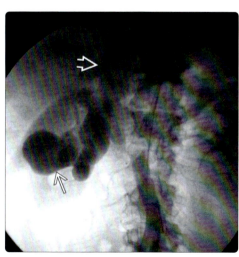

(Left) *CECT of a patient with hypertension, hematuria, and congestive heart failure shows early filling of the huge draining vein* ➡ *of a congenital arterial venous fistula. Note the relatively delayed right renal nephrogram due to extensive renal arterial-venous shunting* ➡. **(Right)** *Angiography performed in the same patient shows early filling of the inferior vena cava* ➡ *and a massively dilated draining vein* ➡. *Embolization of such a large, complex AVF may be impossible, and in this case, nephrectomy was performed.*

TERMINOLOGY

- Obstruction of renal vein (RV) by thrombus

IMAGING

- RV thrombus with renal enlargement and delayed renal function
- Renal enlargement in 75% of cases
- Doppler findings
  - Reversal of diastolic flow in intrarenal arteries
  - Absent, or markedly reduced, venous flow
  - Turbulence and ↑ velocity of flow at level of obstruction [in subocclusive RV thrombosis (RVT)]
  - Classic arterial Doppler findings are only seen in setting of acute RVT
- Best imaging tool: CECT, gadolinium-enhanced MR

TOP DIFFERENTIAL DIAGNOSES

- Other causes of unilateral renal enlargement
  - Ureteral obstruction
  - Infiltrating tumor
  - Pyelonephritis

PATHOLOGY

- Nephrotic syndrome and underlying malignancy (usually renal cell carcinoma) are most common etiologies in adults
- Dehydration and sepsis are most common etiologies in children

CLINICAL ISSUES

- More common in adults but also seen in patients < 2 years
- Acute signs/symptoms: Flank pain, nausea, vomiting, palpable kidney, hypertension, hematuria
- Pediatric (neonatal) RVT is characterized by classic triad of palpable abdominal mass, gross hematuria, and thrombocytopenia
- Chronic signs/symptoms: Asymptomatic or thromboembolic disease; fever, edema
- Treatment: Anticoagulation therapy (though efficacy controversial)

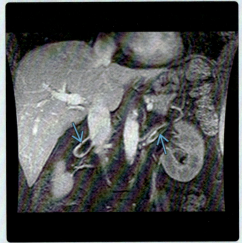
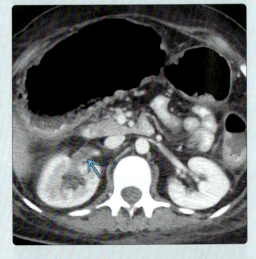

(Left) Coronal postcontrast T1WI MR in a 49-year-old man with history of chronic myeloid leukemia and nephrotic syndrome shows bilateral renal venous thrombosis ➡. (Right) Axial CECT in a 30-year-old man with a history of ulcerative colitis shows right renal vein thrombosis ➡ with associated delayed enhancement of the right kidney. Note the marked dilatation of the transverse colon with mucosal denudation and pseudopolyposis compatible with toxic megacolon.

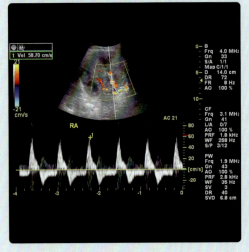
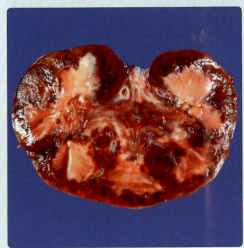

(Left) Spectral Doppler tracing of a renal allograft artery shows reversal of diastolic flow. The allograft was noted to be enlarged. There was no detectable flow in the renal vein. (Right) Longitudinal section through the explanted renal allograft in the same patient demonstrates renal enlargement with areas of hemorrhagic infarction. The renal vein was noted to be completely thrombosed.

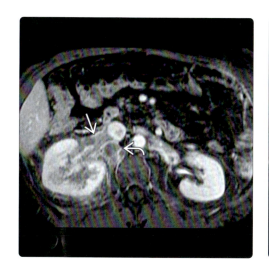
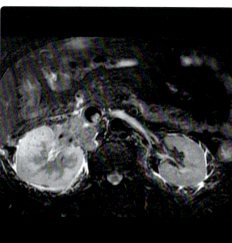

(Left) *Axial postcontrast T1WI MR in a 59-year-old man with history of right renal mass shows expansile thrombosis of the right renal vein* ➡ *with extension into the inferior vena cava and a lumbar branch* ➡. *Note the enlargement of the right kidney and delayed nephrogram secondary to venous thrombosis.* (Right) *Axial T2WI MR in the same patient shows altered T2 signal in the right kidney secondary to venous thrombosis and congestion. Pathology was consistent with clear-cell renal cell carcinoma.*

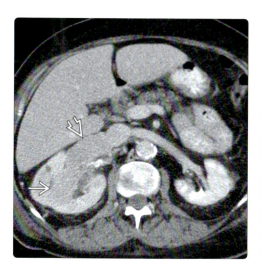
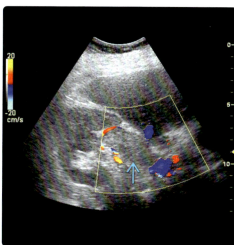

(Left) *Axial CECT in a 60-year-old woman shows an enhancing mass in the interpolar region of the right kidney* ➡ *with tumor thrombosis in the right renal vein* ➡. *Note the marked expansion of the renal vein.* (Right) *Color Doppler ultrasound in the same patient demonstrates an expansile echogenic clot within the right renal vein* ➡.

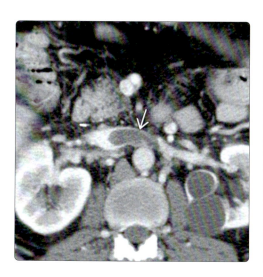
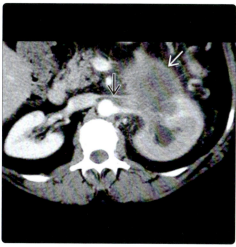

(Left) *Axial CECT in a 46-year-old woman who presented with vague abdominal pain and a history of protein S deficiency demonstrates a thrombus within the inferior vena cava and the left renal vein* ➡. (Right) *Axial CECT in a patient presenting with weight loss and flank pain shows a pancreatic tail mass* ➡ *extending to and encasing the left renal vein with resultant renal vein thrombosis* ➡. *Note the delayed nephrogram and hydronephrosis.*

KEY FACTS

IMAGING

- Best diagnostic clue: Renal parenchymal defect with perirenal hemorrhage ± extravasation of blood/urine
- CT findings
  - Laceration: Linear, hypoattenuating defect
  - Segmental renal infarct: Sharply demarcated, wedge-shaped area of decreased enhancement
  - Global infarction (nonenhancement) and no perinephric hematoma: Renal artery thrombosis
  - Global infarction (nonenhancement) and perinephric hematoma: Renal artery avulsion
- Protocol advice: If renal laceration is evident, obtain 10- to 12-minute delayed scans

TOP DIFFERENTIAL DIAGNOSES

- Hemorrhage from renal tumor
- Hemorrhage from vasculitis

PATHOLOGY

- Blunt, penetrating, and deceleration injuries
- Serious renal injuries usually associated with multiorgan involvement

CLINICAL ISSUES

- Flank pain, ecchymosis, hematuria, shock
- Poor correlation between degree of hematuria and severity of injury
- AAST classification correlates well between surgical and MDCT findings

DIAGNOSTIC CHECKLIST

- Consider possibility of underlying tumor if bleeding seems disproportionate to degree of trauma
- Arterial extravasation usually requires catheter embolization
- Urinary extravasation often requires ureteral stent ± catheter drainage of urinoma

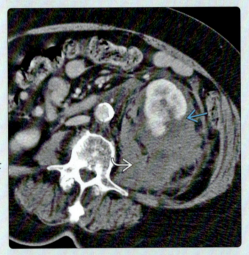
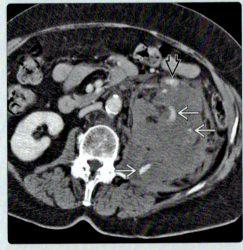

(Left) Axial CECT following a motor vehicle crash shows a contour deformity ➡ of the posterior aspect of the left kidney due to fracture (the shattered fragment is not shown on this image). Note the large perinephric hematoma ➡. (Right) More inferior axial CECT in the same patient reveals multiple sites of active arterial extravasation ➡ & a fragment of the fractured kidney ➡, consistent with a grade V injury. Due to the extensive parenchymal damage & active bleeding, emergent nephrectomy was performed.

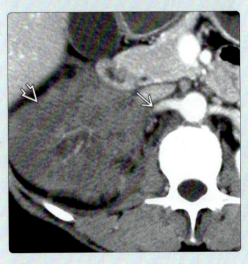
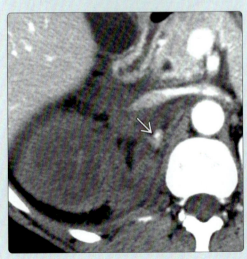

(Left) Axial CECT in a 19-year-old man who sustained blunt abdominal trauma in a motorcycle crash reveals a traumatic renal artery occlusion ➡ due to dissection. Nonenhancement of the right kidney ➡ is consistent with global infarction, consistent with grade V injury. (Right) Axial CECT in the same patient reveals an additional small area of active bleeding from the lumbar artery ➡, which accounted for bleeding into the perirenal and psoas compartments.

IMAGING

Radiographic Findings

- Most commonly used classification system for renal trauma was set forth by American Association for Surgery of Trauma (AAST)
  - AAST classification consists of 5 injury classifications
    - ~ 80-85% of renal injuries are classified as grade I
  - AAST classification strongly correlates with surgical and MDCT findings
  - AAST classification of injury corresponds to clinical outcome

CT Findings

- AAST classification of kidney injuries
- Grade I injury
  - Contusion
    - Poorly defined region of decreased parenchymal enhancement
    - NCCT: Contusions may be iso- to hyperattenuating relative to adjacent normal renal parenchyma
  - Hematoma
    - Nonexpanding, subcapsular collection that has crescentic shape and follows renal contour when small
    - When large, subcapsular hematomas are convex and exert mass effect on kidney
    - No associated laceration in grade I injuries
- Grade II injury
  - Hematoma
    - Nonexpanding hematoma confined to perinephric space
    - Blood dissecting along perinephric septa results in "stranding" or "cobwebbing"
    - Acute to subacute hematomas are iso- to hyperattenuating (~ 35-70 HU)
    - Chronic hematomas evolve and may approach near water attenuation (0-15 HU) as blood products become resorbed
  - Laceration
    - Superficial cortical defect (≤ 1 cm)
      - Typically linear and hypoattenuating
    - No associated collecting system injury
- Grade III injury
  - Laceration
    - > 1 cm in depth
    - Laceration does not affect collecting system
- Grade IV injury
  - Laceration
    - Extends through renal cortex, medulla, and collecting system
  - Vascular
    - Injury of main renal artery or vein with contained hematoma
    - Segmental infarctions due to segmental vessel injury
- Grade V injury
  - Laceration
    - Shattered kidney
      - Islands of vascularized or devascularized tissue
    - Avulsion of ureteropelvic junction

- Urine leak/urinoma: Extravasation of contrast-opacified urine during excretory phase
  - Vascular
    - Avulsion or thrombosis of main renal artery or vein with renal devascularization
      - Avulsion: Brisk extravasation of contrast and massive hematoma
      - Thrombosis: Abrupt termination of renal vessel
- AAST classification does not specifically address active hemorrhage
  - Active hemorrhage is more commonly associated with high-grade injuries (grades IV and V) but can occur with lower grade injuries (grades II and III)

Imaging Recommendations

- Protocol advice
  - Multiphasic CECT is preferred modality
  - If renal laceration is evident on CT, mandatory 10- to 12-minute delayed scan (to evaluate for urine extravasation)
- Retrograde pyelogram: Assess ureteral and renal pelvic injuries

MR Findings

- MR typically plays no role in evaluation of acute renal injury
- MR can be useful for detection of complications
- Hematoma: Varies with age of blood products
  - Acute: ↑ signal intensity (SI) on T1WI; ↓ SI on T2WI
  - Subacute: ↑ SI on T1WI and T2WI
  - Chronic: ↓ SI on T1WI and T2WI

Angiographic Findings

- Active hemorrhage: Ill-defined blush of extravasated contrast material
- Pseudoaneurysm: Contained, smoothly marginated outpouching of contrast
- Dissection: Linear, intraluminal flap due to intimal injury
- Occlusion: Lack of flow through lumen due to traumatic dissection or embolus
- Arteriovenous fistula: Early opacification of vein during arterial-phase injection

Ultrasonographic Findings

- No significant role in acute renal injury
- Hematoma: Varies with age of blood products
- Pseudoaneurysm: Swirling of blood ("yin yang" sign)
  - To and fro spectral pattern at neck of pseudoaneurysm
- Arteriovenous fistula: Turbulent, low-resistance waveform (high diastolic flow)

DIFFERENTIAL DIAGNOSIS

Renal Tumor

- Spontaneous bleed/rupture may be seen
- Perinephric fluid collection of blood density
- Underlying renal mass lesion
  - Renal cell carcinoma vs. angiomyolipoma

Vasculitis

- Wedge-shaped defects or striated nephrogram
- Microaneurysms of small vessels

(Left) Coronal CECT during the nephrographic phase following a gunshot wound through the left flank reveals fracture of the left kidney, consistent with grade V injury; the superior ➡ and inferior ➡ fragments are perfused but are separated and surrounded by intermediate attenuation "fluid" ➡. (Right) Coronal CECT during the excretory phase in the same patient reveals extravasation ➡ of contrast-opacified urine due to disruption of the renal pelvis.

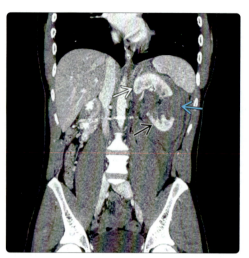
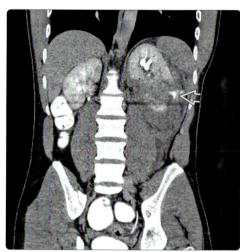

(Left) Coronal CECT during the corticomedullary phase demonstrates fracture ➡ of the right kidney and a traumatic pseudoaneurysm ➡ within the hematoma that separates the superior and inferior fragments. (Right) AP view during digital subtraction angiography shows a catheter in the right renal artery and the pseudoaneurysm ➡ adjacent to the avascular plane of the renal fracture. The pseudoaneurysm was subsequently treated with coil embolization.

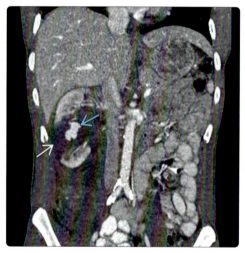
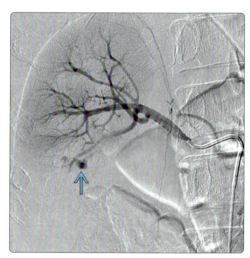

(Left) Axial CECT following trauma reveals hematoma ➡ in the left perinephric space and multiple peripheral areas of nonenhancement due to sites of contusion ➡. The patient was treated conservatively and did not experience any long-term sequelae. (Right) Axial CECT was performed after a patient developed right flank pain following minor trauma. There is a large hematoma ➡ within an angiomyolipoma (AML) and a small amount of perinephric hematoma ➡. The patient had bilateral AMLs due to tuberous sclerosis.

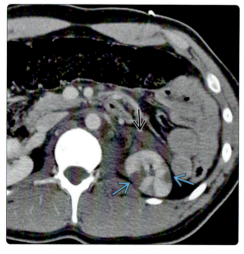
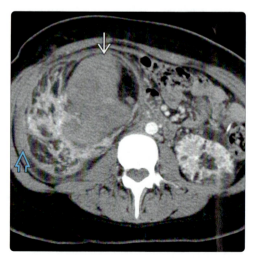

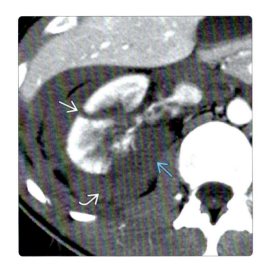 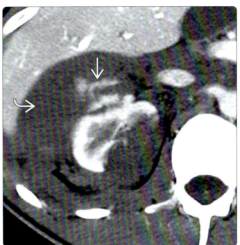

(Left) Axial CECT following trauma demonstrates a deep laceration ➡ that extends through the renal cortex and medulla and a large volume of perirenal hematoma ➡. The lack of enhancement of the posteromedial aspect of the kidney is due to a segmental infarction ➡. (Right) Axial CECT in the same patient reveals active arterial extravasation ➡ into the perirenal hematoma ➡. The patient subsequently underwent an urgent nephrectomy due to the active hemorrhage.

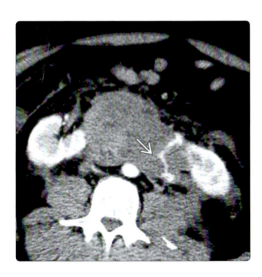 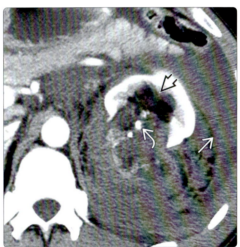

(Left) Axial CECT shows injury to the isthmus of a horseshoe kidney. Note the midline hematoma, which contains a high-attenuation area of active arterial extravasation from the isthmus ➡. (Right) Axial CECT in a 69-year-old woman presenting with severe left flank pain 24 hours after a minor fall reveals a large perirenal hematoma ➡ as well as areas of pseudoaneurysm formation ➡ in a fat-containing AML ➡.

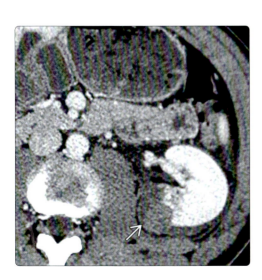 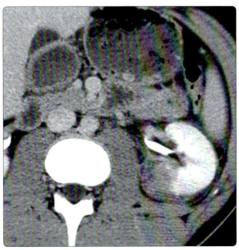

(Left) Axial CECT during the corticomedullary phase of enhancement in a 25-year-old woman who was involved in a high-speed motor vehicle crash reveals a hematoma ➡ in the left kidney, representing a grade II injury. (Right) Axial CECT during the excretory phase in the same patient reveals no injury to the collection system; the patient recovered uneventfully. This case illustrates that the majority of patients with minor renal trauma can be managed without surgery.

KEY FACTS

TERMINOLOGY

- Loculated collection of urine from urinary leak

IMAGING

- Location
  - Along course of urinary tract: Perinephric space, retroperitoneum along ureter, extraperitoneal pelvis adjacent to bladder
  - Pelvic intra- or extraperitoneal location secondary to bladder rupture
- Best imaging tool: CECT or MR; cystogram if bladder leak suspected
  - Typically appears as well-marginated, homogeneous fluid collection
  - Thin rim enhancement with near-water attenuation interior
  - ↓ signal intensity (SI) on T1WI; ↑ SI on T2WI
  - Consider US for assessment and image-guided drainage
- Protocol advice

- CECT or MR with additional imaging during excretory phase (10-minute delay)
- Cystogram: Distend bladder with at least 350 mL of contrast under fluoroscopy to visualize leak as bladder is being filled
- CT cystogram: More sensitive than x-ray cystogram
  - Eliminates need for postdrainage imaging

TOP DIFFERENTIAL DIAGNOSES

- Hematoma
- Abscess
- Lymphocele

CLINICAL ISSUES

- Most common signs/symptoms: Pain due to mass effect; fever if infected
  - Consider superinfection if imaging appearance is complex
- Small urinomas typically resolve spontaneously; large urinomas require percutaneous or surgical drainage

(Left) *Axial NECT following partial nephrectomy is shown. A large urinoma ➡ is encapsulated and has homogeneous near-water attenuation. Note anterior displacement of the left kidney ➡ and hydronephrosis due to mass effect.* (Right) *Axial T2WI MR with fat saturation shows homogenous high signal intensity within the urinoma ➡; a few thin septa ➡ are noted. The lack of complexity (i.e., thick septa, heterogeneous signal intensity, and layering debris) argues against an abscess.*

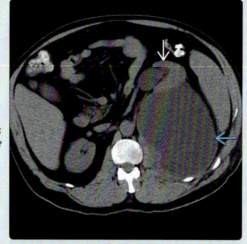
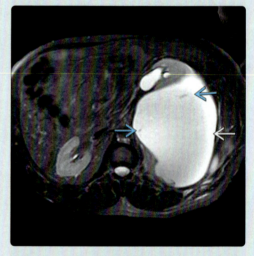

(Left) *Axial postcontrast T1WI MR with fat saturation shows enhancement of the rim of the urinoma ➡.* (Right) *Coronal T1WI MR with fat saturation during the excretory phase shows accumulation of contrast material ➡ layering within the urinoma ➡. Excretory-phase imaging is the key to differentiating urinomas from other fluid collections since excreted contrast will accumulate in the urinoma. The excretory phase is acquired ~ 8-12 minutes after the initial contrast injection.*

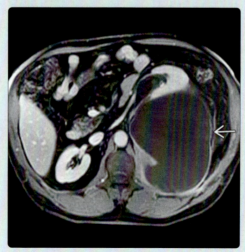
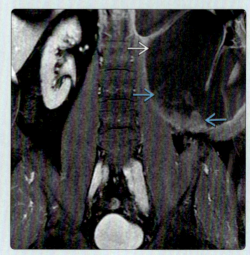

Perinephric Hematoma

TERMINOLOGY

- Hemorrhagic collection in perinephric spaces: Subcapsular, perirenal, anterior and posterior pararenal

IMAGING

- Avascular solid or cystic masses in 1 or more perinephric spaces
- Echogenicity of blood changes over time
- Sonographic features vary over time
  - Acute: Highly echogenic perinephric mass
  - Subacute: Partial liquefaction, echogenic debris, retractile clot with thick septa
  - Chronic: May be almost anechoic
- Useful to assess perfusion in compressed kidney
- Sometimes reveals etiologies such as pseudoaneurysm

TOP DIFFERENTIAL DIAGNOSES

- Lymphoma infiltration
- Cystic lymphangioma

- Perinephric abscess

PATHOLOGY

- Causes include trauma, renal biopsy, renal cyst or tumor rupture, anticoagulation, aneurysm rupture

CLINICAL ISSUES

- Treatment varies with etiology
- Hematoma without underlying significant pathology usually resolves spontaneously
- Flank pain, often severe, palpable mass, shock
- Diminished hematocrit may prompt evaluation
- Subcapsular hematoma may cause hypertension

DIAGNOSTIC CHECKLIST

- Must identify underlying etiology in spontaneous perinephric hematoma to exclude malignancy

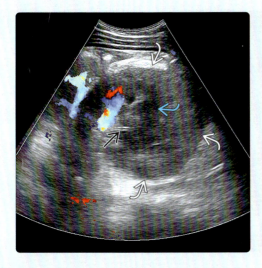
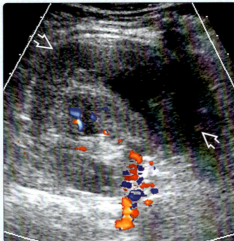

(Left) Transverse color Doppler US of a 6 year old after stent placement ➡ shows a grossly enlarged renal contour ➡ due to large echogenic perinephric hematoma. The relatively hypoechoic kidney is seen in the center of the mass ➡, demonstrating how hyperechoic acute blood can obscure normal structures. (Right) Transverse color Doppler US shows a large, spontaneous perinephric hematoma with mixed echogenicity ➡. Note occult RCC must be considered in spontaneous hemorrhage.

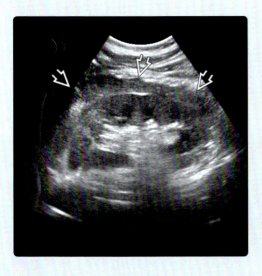
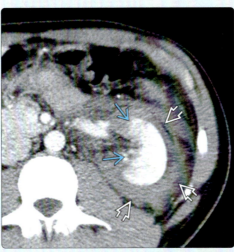

(Left) Longitudinal US in a young man with left flank pain after collision during a soccer game illustrates a thick, irregular soft tissue rind ➡ of blood surrounding the left kidney. (Right) CT confirms an extensive perinephric hematoma ➡ in the same patient, with associated renal lacerations ➡.

IMAGING

- CTA is modality of choice for preoperative evaluation of potential renal donors
- Doppler US: Frontline modality for identification of potentially correctable causes of transplant dysfunction
  - Parenchymal disease (rejection, acute tubular necrosis, drug toxicity pyelonephritis, etc.): Clinical correlation and biopsy often needed given nonspecific US appearance
  - Collecting system dilatation
    - Mild nonobstructive pelvicaliectasis common: Reflux and denervated collecting system
    - Obstructive pelvicaliectasis due to stricture at ureteroneocystostomy, calculi, clot, fungus balls
  - Perinephric fluid collections
    - Hematoma, urinoma, lymphocele, abscess: Time interval post transplantation helps differentiate
    - Appearance often nonspecific, and aspiration is typically necessary for definitive diagnosis
  - Renal artery stenosis
    - Most common renal vascular complication: Unexplained graft dysfunction, hypertension
    - Color aliasing at renal arterial anastomosis: Renal arterial/external iliac artery velocity gradient (> 1.8)
  - Renal vein thrombosis
    - Anuria, graft swelling in immediate postoperative period
    - Doppler: Reversal of intrarenal arterial diastolic flow and absent renal venous flow
  - Pseudoaneurysm
    - Contained biopsy injury of intrarenal artery: "Yin-yang" color flow within intrarenal cyst; to-and-fro flow within neck
  - Arteriovenous fistula
    - Iatrogenic communication between intrarenal artery and vein post biopsy
    - Focal color flurry, high-velocity, "low-resistance" flow within feeding artery and pulsatile flow within draining vein

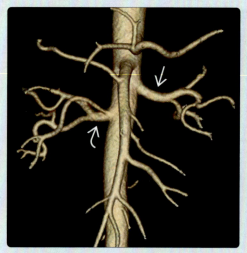
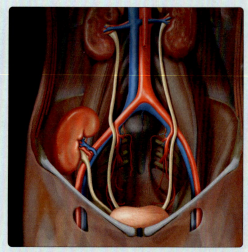

(Left) Volume rendered CTA performed on a potential donor shows a single left renal artery ➡ and a right perihilar branching pattern ➡. The number and branching pattern of renal arteries and veins are detailed so that prohibitive anatomy is not encountered during laparoscopic organ harvesting. (Right) Graphic shows typical renal transplant anatomy. The kidney is placed in the right iliac fossa. The ureter is tunneled through the dome of the bladder. The renal artery and vein are anastomosed end to side with the external iliac vessels.

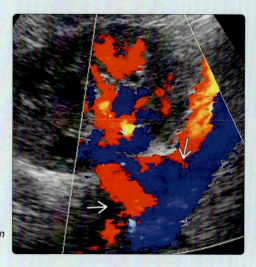
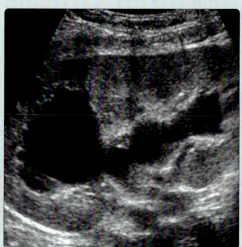

(Left) Color Doppler map of vascular anatomy is initially created to identify potential vascular complications. Flow disturbances (aliasing) are quantified with pulse wave Doppler. Note end-to-side arterial and venous anastomoses ➡. (Right) Ultrasound shows marked hydronephrosis. It is often impossible to differentiate between obstructive and nonobstructive pelvicaliectasis, but improvement in hydronephrosis after bladder emptying suggests reflux (as in this case).

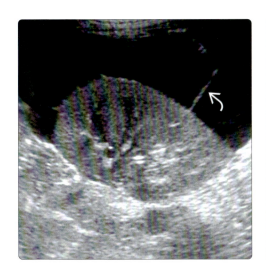

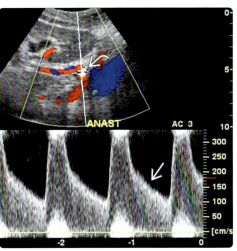

(Left) *Ultrasound performed 4 months post transplantation shows a large, anechoic, perinephric fluid collection. The time course and septation* ➡ *suggest a lymphocele, but aspiration is needed for definitive diagnosis.* (Right) *Renal Doppler was performed for graft dysfunction and hypertension. The Doppler gate is placed on an area of color aliasing* ➡*. Pulse wave Doppler shows anastomotic velocities of > 3.5 m/s and marked diastolic broadening* ➡*, features compatible with a high-grade arterial stenosis.*

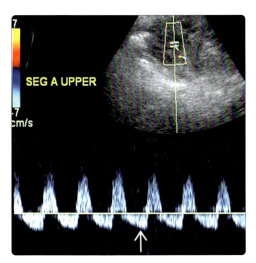

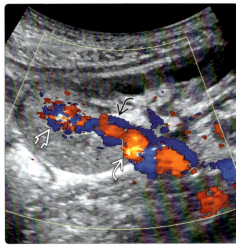

(Left) *Doppler interrogation of a segmental artery in an anuric patient 1 day post transplantation shows reversed diastolic flow* ➡*. Renal venous flow was also absent, and nephrectomy was performed after unsuccessful thrombectomy.* (Right) *Color Doppler ultrasound performed on a patient with renal insufficiency 3 weeks post biopsy shows a focal flurry* ➡ *(due to tissue vibration at an arteriovenous fistula), a feeding artery* ➡*, and a draining vein* ➡*.*

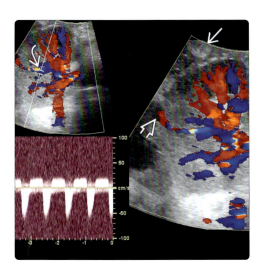

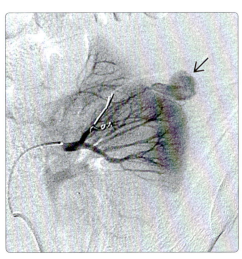

(Left) *Color Doppler ultrasound performed in a patient with pain and a ↓ hematocrit post biopsy shows echogenic perinephric clot* ➡ *and a small pericapsular pseudoaneurysm (PA)* ➡*. Interrogation of the neck shows to-and-fro flow* ➡*.* (Right) *DSA during an ultimately successful embolization procedure on the same patient shows an extrarenal PA* ➡*. PAs are typically due to needle biopsy. Small, incidental intrarenal PAs may resolve over time; enlarging or extrarenal PAs should be embolized.*

KEY FACTS

TOP DIFFERENTIAL DIAGNOSES

- **Total nephrectomy**
  - **Radical nephrectomy**: Total nephrectomy with excision of adrenal gland and regional lymph nodes (performed for malignant tumors)
  - Indications
    - High-grade traumatic injury: Such as devascularization, shattered kidney
    - Irreversible kidney damage in setting of chronic infection and congenital causes
    - Nonfunctioning kidney resulting in renovascular hypertension
    - Symptomatic nephrolithiasis in setting of nonfunctioning kidney (< 10% split function)
    - Kidney donor
    - Large, locally advanced malignant tumors
- **Partial nephrectomy**
  - Resection of part of kidney, a.k.a. nephron-sparing surgery

- Performed for both benign and neoplastic conditions
  - **Trauma**: In setting of low-/intermediate-grade traumatic renal injury; to control hemorrhage or urinary leak
  - **Benign tumors**: Such as renal angiomyolipoma
  - **Malignant tumors**
  - Site of resection is often packed with fat tissue, which can resemble fat-containing lesion on CT
  - Absorbable hemostat material (such as Gelfoam or Surgicel) may be placed at surgical resection site to control bleeding
- **Renal tumor ablation**
  - Radiofrequency (heat) or cryoablation (freezing)
    - Both are effective in eradication of small tumors
  - Morbidity is lower than surgery, although recurrence rate is slightly higher
  - May cause release of gas at site of ablation from sudden death of tumor mass

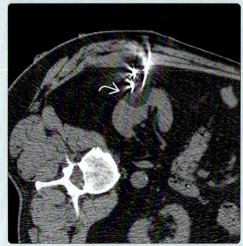
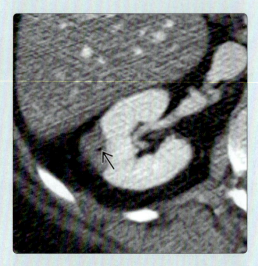

(Left) CT obtained during percutaneous cryoablation of an exophytic papillary-type renal cell carcinoma shows formation of an ice ball ⇗ around the cryoablation probes. (Right) Axial CECT, following cryoablation, shows posttreatment changes with no residual enhancing tissue seen. Note the small bubble of gas at the cryoablation site ⇗, which should not be considered indicative of infection in this setting.

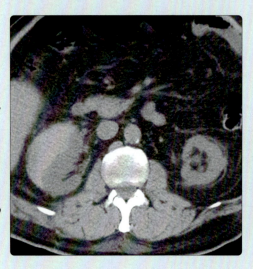
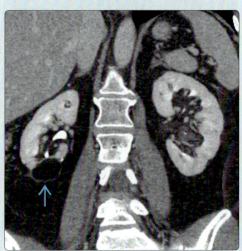

(Left) Axial CT through the kidneys, obtained 2 days following right partial nephrectomy for clear cell-type renal cell carcinoma, shows a large subcapsular hematoma with significant mass effect on the kidney. The patient was taken back to the operating room for drainage of the hematoma. (Right) Coronal CT urography in a 68-year-old woman with history of right partial nephrectomy shows packing of perinephric fat into the surgical bed ⇒, to achieve hemostasis, which could be mistaken for an angiomyolipoma.

Radiation Nephritis

TERMINOLOGY
- Renal injury caused by ionizing radiation

IMAGING
- Sharply demarcated area of decreased attenuation and parenchymal atrophy on CECT (corresponding to irradiated portion of kidney)
- Partial kidney radiation
  - Irradiated portion is sharply demarcated and has smooth surface
- Whole-kidney radiation
  - Progressive atrophy of kidney (most pronounced in outer cortex)
  - Bilateral radiation nephritis is indistinguishable from other causes of chronic renal failure

TOP DIFFERENTIAL DIAGNOSES
- Pyelonephritis

  - Usually has wedge-shaped or striated nephrogram and perirenal infiltration
- Renal infarction
  - Usually has wedge-shaped or global distribution
  - Cortical rim sign
- Chronic renal failure (other causes)

PATHOLOGY
- Etiology: Ionizing radiation → oxidative injury to DNA → cell damage/death
- **Total dose** and **volume** of irradiated kidney are most important predictors of degree of renal injury
- Patients receiving total dose of > 20 Gy (2000 rad) have highest risk (when kidneys included in field of radiation)

CLINICAL ISSUES
- Only 20% of patients receiving > 25 Gy to kidneys develop renal dysfunction
- Proteinuria, azotemia, and hypertension are most common signs/symptoms

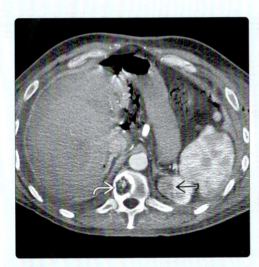
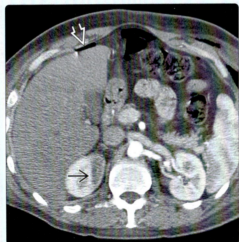

(Left) *Middle-aged man is shown post recent resection of colon carcinoma and radiation therapy for a vertebral metastasis. Axial CECT shows a sharply demarcated hypoenhancing area in the left kidney ➡. Note the vertebral metastasis ➡ that was the target of the radiation therapy.* (Right) *A more caudal section in the same patient shows evidence of the radiation nephritis ➡ in the right kidney as well. Note the free air ➡ related to recent laparotomy.*

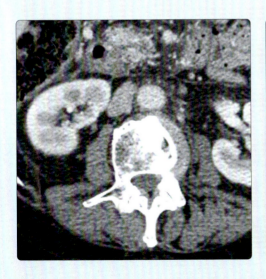
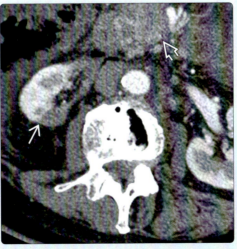

(Left) *This 72-year-old woman with a history of unresectable pancreatic adenocarcinoma underwent external beam radiation. Axial CECT through the kidneys, 5 months following radiation, does not show any discernible changes.* (Right) *Repeat imaging 15 months following external beam radiation shows atrophy and markedly decreased perfusion of the medial aspect of the right kidney along the radiation port. Note sharp demarcation ➡ between the normal and affected parts of the kidney. Note the pancreatic mass ➡.*

TERMINOLOGY

- Acute kidney injury (AKI) within 24-48 hours following intravascular administration of contrast material (CM); must exclude other causes of AKI
  - AKI: Absolute increase in serum creatinine of 0.5 mg/dL or relative 25% increase from baseline value

IMAGING

- Delayed nephrogram on subsequent CT or KUB

TOP DIFFERENTIAL DIAGNOSES

- AKI
  - Other causes of AKI, such as nephrotoxic drugs, prerenal azotemia, urinary obstruction, etc.
  - It may be difficult to recognize exact cause of acute tubular necrosis (ATN) in inpatients since they are exposed to multiple risk factors
- Acute interstitial nephritis
- Renal atheroembolic phenomena

PATHOLOGY

- Animal models have indicated that ATN is underlying pathogenesis, but mechanism by which ATN occurs is not well understood
  - Renal vasoconstriction
  - Direct tubular injury
- Risk of CIN is deterministic (dose dependent)

CLINICAL ISSUES

- **Prophylaxis**
  - Consider alternative imaging methods not requiring CM
  - Use lower dose of CM; avoid closely spaced contrast-enhanced studies
    - Hypoosmolar and isoosmolar nonionic CM have been shown to be superior to hyperosmolar ionic agents
  - Intravenous hydration
  - N-acetylcysteine, orally or IV
  - Discontinuing nephrotoxic drugs
  - No benefit in prophylactic hemodialysis

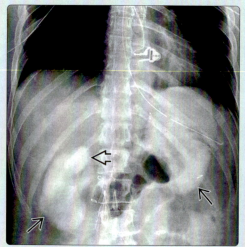

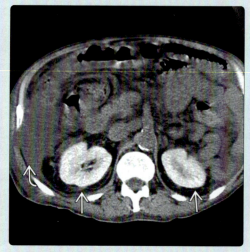

(Left) *Radiograph taken 18 hours after a coronary angiogram shows persistent nephrograms ➡, a finding indicating acute tubular necrosis. The densely opacified bile within the gallblader ➡ is due to vicarious excretion of contrast through the hepatobiliary system to compensate for the decreased renal excretion.* (Right) *Axial NECT shows dense bilateral nephrograms ➡ with otherwise normal-appearing kidneys in a patient with acute renal failure following angiography. Ascites is also present ➡.*

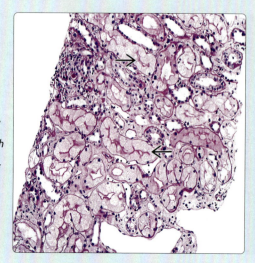

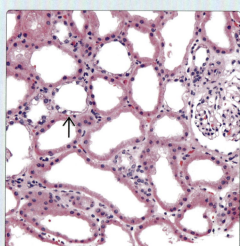

(Left) *Photomicrograph in a patient with osmotic tubulopathy associated with use of iodinated contrast shows tubular profiles that have cytoplasmic swelling, vacuolization, and preservation of the brush borders ➡. (From DP: Kidney, 2e.)* (Right) *Photomicrograph, H&E staining, in a patient with acute tubular necrosis shows epithelial attenuation, loss of apical cytoplasm, prominent dilated tubules, and focal, largely distal, tubular epithelial vacuolization ➡. (From DP: Kidney, 2e.)*

TERMINOLOGY

Definitions

- Acute kidney injury (AKI) within 24-48 hours following intravascular administration of contrast material (CM); must exclude other causes of AKI

DIFFERENTIAL DIAGNOSIS

AKI

- Other causes of AKI, such as nephrotoxic drugs, prerenal azotemia, urinary obstruction, etc.
- It may be difficult to recognize exact cause of acute tubular necrosis (ATN) in inpatients since they are exposed to multiple risk factors
  - In large retrospective study (Newhouse et al, AJR 2008) of 32,161 inpatients who were not exposed to CM, > 50% of them developed AKI

Acute Interstitial Nephritis

- History of drug hypersensitivity
- White blood cell casts on urinalysis

Renal Atheroembolic Phenomena

- Decline in renal function after angiography secondary to renal infarction in setting of thromboembolic and atheroembolic phenomena
- Its onset is usually delayed for days to weeks; protracted course with little or no recovery

PATHOLOGY

General Features

- Etiology
  - Animal studies have shown that ATN is critical unifying precipitating event, but mechanism by which ATN occurs is not well understood
  - Hypothesized mechanisms include
  - **Renal vasoconstriction**
  - **Direct tubular injury**
  - **Risk of contrast-induced nephropathy (CIN) is deterministic (dose dependent)**
  - CIN almost never occurs if renal function is normal
  - Risk factors
    - **Underlying renal dysfunction** (glomerular filtration rate < 60 mL/min): Most important risk factor
    - Decreased renal perfusion: Heart failure, hypotension, or dehydration
    - Age > 70 years
    - Diabetes mellitus
    - Concomitant use of nephrotoxic drugs (NSAIDs, aminoglycosides, cyclosporine, etc.)
    - Multiple myeloma
    - **Procedure-related risk factors**
      - □ Large CM volume
      - □ High osmolarity ionic (1st generation) CM
      - □ Type of study: Much higher prevalence with coronary angiography

CLINICAL ISSUES

Demographics

- Age

  - ↑ incidence in elderly due to ↓ ability to accommodate to oxidative injury
- Epidemiology
  - 3rd leading cause of acute renal failure in hospitalized patients
  - Incidence: Negligible (< 1%) in patients without risk factors; ~ 10% in patients > 70 years old; can increase to 50% in patients with multiple risk factors
    - Decreased incidence of CIN in past decade might be due to use of nonionic isoosmolar and hypoosmolar CM
  - In general, risk of CIN after coronary angiography is much higher than after CT (due to comorbidities and the higher administered dose)

Natural History & Prognosis

- Serum creatinine rises within 24 hours, peaks in 2-3 days, and usually returns to baseline within 7-10 days
- Majority of cases have mild decline in GFR
  - In prospective study of 353 patients with moderate to severe renal dysfunction who underwent coronary angiography (Brar et al, JAMA 2008), < 1% had severe AKI requiring dialysis
- In retrospective study of 21,346 hospitalized patients (McDonald et al, Radiology 2014), CM was **not** found to be independent risk factor for AKI, emergent dialysis, or 30-day mortality.

Treatment

- In patients at risk for CIN, serum Cr or estimated GFR should be measured before study and 24-48 hours after administration of CM
- **Prophylaxis**
  - Use lower dose of CM; avoid closely spaced contrast-enhanced studies
    - Hypoosmolar and isoosmolar nonionic CM have been shown to be less nephrotoxic than hyperosmolar ionic agents
  - Intravenous hydration
    - No consensus regarding optimal solution and rate of administration
      - □ Isotonic solutions were shown to be superior to hypotonic ones
      - □ Several studies have suggested that serum alkalinization with sodium bicarbonate may be beneficial
    - Suggested rate: Isotonic saline or sodium bicarbonate (1 mL/kg/hour, starting 12 hours before study until 12 hours afterward)
    - No evidence-based benefit to oral hydration with water
  - N-acetylcysteine, orally or IV
    - Theoretically can prevent CIN by ↓ vasoconstriction and ↓ production of oxygen free radicals
    - Due to lack of convincing data, use of IV acetylcysteine is not generally recommended
  - Discontinuing nephrotoxic drugs
  - **No** benefit in prophylactic hemodialysis
- Performing hemodialysis immediately after CM administration does not prevent CIN

SECTION 5
Ureter

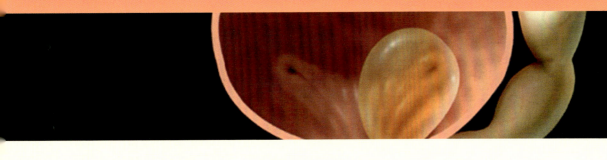

Anatomy

The ureter is a muscular tube extending from the ureteropelvic junction (UPJ) to the bladder for a length of 25-30 cm. The proximal ureter is in the perirenal space, passing posterior to the gonadal vessels and traveling along the psoas muscle to cross over the iliac vessels at the pelvic brim.

The ureters continue inferiorly along the pelvic wall to ~ the level of the ischial spines where they curve anteromedially to enter the bladder. This occurs at the level of the seminal vesicles in men and cervix in women. This anatomic proximity has important implications in women with invasive cervical cancer in whom ureteral obstruction is a common and important complication.

At the ureterovesical junction (UVJ), the ureters pass obliquely through the bladder wall creating a valve effect and therefore preventing reflux. The UVJ, along with the UPJ and pelvic brim, are all physiologic points of narrowing and are often the sites where ureteral stones may be lodged.

Imaging Techniques and Indications

Radiography

With the advent of multidetector CT and advancing MR techniques, excretory urography (also referred to as intravenous pyelography or IVP) has largely been replaced. Modern CT and MR provide a comprehensive assessment of both the renal parenchyma and now, with excretory-phase protocols, the urinary tract. Although retrograde urography is still performed, it is usually undertaken in conjunction with a procedure, such as stone retrieval or biopsy of a mass and less commonly as a primary diagnostic procedure (particularly in patients with renal insufficiency).

CT Urography

There is no universally accepted technique for performing a CT urography. An unenhanced phase is necessary for detection of calculi, a nephrographic phase is best for identifying renal masses, and an excretory phase best detects urothelial lesions.

The goal in evaluating the ureter is to view it distended and opacified throughout its entire course, but as in the days of the conventional excretory urogram, peristalsis may result in unopacified ureteral segments. Because the ureters taper as they enter the bladder, the distal portions are particularly difficult to completely opacify.

While many protocols exist, it is clear that the ureter is best evaluated when the patient is well hydrated. Hydration can be achieved orally (750-1,000 mL of water ~ 30 minutes prior to the exam) or by a combination of oral and intravenous approaches (for example: 500 mL of water ~ 30 minutes prior to the exam and then 250 mL of intravenous 0.9% saline just before scanning the patient). Several investigators have advocated intravenous administration of 10 mg of furosemide 2-3 minutes prior to the procedure to further increase the flow rate of opacified urine.

Excretory-phase images are obtained 10-15 minutes after the initial contrast administration with thin beam collimation and low-pitch scanning. Since radiation dose is a paramount consideration, particularly in young patients, various protocols, including split-bolus and triple-dose techniques, have been designed to reduce the number of scans. Inconsistent results, however, with the split-bolus technique have prompted many centers to employ 3-phase protocols for all referred patients or to selectively employ split-bolusing in low-risk, younger patients. Novel reconstruction algorithms (i.e., statistical and model-based iterative algorithms) allow for significant dose reduction without affecting the diagnostic quality of 3-phase exams.

The ureters should be reviewed routinely in both the axial and coronal planes. Further postprocessing reconstructions, including maximum intensity projections, curved planar reformations, and 3D volume rendering, give the "big picture," simulating the old excretory urogram. The result is an excellent evaluation of ureters, which is equivalent to retrograde urography for the detection of urothelial tumors.

MR Urography

MR is more technically challenging than CT and is primarily used to limit radiation dose in children, younger patients, and pregnant women. Two basics techniques can be used to view the ureter: Static-fluid MR urography and contrast-enhanced excretory MR urography.

Static-fluid MR urography uses heavily T2-weighted images with suppression of background tissues, similar to that done in MR cholangiography. This technique is useful when the collecting system is dilated, but it may be difficult to completely visualize normal ureters. Multiple thick-slab, single-shot, fast spin-echo images can be obtained and viewed in a cine loop to improve visualization of nondilated ureters and avoid mistaking ureteral peristalsis for a stricture of filling defect.

Excretory MR urography is performed after the administration of gadolinium. This technique is technically challenging. Gadolinium initially appears bright on T1-weighted images. As it becomes concentrated, however, the signal intensity of urine decreases. Administration of a diuretic greatly improves the quality of MR urography by both distending the collecting system and diluting the gadolinium concentration.

Approach to Abnormal Ureter

Structural abnormalities of the ureter can be divided into 3 simplified categories: **Dilatation**, **stricture**, and **filling defect (masses)**. Clearly there is overlap in these categories.

Ureteral dilatation can be structural (due to downstream obstruction) or functional. **Obstructive etiologies** include ureteral calculi (the most common etiology, particularly in the acute setting), obstructing masses, downstream strictures, extrinsic compression, and ureteroceles. **Functional etiologies** include reflux, primary megaureter, and ureterectasis of pregnancy.

Ureteral strictures may be caused by neoplastic, infectious, or inflammatory processes. Neoplastic strictures include urothelial tumors or encasement by an extrinsic tumor, such as colon or cervical cancer. Infections (TB, schistosomiasis) or inflammatory/infiltrative processes (Crohn disease, endometriosis) also may involve and constrict the ureter. Many of these entities also cause ureteral wall thickening. When wall thickening is profound, always consider lymphoma.

The most common **ureteral filling defects** are calculi and urothelial tumors. Other differential considerations include blood clot, mycetoma, fibroepithelial polyp, papilloma, ureteritis cystica, and malakoplakia.

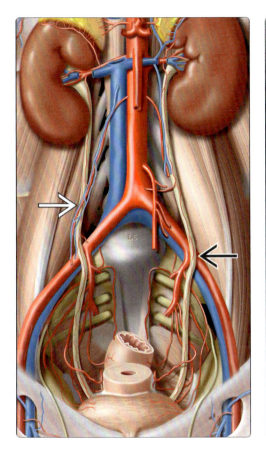

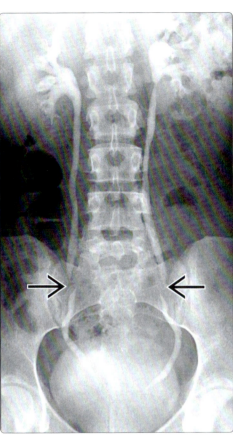

(Left) Graphic illustrates the normal course of the ureters, which extend from the renal pelvis to the urinary bladder. The ureters travel along the psoas muscle, passing posterior to the gonadal vessels ➡. Near the pelvic brim, the ureter ➡ passes over the iliac vessels, which can cause extrinsic impression on the ureter on imaging studies. (Right) Excretory urogram shows mild extrinsic compression and medial deviation of the ureters ➡ where they pass over the iliac vessels. Excretory urography has essentially been replaced by CT and MR urography, which provide a comprehensive assessment of the kidney, urinary tract, and surrounding structures.

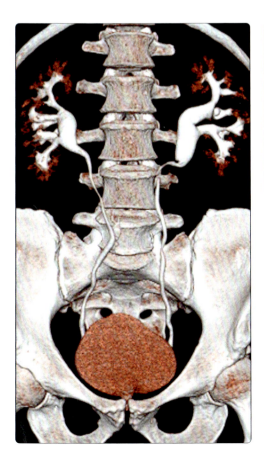

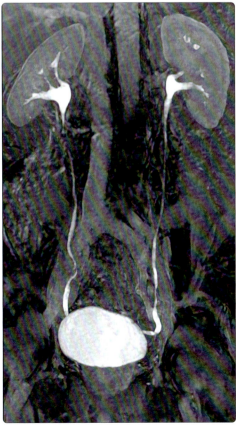

(Left) In this 3D surface-rendered reconstruction of the urinary tract, the windowing has been optimized to display the renal collecting system. The color scale is arbitrary, and in this case, opacified urine is displayed as white. Less dense urine, within the renal tubules of the pyramids and the diluted urine within the bladder, is displayed in shades of red. (Right) Coronal MIP postcontrast T1WI MR (MR urography) in a 48-year-old man with a history of microscopic hematuria shows opacification of renal collecting systems, ureters, and bladder. This method is especially useful in children (for evaluation of congenital anomalies).

Duplicated and Ectopic Ureter

TERMINOLOGY

- **Ectopic ureter**: Ureteral orifice below normal insertion in trigone; commonly associated with duplex collecting system
- **Duplicated ureter**: 2 ureters drain duplex kidney and remain separate down to bladder insertion or beyond

IMAGING

- Location
  - Males: Ectopic insertion of ureter is always above external sphincter
    - Insertion sites: Prostatic urethra (54%), seminal vesicles (28%), vas deferens (10%), ejaculatory duct (8%)
  - Females: Ectopic insertion is usually below sphincter resulting in urinary incontinence
    - Insertion sites: Bladder neck and upper urethra (33%), vestibule (33%), vagina (25%), cervix and uterus (5%)

- 75-90% of ectopic ureters occur in setting of duplication (in Western world)
- 85% of duplicated ureters obey Weigert-Meyer rule
- **Weigert-Meyer rule**: Upper pole ureter inserts medial and caudal to lower pole ureter

TOP DIFFERENTIAL DIAGNOSES

- Bifid ureters
- Ureterocele
- Seminal vesicle cyst
- Gartner duct cysts

CLINICAL ISSUES

- Often asymptomatic in males
- Incontinence is only seen in females due to insertion of upper pole ureteral orifice below bladder sphincter
- Management depends on presence of duplication and on function of involved kidney (moiety)

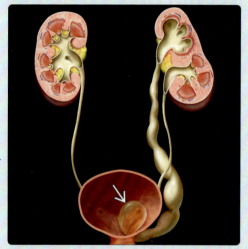
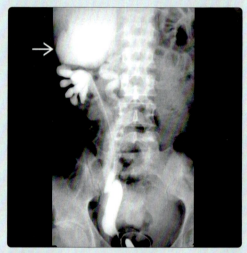

(Left) *Graphic illustrates a duplex left kidney and the Weigert-Meyer principle. The ureter from the upper pole inserts medial and caudal to the lower pole ureter, ending in a ureterocele* ➡ *in this case.* (Right) *AP projection from intravenous urograph (IVU) shows duplex right kidney and complete duplication of ureters with marked dilatation of the upper pole moiety collecting system* ➡*, due to an obstructing ureterocele. The lower moiety ureter is stented due to an obstructing ureterovesical junction stone (not shown).*

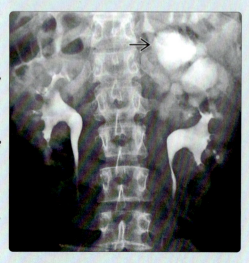
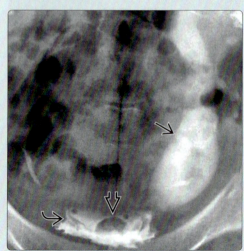

(Left) *AP projection from IVU shows marked dilation of the pelvocalyceal system in the left upper pole moiety* ➡ *displacing the lower pole calyces inferiorly (drooping lily sign).* (Right) *Excretory image from IVU in the same patient shows dilated upper-pole ureter* ➡ *just above its ectopic insertion near the base of the bladder, where it terminates in a ureterocele, seen as a filling defect* ➡ *in the bladder. Note the ureter from the right kidney and its normal insertion in the trigone* ➡.

Ureteritis Cystica

TERMINOLOGY

- Reactive proliferative changes of urothelium with formation of multiple small, subepithelial cysts

IMAGING

- More common in proximal 1/3 of ureter
- May also occur in renal pelvis (pyelitis cystica) and urinary bladder (cystitis cystica)
- Ureterogram (intravenous or retrograde/antegrade)
  - Nodular, mural-based, radiolucent small filling defects in ureteral lumen
  - Scalloping of ureteral margins (in profile view)

TOP DIFFERENTIAL DIAGNOSES

- Blood clots, radiolucent stones
- Air bubbles
- Multifocal transitional cell carcinoma or papillary tumors
- Metastatic melanoma
- Impression from crossing vessels

- Chronic infectious ureteritis

PATHOLOGY

- Likely response to chronic inflammation or irritation
  - Seen in association with UTI, urolithiasis, chemotherapy, radiation, schistosomiasis, and instrumentation
- Theory of pathogenesis: **von Brunn cell nest**
  - Inflammatory stimulation → proliferation of urothelium → invagination of urothelial cells
  - Cells become isolated within lamina propria → metaplastic transformation into glandular structures (**ureteritis glandularis**) → cystic dilation of von Brunn nests (**ureteritis cystica**)

CLINICAL ISSUES

- Usually inconsequential; should rule out UTI
- No risk of malignant degeneration
  - Predisposing factors for ureteritis cystica (such as chronic infection) may act as risk factors for urothelial malignancy

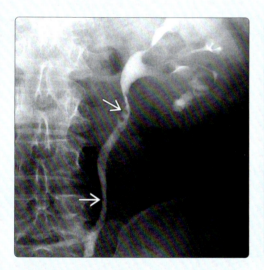

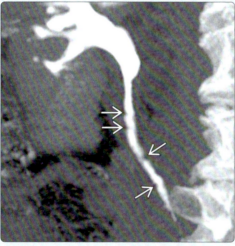

(Left) Frontal projection from excretory-phase IVP shows several small, mural-based filling defects in left proximal and mid ureter ➡, typical findings of ureteritis cystica. (Right) Coronal reformat from CT urogram shows several smooth filling defects ➡ along the right ureter in this elderly man with dysuria and prior infections. Endoscopy confirmed the submucosal location of these lesions, and biopsy specimens were negative for transitional cell carcinoma.

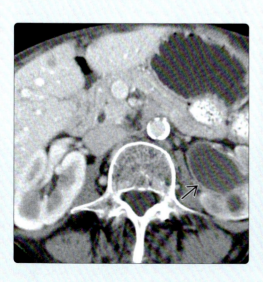

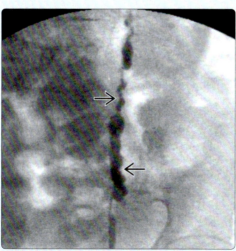

(Left) Axial contrast-enhanced CT shows left-sided hydronephrosis and a delayed nephrogram in this elderly man with pyuria and fever. The walls of the left ureter and renal pelvis are thickened and enhance with contrast ➡, indicating inflammation. Pyonephrosis was confirmed at nephrostomy. (Right) Antegrade ureterography in the same patient shows an irregular contour of the left ureter ➡, compatible with ureteritis. Ureteral spasm may also play a part in this patient, as active infection is present.

Ureteral Stricture

TERMINOLOGY

- Narrowing of ureteral lumen due to intraluminal, intramural, or extrinsic process

IMAGING

- Segmental narrowing of ureter with dilation of upstream ureter on pyelography
- Best imaging tool
  - Retrograde pyelography for best resolution of length and degree of stenosis
- CT or MR for extrinsic processes
  - e.g., retroperitoneal fibrosis or malignancy

TOP DIFFERENTIAL DIAGNOSES

- Iatrogenic stricture
  - Most common etiology
  - Seen after lithotomy, ureteroscopy, ureteral catheterization, or radiation therapy
- Postoperative stricture

- Most commonly at site of anastomosis of ureter to bladder, neobladder, or ileal conduit
- Urolithiasis
  - 25% of patients with prolonged stone impaction (> 2 months) develop stricture
  - Most strictures are secondary to edema and are transient, resolving in 6-12 weeks
- Malignant stricture
  - Urothelial carcinoma, metastases, and lymphoma
- Retroperitoneal fibrosis
- Malakoplakia
- Tuberculosis
- Congenital ureteral stricture
- Vascular compression

CLINICAL ISSUES

- Most strictures are benign and are treated by catheter balloon dilation &/or stent placement

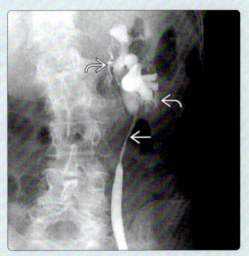
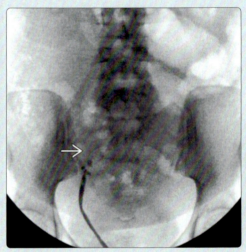

(Left) Retrograde pyelography shows a long segment stricture ➡ of the proximal ureter with dilation of the calyces. Note the intravasation of contrast ➡, an indication of overdistention of the collecting system under pressure. This resulted from the surgical extraction of a ureteral stone. (Right) Retrograde pyelogram shows complete obstruction of the right ureter in the pelvis ➡ due to a ureteral injury from gynecologic surgery. The findings were confirmed on antegrade pyelogram (not shown).

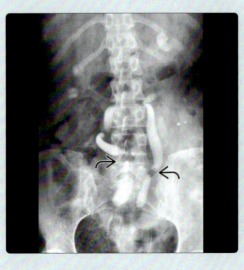
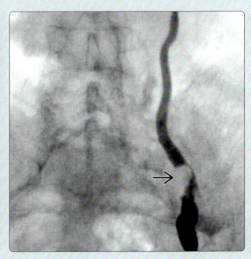

(Left) Retrograde pyelogram shows medial deviation and partial obstruction of both ureters ➡, a classic feature of retroperitoneal fibrosis. The diagnosis was confirmed on CECT (not shown) as a mantle of tissue surrounding the aorta, inferior vena cava, and distal ureters. (Right) Retrograde pyelogram shows an eccentric filling defect ➡ and stricture in the distal ureter with both a smooth and an irregular surface component. This proved to be a malignant stricture from urothelial carcinoma.

TERMINOLOGY

- Rare chronic granulomatous condition affecting urinary tract
- Malacoplakia = soft plaque

IMAGING

- Bladder is most frequently involved organ (40%) followed by renal parenchyma, upper urinary tract, prostate, and urethra
- Variable appearance ranging from flat plaques to nodules and masses ± ulceration
- In rare cases, lesion can act aggressively and extend beyond ureter and bladder

TOP DIFFERENTIAL DIAGNOSES

- Transitional cell carcinoma
- Leukoplakia
- Ureteritis cystica
- Chronic granulomatous ureteritis (tuberculosis)

PATHOLOGY

- Thought to be due to impaired host response and defective phagocytosis
- Highly associated with *Escherichia coli* and other gram-negative bacilli
- More common in immunosuppressed and diabetic patients
- Distinctive histologic appearance
  - Mass-forming histiocytic infiltrate with granular eosinophilic cytoplasm (von Hansemann cells)
  - Characteristic basophilic intracytoplasmic inclusions (Michaelis-Guttman bodies)

CLINICAL ISSUES

- No malignant potential
- Predominantly seen in women (F:M = 4:1)

DIAGNOSTIC CHECKLIST

- Imaging manifestations are nonspecific, and there is overlap with other inflammatory and neoplastic conditions

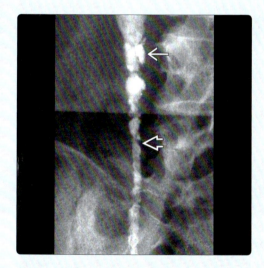

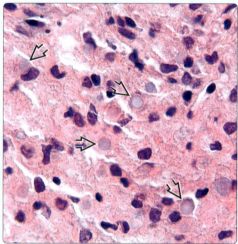

(Left) *Coned-down view of the right ureter in a case of malakoplakia shows diffuse irregularity with small plaques* ⮕ *and ulcerations* ⮕. *Urinary tract involvement can be quite variable from a focal lesion to diffuse abnormality.* (Right) *High-power H&E stain shows sheets of histiocytes (von Hansemann cells) with lamellated intracytoplasmic inclusions (Michaelis-Gutman bodies)* ⮕. *Malakoplakia is felt to be the result of defective phagolysosomal activity in patients with recurrent E. coli infections. (From DP: Genitourinary.)*

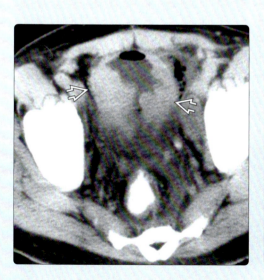

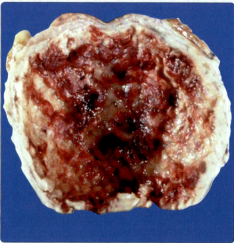

(Left) *CECT at the level of the bladder shows irregular, mass-like thickening of the bladder wall* ⮕. *This appearance is indistinguishable from urothelial carcinoma and requires biopsy.* (Right) *Photograph of the cut, resected specimen shows a friable, hemorrhagic surface and dramatic wall thickening. The bladder is the most frequent site of malakoplakia followed by the renal parenchyma, upper urinary tract, prostate, and urethra.*

Ureteral Trauma

TERMINOLOGY

- Injury of ureter from blunt, penetrating, or iatrogenic trauma

IMAGING

- Best imaging tools: CECT with CT urography for global view of abdomen & urinary tract
  - Antegrade or retrograde pyelography for detailed analysis of site & character of injury
- Sites of urine accumulation
  - Perirenal or subcapsular from blunt renal injury
  - Medial to ureteropelvic junction (UPJ) for proximal ureteral & UPJ leaks
  - May enter peritoneal cavity (after penetrating trauma or laparotomy/laparoscopy)
- Ureteral strictures less accurately diagnosed by CT
  - Difficult to distinguish segments of stricture from ureteral spasm & peristalsis due to stricture

- Indirect signs of ureteral stricture: Delayed nephrogram, hydronephrosis

TOP DIFFERENTIAL DIAGNOSES

- Abdominal abscess
- Postoperative hematoma or seroma
- Postoperative edema

CLINICAL ISSUES

- > 80% of trauma affects inferior 3rd of ureter
- Distal ureteral injury repaired with ureteroneocystotomy ± psoas hitch ± Boari flap
- Mid-/proximal ureteral injury repaired with ureteroureterostomy
- For extensive injury, can perform transureteroureterostomy, ileal ureter, buccal ureter, or kidney autotransplant
- Best imaging protocol: CECT with CT urography
  - Includes excretory phase (10-12 minutes post IV injection)

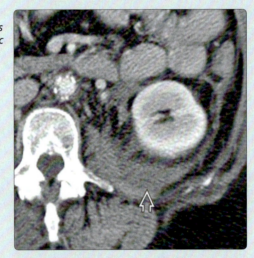
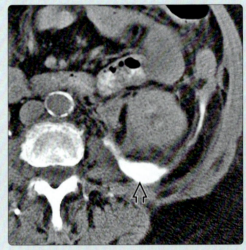

(Left) Axial CECT in a patient following spine surgery shows fluid ⇒ in the left perinephric space. Differential considerations include hematoma and urinoma. CT was performed due to aberrant spinal screw placement and concern for retroperitoneal hemorrhage. (Right) Axial CECT during the excretory phase in the same patient demonstrates opacification of the perinephric fluid consistent with extravasated urine ⇒ due to ureteral injury.

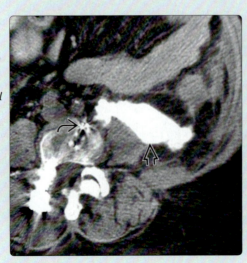
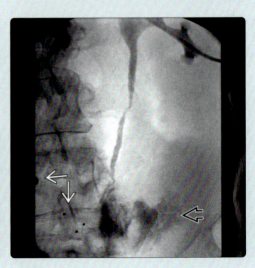

(Left) More inferiorly, axial CECT during the excretory phase in the same patient shows increased accumulation of the extravasated urine ⇒. Note the metallic spinal hardware ⇒ along the ventral margin of the vertebral body. (Right) AP image during antegrade nephrostogram demonstrates transection of the distal aspect of the left ureter and extravasation of contrast material ⇒ into the retroperitoneum. Note the spine hardware ⇒ at the same level.

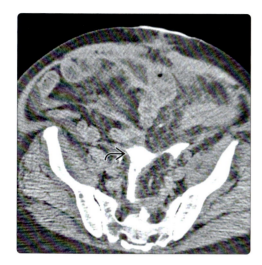
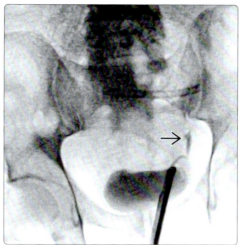

(Left) *Axial CECT during the excretory phase following subtotal colectomy demonstrates extravasation of contrast-opacified urine* ⇒ *into a collection near the site of the colonic anastomosis due to ureteral transection.* **(Right)** *Retrograde pyelogram in the same patient shows truncation of the left ureter and subtle extravasation* ⇒. *A ureteral transection was confirmed at reoperation.*

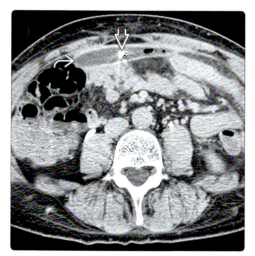
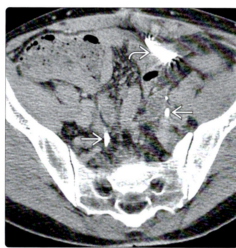

(Left) *Axial CECT shows an elliptical fluid collection* ⇒ *in the ventral aspect of the abdomen following partial colectomy. A portion of a percutaneous drainage catheter* ⇒ *is shown in the center of the fluid collection; the aspirated contents were suspicious for infected urine.* **(Right)** *Excretory-phase CECT shows a more caudal section in the same patient. Note the dense opacification of the ureters* ⇒ *and contrast material filling the fluid collection* ⇒ *around the catheter.*

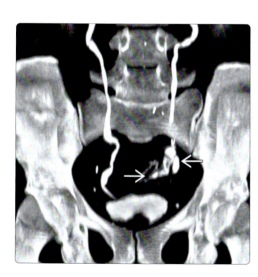
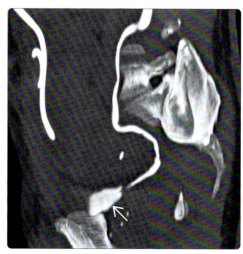

(Left) *Coronal multiple intensity projection from excretory-phase CECT in the same patient shows extravasation of contrast-opacified urine* ⇒ *from the transected left ureter. Note that the more distal ureter is not opacified. The extravasated urine collected within the previously identified elliptical collection.* **(Right)** *Coronal oblique reformatted image from an excretory-phase CECT in the same patient clearly shows the extravasation of urine* ⇒ *from the distal left ureter.*

TERMINOLOGY

- Synonym: Ureteral fibroepithelial polyp
- Definition: Benign mesodermal lesion with hyperplastic fibroconnective stromal core and normal urothelial lining

IMAGING

- Elongated soft tissue-density intraluminal mass with smooth surface
- Shows enhancement
- CT or US may show protrusion of polyp through ureteral orifice into bladder
- ± hydroureter/hydronephrosis
- Delayed imaging (CT urography) helps to better delineate shape and contour of lesion
- CT is helpful in excluding other causes of obstruction, such as stone, etc.

TOP DIFFERENTIAL DIAGNOSES

- Urothelial neoplasms
  - Papillary urothelial neoplasms have exophytic growth and may have polypoid morphology
  - Papillary urothelial neoplasms are usually smaller and fixed
- Other mesenchymal ureteral tumors
  - Leiomyoma, neurofibroma, lymphangioma, hemangioma
- Intraluminal filling defects
  - Stone, blood clot, debris, sloughed papillae, fungus ball, and foreign body
  - CT is particularly helpful to differentiate: Evaluate morphology and attenuation

PATHOLOGY

- Exact etiology is unknown
- Congenital factors and chronic inflammation play role

CLINICAL ISSUES

- Ureteroscopic excision

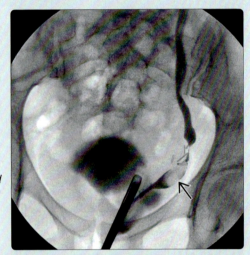
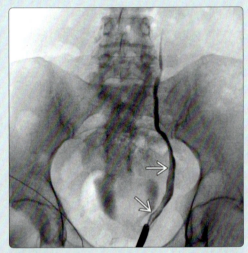

(Left) *AP retrograde urography shows a well-delineated intraluminal filling defect in the distal left ureter* ➡️. *Pathology was consistent with a fibroepithelial polyp. The surgical clips in the left pelvis are related to a prior hysterectomy.* (Right) *AP retrograde urogram shows a well-delineated, elongated intraluminal filling defect in the distal left ureter* ➡️. *Cystoscopy showed a polypoid lesion with a long stalk, which intermittently protruded through the ureteral orifice.*

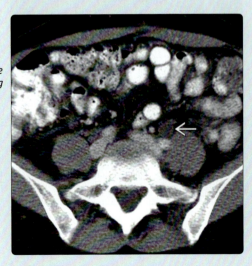
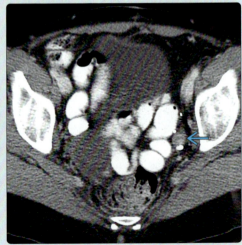

(Left) *Axial CT at the pelvic brim shows moderate dilatation of the left ureter* ➡️. (Right) *CECT section through the lower pelvis in the same patient shows enhancing soft tissue within the distal left ureter* ➡️. *Subsequent retrograde urography and cystoscopy confirmed an intraluminal polypoid lesion. The patient underwent ureteroscopic excision of a polyp, and pathology was consistent with a fibroepithelial polyp.*

Ureteral Urothelial Carcinoma

TERMINOLOGY

- Carcinoma arising from transitional epithelium of ureter
  - 5% of all urothelial malignancies
  - 90% of ureteral tumors are urothelial carcinoma

IMAGING

- Intraluminal soft tissue mass with dilation of ureter upstream
- More common in distal ureter (70%); presumably due to stasis
- CT urography is best noninvasive imaging tool for diagnosis and staging
  - ↑ sensitivity/specificity and ↑ accuracy compared with IVP
- MR urography is noninvasive alternative to CT urography in patients with contraindication for intravenous iodinated contrast
- Bilateral ureteral urothelial carcinoma seen in 2-5%

TOP DIFFERENTIAL DIAGNOSES

- Urolithiasis
- Blood clot
- Sloughed papilla (papillary necrosis)
- Fibroepithelial polyp
- Ureteritis cystica
- Tuberculosis
- Ureteral malakoplakia

PATHOLOGY

- Risk factors
  - Smoking, dose dependent
  - Occupational exposure: Aniline, benzidine, aromatic amine (used in textile industry)
- ~ 50% of patients with upper urinary tract urothelial cancer will develop metachronous bladder cancer
- 12% will develop metachronous urothelial carcinoma of upper urinary tract within 28 months

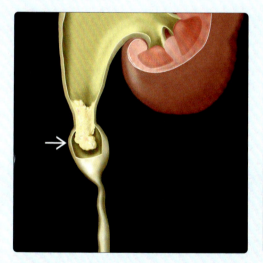
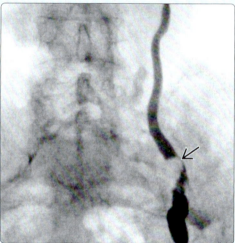

(Left) Graphic shows urothelial carcinoma of the proximal ureter with dilation of the renal pelvis. Note the focal expansion of the lumen ➡ at the site of the tumor, the origin of the goblet sign seen on pyelography and sometimes on urography as well. (Right) Retrograde pyelogram in an 87-year-old man shows an eccentric filling defect ➡ in the distal ureter with both a smooth and an irregular surface component.

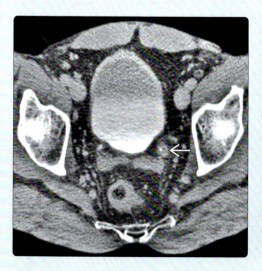
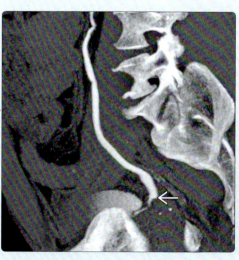

(Left) Axial CECT in an elderly man with hematuria shows circumferential wall thickening and luminal narrowing of distal left ureter ➡ just proximal to the ureterovesical junction. (Right) Volume-rendered 3D image from the excretory phase of CECT in the same patient shows the filling defect ➡ within the distal ureter that proved to be urothelial carcinoma of the ureter. Such reformations are complementary to the axial sections and should not be viewed in isolation.

TERMINOLOGY

- Reported in setting of breast carcinoma, colorectal carcinoma, gastric carcinoma, melanoma, lymphoma, and prostate cancer
- Majority of cases are asymptomatic and only detected on autopsy
  - In 1 autopsy series in patients with disseminated breast cancer, 6% had ureteral metastasis
- While hematogenous metastases are rather rare, involvement of ureters by direct invasion of tumor is not uncommon (seen in setting of colorectal, prostate, and gynecologic malignancies)

IMAGING

- Lesion tends to be enhancing and mass-like, typically larger than urothelial carcinoma
- Most cases manifest as discrete mass along course of ureter (rather than stricture or intraluminal mass, as seen in case of urothelial carcinoma)

- Many cases in fact represent enlarged node or tumor deposit along periureteral lymphatic plexus invading into ureter rather than true ureteral seeding

TOP DIFFERENTIAL DIAGNOSES

- **Ureteral Urothelial Carcinoma**
  - Urothelial carcinoma arises in urothelium whereas most metastatic lesions are centered in periureteral plexus or in ureteral wall
  - Most reported ureteral metastasis are large intramural/periureteral masses at time of diagnosis

PATHOLOGY

- Proposed patterns of secondary involvement of ureters
  - Homogeneous spread
  - Lymphatic dissemination through periureteral plexus
  - Direct invasion (mostly in case of cervical cancer)
  - Drop metastasis (in patients with urothelial carcinoma elsewhere)

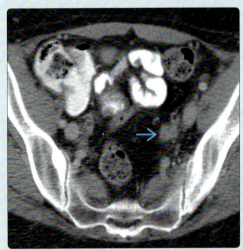
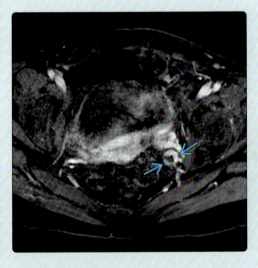

(Left) Axial CECT in a patient with a history of metastatic cholangiocarcinoma shows an enhancing tumor deposit ➡ in the retroperitoneum centered around, and encasing, the left ureter. (Right) Axial contrast-enhanced T1WI MR shows eccentric mass-like wall thickening of distal left ureter ➡. The wall thickening was contiguous with a small ossified retroperitoneal mass (not shown). Biopsy was consistent with osteosarcoma.

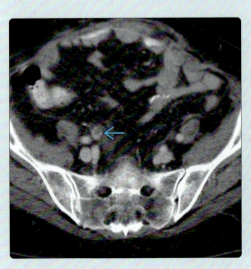
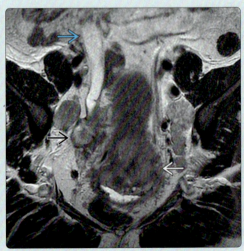

(Left) Axial CECT in a patient with a history of metastatic breast cancer shows mass-like eccentric ureteral wall thickening ➡ and abnormal wall enhancement representing metastatic focus. (Right) Coronal oblique T2WI MR in a 36-year-old woman with a history of locally advanced cervical cancer ➡ shows tumor implant in the right parametrium ➡ with invasion into the distal right ureter and resultant hydronephrosis ➡.

Ureterectasis of Pregnancy

TERMINOLOGY

- Physiologic dilatation of ureter and renal collecting system during pregnancy

IMAGING

- Ureteral dilatation down to point of compression (where ureter crosses iliac vessels)
- Ureter should taper to normal diameter below pelvic brim; failure to do so is highly suggestive of pathologic obstruction
- Predominantly on right side (**80-90%**)
- Bilateral ureteral jets present
  - Ureteral jet might not be visible in supine position; turning patient into contralateral decubitus position helps to see jet
  - Absent unilateral ureteral jet is suggestive of high-grade obstruction (usually due to stone)

TOP DIFFERENTIAL DIAGNOSES

- Urolithiasis (renal calculi)
  - Obstruction is abrupt and is usually above or below level of common iliac arteries
  - ± posterior shadowing, ± twinkling artifact
  - Unilateral absence of ureteral jets

PATHOLOGY

- Caused by combination of extrinsic compression on ureter (more important factor) and intrinsic changes in ureters
- **Extrinsic compression**: Mainly by enlarged gravid uterus and, to lesser extent, by engorged parauterine vessels
- **Intrinsic changes**: ↓ ureteral tone and ↓ peristalsis caused by increased progesterone and gonadotropin levels

CLINICAL ISSUES

- Seen in ~ 90% of pregnant women in 3rd trimester
- Prevalence and severity increase as pregnancy advances
- Usually regresses within 8 weeks postpartum

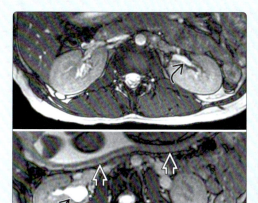

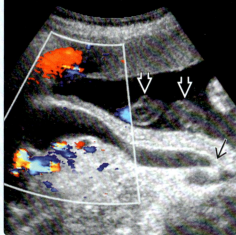

(Left) *Axial T2WI MR performed for evaluation of a fetal mass shows incidental mild dilatation of the right maternal collecting system ➡, which extended to the pelvic brim. The left collecting system ➡ is normal. Note the posterior uterine wall ➡.* (Right) *Longitudinal color Doppler US through the retroperitoneum shows significant right ureteral dilatation. The ureter tapers where it crosses the iliac vessels ➡. Ureterectasis is more common on the right. Note the loops of umbilical cord ➡.*

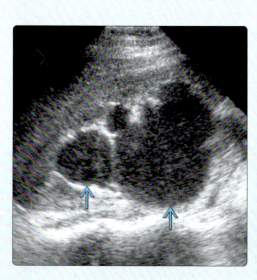

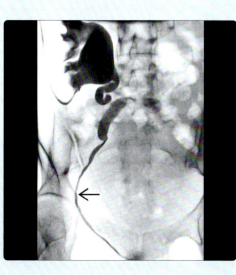

(Left) *Longitudinal US through the right kidney shows unusually marked dilation of the right renal pelvis and calyces ➡ in a pregnant woman.* (Right) *Antegrade nephrostogram performed after delivery in the same patient shows lateral displacement of the distal right ureter ➡ by the enlarged uterus. Note the persistent dilation of the proximal right ureter and right collecting system despite placement of a nephrostomy catheter.*

SECTION 6
Bladder

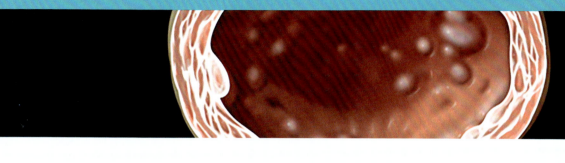

Embryology and Anatomy

The bladder is a hollow distensible viscus with a strong muscular wall. Embryologically, it forms from the urogenital sinus, which is contiguous with the allantois (a hindgut diverticulum that extends to the umbilicus). The allantois normally involutes by the 2nd month of gestation, forming the median umbilical ligament. Any persistent segments of the allantoic channel are called urachal remnants.

The distal ureters are incorporated into the posterolateral portion of the bladder wall at the trigone. The urethral orifice forms the distal apex of the trigone at the bladder base.

The bladder wall consists of 4 layers. The lumen is lined by uroepithelium, which consists of 3-7 layers of stratified flat cells. These cells are flexible and can change shape from cuboidal to flattened as the bladder distends (hence the term transitional epithelium). The 2nd layer is the lamina propria, which is very vascular. The 3rd layer is the detrusor muscle (muscularis propria). The detrusor muscle is a complex network of interlacing smooth muscle fibers. The inner and outer muscle fibers tend to be oriented in a longitudinal fashion, but distinct layers are usually not discernible. Fibers from the detrusor muscle merge with the prostate capsule (or anterior vagina in females) and pelvic floor muscles. A 4th adventitial layer is formed by connective tissue. A serosal covering, formed by the peritoneum, is present only over the bladder dome.

The bladder is located within the extraperitoneal space and is surrounded by loose connective tissue and pelvic fat. The perivesical space contains the bladder and urachus. The prevesical space (also called space of Retzius) extends anteriorly to the pubic symphysis and communicates posteriorly with the presacral space. These spaces can expand to contain large amounts of fluid as in an extraperitoneal bladder rupture or hemorrhage from pelvic fractures.

Imaging Techniques and Indications

Conventional Cystogram

Conventional cystography is primarily used to evaluate for bladder leak (either abdominal trauma or iatrogenic injury) or for fistulae (vesicocolic, vesicoenteric, vesicovaginal). Cystography has an accuracy rate of 90-100% for detecting bladder injury if performed properly.

A scout film should be performed in all cases before infusion of contrast. It is imperative that adequate bladder distention is obtained with a minimum of 300 cc of contrast. Small leaks are easily missed if the bladder is not appropriately distended. Ideally, the study should be performed under fluoroscopy with oblique images. However, in practice, these patients often have pelvic fractures and are not mobile. Diagnostic images can still be obtained in this situation, but it is imperative to obtain images of a maximally filled bladder and a postdrainage film. The importance of the postdrainage film cannot be overemphasized because in ~ 10% of cases, the injury is only seen on the postdrainage film.

Leaks may occur in the extraperitoneal space, and appear as focal collections of contrast, or in the intraperitoneal space, in which the contrast is free flowing and outlines bowel loops. Fistulae are also well demonstrated with contrast accumulating in the small bowel, colon, or vagina.

CT Cystogram

CT cystography has an equal sensitivity and specificity to conventional cystography for bladder leaks and can be performed at the time of the initial trauma CT. Note that merely clamping the Foley catheter during a routine abdominopelvic CT is inadequate for evaluating bladder injury.

After routine CT, the bladder should be drained and a minimum of 350 cc of dilute contrast instilled followed by a repeat scan through the bladder. Multiplanar reformations in the coronal and sagittal plane have been shown to be helpful delineating the precise point of injury. Unlike with conventional cystography, a postdrainage film is not required.

CT and MR

Both modalities are suboptimal in evaluating the bladder wall. Underdistention can erroneously simulate wall thickening, and small, sessile masses can be obscured with overdistention. The depth of mural invasion by tumors cannot currently be accurately determined with either modality. MR has moderate accuracy in assessment of T stage. Currently, the predominant role of imaging in bladder tumor evaluation is to differentiate organ-confined from nonorgan-confined disease and to look for lymphadenopathy and distant metastasis. Continued advancements in multiparametric MR techniques may result in improved accuracy in T staging in the near future.

Ultrasound

The bladder is easily seen with transabdominal imaging, but such imaging is fraught with potential pitfalls. It is easy to overidentify bladder wall thickening, unless the bladder is adequately distended. In addition, the anterior wall is poorly evaluated secondary to reverberation artifact. Color Doppler is useful to evaluate the vascularity of masses and presence of ureteral jets. Postvoid residuals are also easily calculated.

Approach to Bladder Mass

Pathologic conditions of the bladder can manifest as either a focal bladder mass or diffuse wall thickening. Focal masses are most commonly neoplastic but may develop secondary to congenital, inflammatory, or infectious processes. Some focal defects, such as ureteroceles, have a very diagnostic appearance. Extrinsic inflammatory diseases, such as Crohn disease and diverticulitis, may be associated with fistulae to the bladder and cause a focal bladder wall abnormality. In many cases, the clinical, macroscopic, and radiologic findings for these masses may overlap; thus, histologic evaluation is often required.

Bladder neoplasms can arise from any of the bladder layers. They are broadly classified as either epithelial or nonepithelial (mesenchymal) neoplasia. Greater than 95% of bladder neoplasms are epithelial. Epithelial tumors that differentiate from normal urothelium are urothelial cell carcinomas. The spectrum of neoplasia ranges from benign papilloma, to carcinoma in situ, to invasive carcinoma. Other primary epithelial tumors include squamous carcinoma and adenocarcinoma. Because epithelial masses derive from the most superficial layer of the bladder wall, they often appear as irregular, intraluminal filling defects.

Neoplasms derived from mesenchymal tissue differentiate toward muscle, nerve, cartilage, fat, fibrous tissue, and blood vessels. Benign tumors include leiomyoma, paraganglioma, fibroma, hemangioma, solitary fibrous tumor, neurofibroma, and lipoma. Malignant tumors include rhabdomyosarcoma, leiomyosarcoma, lymphoma, and osteosarcoma. Because mesenchymal tumors arise from the submucosal portion of the bladder wall, they often appear as smooth intramural lesions. If large, however, they can ulcerate and be confused with a mucosal mass.

Some neoplasms can cause diffuse wall thickening (adenocarcinoma and lymphoma most commonly), but this is more typically seen in nonneoplastic disorders. Diffuse bladder wall thickening can develop secondary to many conditions, including infection with bacteria or adenovirus, schistosomiasis, tuberculosis, and inflammatory conditions, such as cystitis cystica, cystitis glandularis, or eosinophilic cystitis. Exposure to chemotherapy (particularly with cyclophosphamide) or irradiation also cause diffuse wall thickening. Although the radiologic characteristics of these disorders are less specific, radiologic evaluation is still valuable.

Cystitis appears as a thick-walled bladder with enhancing mucosa and perivesicular inflammatory changes. The various types of cystitis require pathologic diagnosis. Bladder infection with tuberculosis and schistosomiasis produce nonspecific bladder wall thickening and ulceration in the acute phase and should be suspected in patients who are immunocompromised or from regions where these infections are common. In the chronic phase, the bladder wall may calcify; wall calcification is a characteristic finding of chronic schistosomiasis. The diagnosis of chemotherapy cystitis and radiation cystitis should be clinically evident, but imaging may be used to determine severity and to assess complications.

Selected References

1. Rajesh A et al: Bladder cancer: evaluation of staging accuracy using dynamic MRI. Clin Radiol. 66(12):1140-5, 2011
2. Ramchandani P et al: Imaging of genitourinary trauma. AJR Am J Roentgenol. 192(6):1514-23, 2009
3. Wong-You-Cheong JJ et al: From the archives of the AFIP: inflammatory and nonneoplastic bladder masses: radiologic-pathologic correlation. Radiographics. 26(6):1847-68, 2006
4. Wong-You-Cheong J et al: Neoplasms of the urinary bladder: radiologic-pathologic correlation. RadioGraphics 26: 553-580',2006
5. Tekes A et al: Dynamic MRI of bladder cancer: evaluation of staging accuracy. AJR Am J Roentgenol. 184(1):121-7, 2005

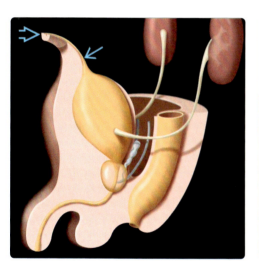

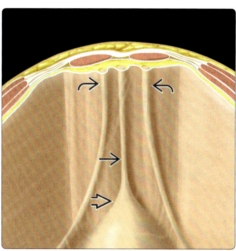

(Left) *Graphic of a developing male fetus shows the urachus ➡ extending from the bladder dome to the umbilicus ➡. Normally, this involutes to form the median umbilical ligament. Failure to do so leads to a host of urachal anomalies.* (Right) *Posterior view of the anterior pelvic wall shows the median umbilical ligament ➡ as a midline structure extending cephalad from the bladder dome ➡. On either side are the medial umbilical folds ➡, which cover the obliterated umbilical arteries.*

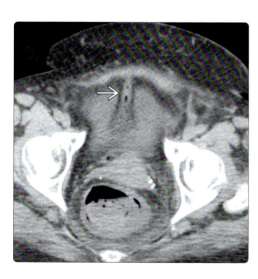

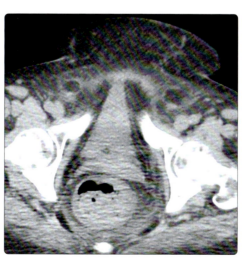

(Left) *Axial NECT shows gas within a small urachal diverticulum ➡. This diverticulum is outlined by ascites on either side. This continued superiorly to the umbilicus as a fibrous cord, the median umbilical ligament.* (Right) *More inferior NECT in the same patient shows a triangle-shaped bladder due to the urachal diverticulum.*

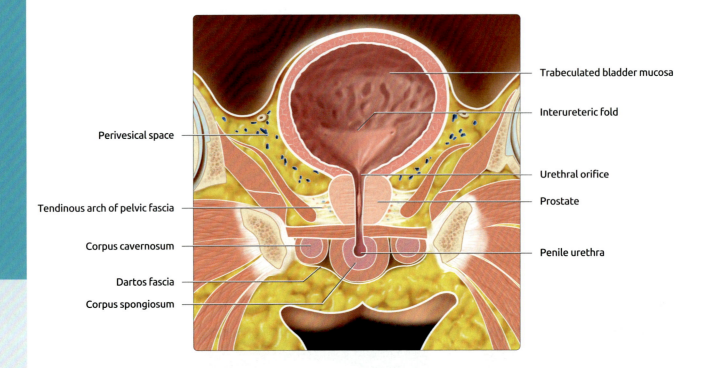

Trabeculated bladder mucosa

Interureteric fold

Urethral orifice

Prostate

Penile urethra

Perivesical space

Tendinous arch of pelvic fascia

Corpus cavernosum

Dartos fascia

Corpus spongiosum

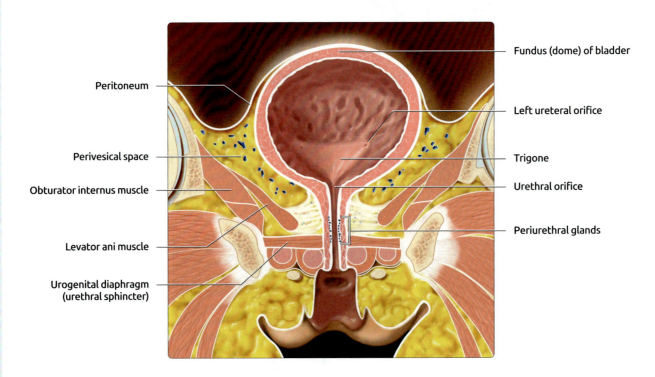

Fundus (dome) of bladder

Left ureteral orifice

Trigone

Urethral orifice

Periurethral glands

Peritoneum

Perivesical space

Obturator internus muscle

Levator ani muscle

Urogenital diaphragm
(urethral sphincter)

(Top) *Coronal section of the male bladder shows that it rests on the prostate. The bladder wall is muscular, strong, and very distensible. The ureters enter the bladder through an oblique anteromedial course that helps to prevent urinary reflux into the ureters.* (Bottom) *Coronal section of the female bladder shows that it rests almost directly on the muscular floor of the pelvis. The dome of the bladder is covered with peritoneum. The trigone is a distinct triangular structure at the base of the bladder whose apices are formed by the ureteral and urethral orifices. The bladder is surrounded by a layer of loose fat and connective tissue (perivesical space) that communicates with the retroperitoneum.*

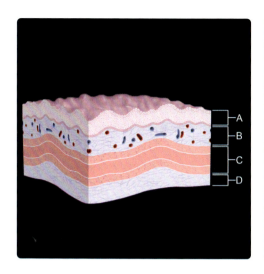 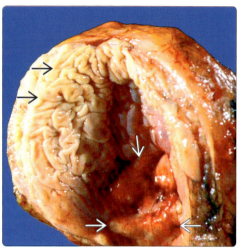

(Left) *Graphic of the 4 layers of the bladder wall shows the urothelium (A), lamina propria (B), muscularis propria (detrusor muscle) (C), and adventitia (D). A 5th layer, the peritoneum, is present only over the dome of the bladder.* (Right) *Gross specimen shows the opened bladder. Note the redundancy of the normal urothelium ⇒ in its collapsed state. A hemorrhagic, fungating urothelial tumor (urothelial cell carcinoma) ➡ is seen at the bladder base protruding into the lumen.*

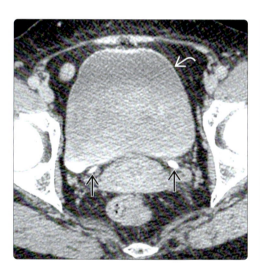 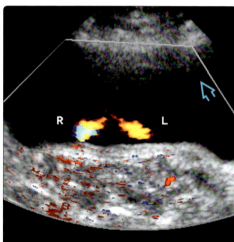

(Left) *Axial CECT of a well-distended bladder shows the ureters ➡ entering the bladder. This marks the level of the bladder trigone. Note the very uniform, thin bladder wall ➡.* (Right) *Transverse color Doppler ultrasound shows bilateral ureteral jets indicating patency of the ureters. Note reverberation artifact ➡ off the anterior bladder wall. This is a major pitfall when using ultrasound to evaluate the bladder.*

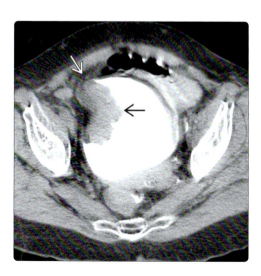 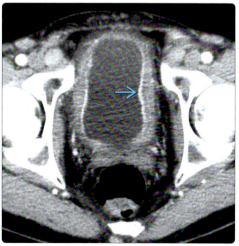

(Left) *Axial CT cystogram show an irregular mucosal mass ➡, which was a urothelial cell carcinoma that had subtle invasion ➡ into the adjacent perivesical fat (T3b lesion). Focal mucosal masses are predominately malignant.* (Right) *Axial CECT shows diffuse bladder wall thickening with mucosal hyperenhancement ➡. This was chemotherapy-related cystitis from cyclophosphamide. Diffuse bladder wall thickening is more commonly benign but can be seen with some malignancies.*

TERMINOLOGY

- **Urachal anomalies**: Spectrum of anomalies due to incomplete obliteration of embryonic connection between bladder dome and allantoic duct
- **Patent urachus**: Entire urachal channel fails to close
- **Urachal cyst**: Umbilical and bladder openings close; channel between remains open and fluid filled
- **Urachal sinus**: Dilatation of urachus at umbilical end; no communication with bladder
- **Urachal diverticulum** (a.k.a. urachal remnant): Dilatation of urachus at vesical end; no communication with umbilicus
- Vestigial obliterated urachus (median umbilical ligament)

IMAGING

- Urachal diverticulum: Midline cystic lesion at anterosuperior aspect of bladder
- Urachal cyst
  - Midline cyst above bladder dome
  - May have rim calcification

- Urachal carcinoma
  - Midline supravesical soft tissue mass
  - Calcification in 70%

TOP DIFFERENTIAL DIAGNOSES

- Cystic lesions near bladder/umbilicus
  - Vitelline cyst: Failure in complete obliteration of omphalomesenteric duct
  - Mesenteric cyst/abdominal abscess
- Bladder tumor
  - Primary dome bladder carcinoma or metastasis

CLINICAL ISSUES

- Complications
  - Stone formation and infection in urachal diverticulum
  - Adenocarcinoma in urachal remnant
    - Poor prognosis related to late presentation: Role of prophylactic surgery for prevention of adenocarcinoma highly controversial

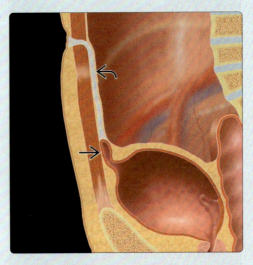

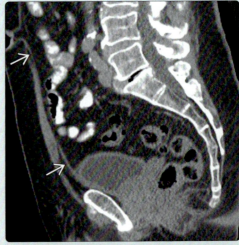

(Left) Sagittal graphic shows a tubular channel ⬑ extending from the dome of the bladder in the midline, which represents a urachal diverticulum. The normal obliterated urachus (median umbilical ligament) ➡ extends to the umbilicus. (Right) Sagittal NECT through the midline shows a normal-appearing obliterated urachus ➡, also known as the median umbilical ligament.

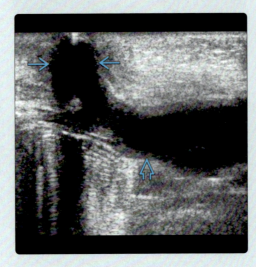

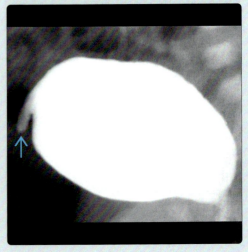

(Left) Midline sagittal ultrasound through the urinary bladder shows a tubular anechoic channel ➡ extending from the bladder dome ⬈, which represents urachal diverticulum. (Right) Lateral view from retrograde cystogram shows a tubular structure ➡ arising from the bladder dome and extending toward the umbilicus, which represents a urachal diverticulum. (Courtesy of G. Friedland, MD.)

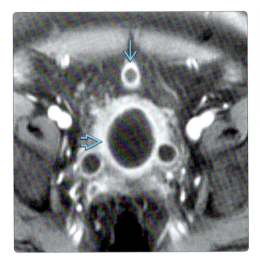

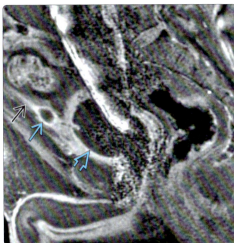

(Left) *Axial contrast-enhanced T1WI MR shows a small cystic structure ➡, anterior and superior to the bladder dome ➡.* (Right) *Sagittal contrast-enhanced T1WI MR in the same patient again shows the cystic structure ➡, superior to the bladder dome ➡. Note the median umbilical ligament ➡ connecting the bladder dome to the umbilicus. A urachal cyst results when the bladder and umbilical ends of the fetal urachus obliterate, while the central part of the tract remains open, as in this case.*

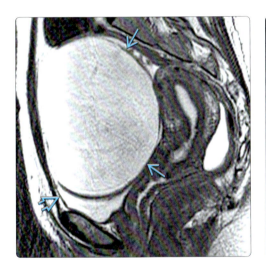

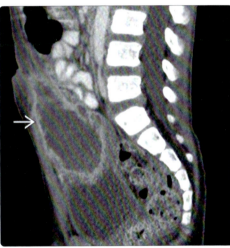

(Left) *Sagittal T2WI MR shows a large urachal cyst ➡ depressing the dome of the urinary bladder ➡ and displacing the uterus posteriorly.* (Right) *Sagittal CECT in a 5-year-old boy with history of incidental cystic mass on ultrasound demonstrates a rim-enhancing complex cyst ➡ superior to the bladder dome and extending toward the umbilicus. The patient underwent exploratory laparotomy, which showed infected urachal cyst.*

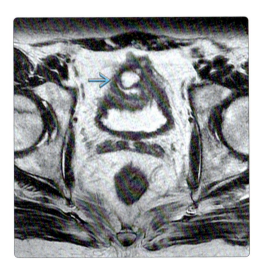

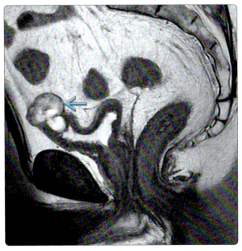

(Left) *Axial T2 SSFSE MR shows a complex solid/cystic mass ➡ attached to the bladder dome.* (Right) *Midline sagittal T2 SSFSE MR in the same patient again demonstrates the complex solid/cystic mass ➡ attached to the bladder dome. The patient could not receive IV contrast due to renal failure. Given its morphology, and vascularity on ultrasound, this lesion was highly concerning for a carcinoma within the urachal remnant. Patient underwent partial cystectomy, and pathology was consistent with adenocarcinoma.*

TERMINOLOGY

- Anorectal malformation of female patients in which rectum, urethra, & vagina converge to form common channel draining to single perineal orifice, which allows clinical diagnosis
- Imaging performed for operative planning & to evaluate associated malformations

IMAGING

- Radiographs: Multiple dilated bowel loops ± Ca²⁺ (from mixing of meconium and urine)
- US: Renal, pelvic, & spine
  - Cystic pelvic mass: Most commonly hydrocolpos (> 35% of all cloaca patients)
    - Rarely dilated bladder, meconium pseudocyst
  - ± hemivaginas/hemiuterus (40%)
  - ± hydroureteronephrosis
  - ± echogenic calcified meconium in dilated bowel or bladder
  - ± spinal anomalies
- Postcolostomy distal colostogram/cloacagram prior to definitive repair

TOP DIFFERENTIAL DIAGNOSES

- Other low/distal neonatal bowel obstructions
- Megacystis-microcolon-intestinal hypoperistalsis syndrome
- Urogenital sinus (GI tract separate)

CLINICAL ISSUES

- Hydrocolpos → ↓ renal function without urgent drainage if causing hydronephrosis
- Prognosis based on common channel length
  - < 3 cm: Most common type (56%), less complex repair, better functional prognosis
  - > 3 cm: Less common type (44%), more complex repair, worse functional prognosis
- Do not confuse with cloacal exstrophy (failed closure of lower abdominal wall in males and females)

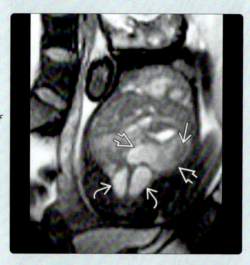 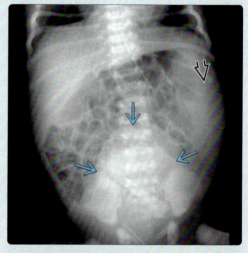

(Left) Coronal SSFP MR in a 31-week-gestation female fetus with a cloaca shows 2 dilated hemivaginas ➡ & a dilated but tapering distal colon ➡. The heterogeneous, low-signal material ➡ within the dilated colon suggests enterolithiasis from mixture of meconium and urine. (Right) AP abdominal radiograph in a 1-day-old girl with cloaca shows a large soft tissue mass arising from the pelvis ➡ displacing bowel, likely representing hydrocolpos. The increased left flank soft tissue is likely due to meconium-filled colon ➡.

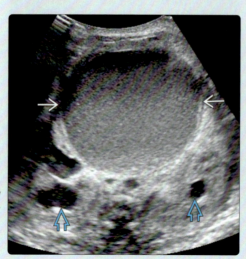 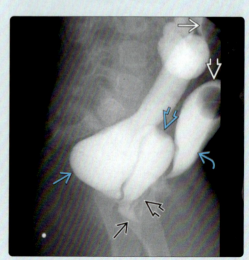

(Left) Transverse US in the same patient shows a markedly distended vagina ➡ filled with echogenic fluid. There is moderate hydroureteronephrosis ➡ of both collecting systems. The urinary bladder (not shown) was compressed by hydrocolpos. (Right) Injection of a mucous fistula ➡ & vesicostomy ➡ shows filling of the rectum ➡, vagina (with cervical impression) ➡, & bladder ➡ plus urethra ➡. All of these structures drain into a common channel (or cloaca) ➡.

Bladder Exstrophy

TERMINOLOGY

- Classic bladder exstrophy (CBE): Low midline abdominal wall defect with exposure of bladder plate & urethra + low-set umbilicus
  - Split lower abdominal skin & rectus abdominis + pubic symphysis diastasis
  - Bifid clitoris in females, epispadias in males
  - Deficient genitalia & pelvic floor muscles
- Epispadias: Abnormal dorsal urethral opening
  - With CBE, entire dorsal urethra open with abnormal bladder sphincter

IMAGING

- Absent urinary bladder by prenatal sonography with normal amniotic fluid
- Pubic symphysis diastasis
- Lobular soft tissue at lower abdominal wall
- High rates of vesicoureteral reflux & dysfunctional bladder prior to ureteral reimplants & bladder neck reconstruction

TOP DIFFERENTIAL DIAGNOSES

- Cloacal exstrophy/OEIS complex: Look for sacral anomalies
- Omphalocele
- Gastroschisis
- Impaired urine production causing absent bladder on prenatal imaging

PATHOLOGY

- Possibly due to cloacal membrane overgrowth prohibiting mesodermal medial migration → results in failed fusion of midline structures below umbilicus & cloacal membrane rupture

CLINICAL ISSUES

- Incidence of 1:10,000-1:50,000 live births
- 2.3-6.0:1.0 = M:F
- Staged repair vs. complete primary repair
  - Continence achieved in up to 81%
  - Most perform clean intermittent catheterization

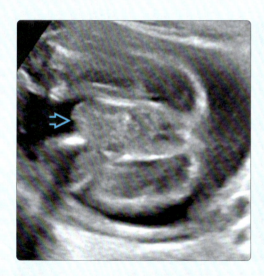
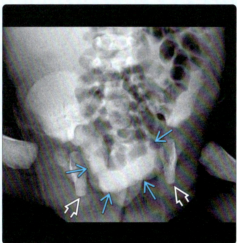

(Left) Axial US in a 32-week gestational age fetus demonstrates abnormal soft tissue ⇨ anterior to the pelvis below the cord insertion (not shown), suspicious for bladder exstrophy. The diagnosis was confirmed postnatally. (Right) AP pelvic radiograph in a neonate with bladder exstrophy shows globular soft tissue of the open bladder plate ⇨ with splayed pubic and ischial ⇨ bones. Note the normal sacrum. This can help differentiate this entity from cloacal exstrophy in which the sacrum is dysplastic or hypoplastic.

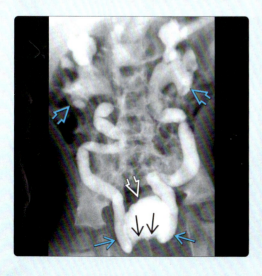
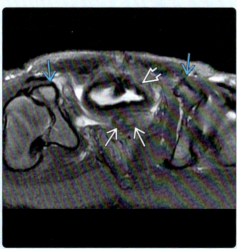

(Left) Frontal VCUG in a 3-year-old girl after bladder exstrophy repair shows a small lobulated bladder ⇨ with elevated bladder base ⇨, J-shaped ureterovesical junctions ⇨, and bilateral high-grade vesicoureteral reflux ⇨. (Right) Axial T2 MR in a 9-month-old girl with bladder exstrophy status post repair with urethroplasty and bladder neck reconstruction shows pubis diastasis ⇨ and bladder irregularity ⇨. Also note 2 cervices of uterine didelphys ⇨.

KEY FACTS

IMAGING

- Acute: Bladder wall thickening, ± hypodense wall (edema), ± perivesical inflammatory changes
- Chronic: Contracted, irregular, thick-walled bladder
- Emphysematous: Gas in bladder wall and lumen

TOP DIFFERENTIAL DIAGNOSES

- Cystitis secondary to adjacent inflammation (such as diverticulitis or salpingitis)
- Bladder underdistention
- Bladder outlet obstruction
- Neurogenic bladder
- Bladder carcinoma

PATHOLOGY

- **Infectious cystitis**
  - Bacterial
  - Schistosomiasis: Inflammatory response to ova deposited in bladder submucosa
  - Emphysematous: Infection with *Escherichia coli*, *Enterobacter aerogenes*, or *Candida* infection; seen in immunosuppressed and diabetic patients
- **Noninfectious cystitis**
  - Mechanical: Local irritation from indwelling catheter, stone, foreign body, etc.
  - Drug related: Cyclophosphamide (hemorrhagic cystitis)
  - Radiation induced
  - Idiopathic interstitial cystitis: Pancystitis causing severe urgency and frequency

CLINICAL ISSUES

- Less common in men due to longer length of urethra and antibacterial properties of prostatic fluid
- **Risk factors**: Sexual intercourse, spermicide use, urogenital anomalies, bladder outlet obstruction, foreign bodies, history of prior urinary tract infections

(Left) Axial CECT shows gas within the bladder lumen and wall ➡ as well as in the renal transplant pelvicalyceal system ➡ compatible with emphysematous cystitis/pyelitis. There was no history of recent instrumentation to account for intravesical/intrarenal gas. (Right) Axial CECT shows eccentric bladder wall thickening with perivesical inflammatory changes ➡ compatible with cystitis, likely due to chronic irritation by an indwelling catheter. Wall hyperemia suggests cystitis, rather than a neoplasm.

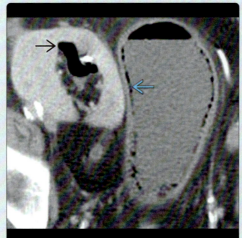
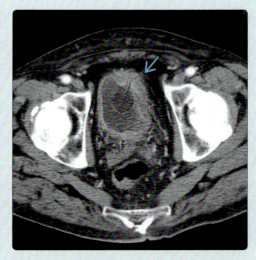

(Left) Axial CT shows marked bladder wall thickening and engorged perivesical blood vessels. The patient was receiving cyclophosphamide, which is excreted in the urine, and these changes were felt to be due to chemical cystitis. Cancer patients are at increased risk of infectious cystitis; urinalysis is helpful in differentiating these 2 entities. (Right) Axial CT in a patient with history of recent external beam radiation for rectal carcinoma ➡ shows bladder wall thickening ➡ representing acute radiation-induced cystitis.

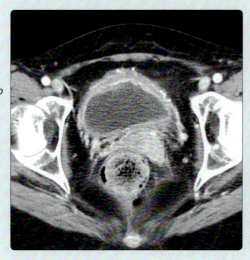
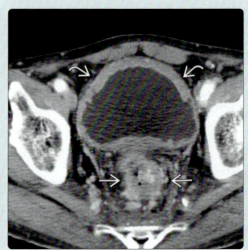

Bladder Schistosomiasis

KEY FACTS

TERMINOLOGY
- Bilharziasis, parasitic infection
- Infection of urinary system by parasite *Schistosoma haematobium*

IMAGING
- Imaging findings mirror pathologic course
  - Acute phase: Nodular bladder wall thickening
  - Chronic phase: Contracted, fibrotic, thick-walled bladder with calcifications
- Calcifications of bladder wall
  - ± calcification of ureter (34%), seminal vesicle (late)
  - Calcification best seen on NECT
- Mucosal irregularity, inflammatory pseudopolyps of bladder
- Ureteritis cystica, cystitis cystica, distal ureteric stricture

TOP DIFFERENTIAL DIAGNOSES
- Bladder calculi
- Bladder carcinoma
- Cystitis
- Emphysematous cystitis (gas can mimic wall calcification on US)

PATHOLOGY
- Clinical manifestations are attributed to host immune response and hypersensitivity reactions
  - Cell-mediated (type IV) immune response: Dominant pathogenetic pathway by forming granulomata (inflammatory and fibrotic phases)
  - Immune-complex-mediated (type III) response: Plays role in glomerulonephritis

CLINICAL ISSUES
- Endemic in Middle East, India, Africa, Central America, and South America
- Confirm diagnosis by identifying ova of parasite in urine
- Squamous cell carcinoma of bladder is late complication

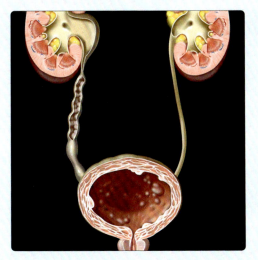
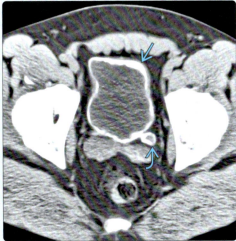

(Left) Schematic drawing shows a markedly thickened urinary bladder wall with mucosal irregularity and mural calcifications. Changes of ureteritis cystica and cystitis cystica are also seen in the bladder and in the dilated right ureter. (Right) Axial NECT shows profound bladder wall calcification ➡, which also extends to involve the left ureter ➡. Calcifications are seen in the chronic phase of the infection and represent calcified granulomata.

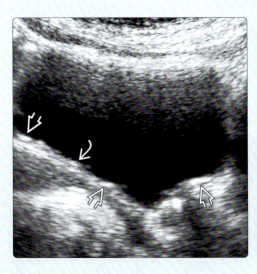
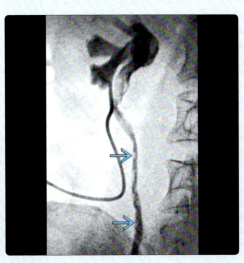

(Left) Longitudinal ultrasound shows multiple echogenic foci of calcifications ➡ and mucosal irregularity ➡ of the posterior bladder wall. Bladder volume is reduced. (Right) Frontal projection from antegrade nephrostogram shows the typical appearance of ureteritis cystica ➡ caused by infection with Schistosoma haematobium.

Bladder

TERMINOLOGY

- Concretions of mineral salts within bladder lumen
- Classified as migrant, primary (idiopathic), and secondary
- Outlet obstruction is primary mechanism for 70% of adult bladder stones

IMAGING

- Round, oval, spiculated, laminated, faceted
- All bladder calculi are radiopaque on CT

TOP DIFFERENTIAL DIAGNOSES

- Other bladder calcifications
  - Urachal carcinoma: Punctate or coarse calcification in mass at bladder dome
  - Schistosomiasis: Calcification in bladder wall
- Other pelvic calcifications
  - Prostate calcification, prostatic and seminal vesicular stones, calcified fibroids
- Filling defect in bladder
  - Blood clot, fungus ball, ureterocele, tumor

PATHOLOGY

- **Stasis**: Bladder outlet obstruction, neurogenic bladder, bladder diverticula
- **Infection**: Especially with *Proteus mirabilis*
- **Foreign bodies**: Nidus for crystal growth
- **Bladder augmentation**: Metabolic derangement and stasis
- Most are mixture of calcium oxalate and calcium phosphate

CLINICAL ISSUES

- Most are asymptomatic
  - Some have suprapubic pain, microhematuria
- Clinical scenarios
  - Elderly man with bladder outlet obstruction
  - Spinal cord injury patient with indwelling Foley catheter
  - Bladder augmentation with ileal or colonic segments
- Complication: Malignant bladder tumors in patients with stones from indwelling Foley catheters

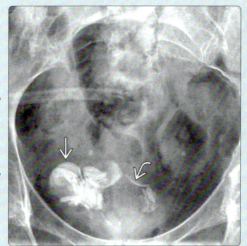
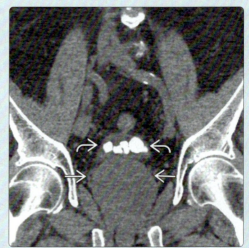

(Left) Plain film frontal radiograph in a 37-year-old woman with paraplegia and microhematuria shows multiple calculi ⟶ within the bladder. Some have a peculiar curvilinear shape ⟶, suggesting that they may have formed around foreign bodies. (Right) Coronal NECT in 90-year-old man with history of benign prostatic hyperplasia shows numerous calcified bladder calculi ⟶, presumably secondary to chronic urinary outlet obstruction. Note the prostate ⟶.

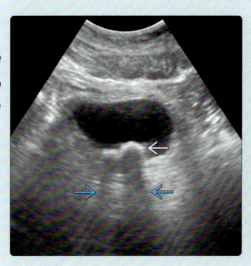
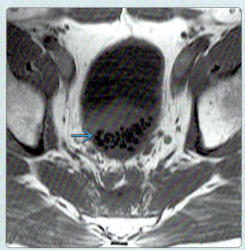

(Left) Transverse US through the bladder shows 2 large intravesical calculi ⟶ with extensive posterior shadowing ⟶. The calculi were mobile. (Right) Axial T1WI MR through the bladder shows innumerable round signal void foci ⟶ in the dependent portion of the bladder, representing calculi in a man with marked prostatic enlargement. Bladder calculi are hypointense on T1WI and T2WI MR due to the diamagnetic property of calcium salts.

Bladder Diverticulum

TERMINOLOGY

- Sac formed by herniation of bladder mucosa and submucosa through muscular wall
- **Hutch diverticulum**: Congenital form due to weakness in detrusor muscle anterolateral to ureteral orifice

IMAGING

- Perivesical cystic mass with connection to bladder
- May be multiple; smooth wall
- May contain debris, calculi, or tumor
- CT: Water-attenuation outpouching from bladder
- MR: Homogeneous low signal on T1WI; high on T2WI
  - May see loss of signal on T2WI due to dephasing with motion of urine between diverticulum and lumen
- US: Anechoic outpouching from bladder with visible neck
  - Check for emptying on postvoid imaging as indicator of degree of stasis
- VCUG: Preferred modality in young children to look for associated vesicoureteral reflux

TOP DIFFERENTIAL DIAGNOSES

- Abdominal abscess
- Postoperative lymphocele
- Everted ureterocele
- Ovarian cystic lesions

PATHOLOGY

- Predisposing conditions: Bladder outlet obstruction, neurogenic bladder, congenital weakness of detrusor muscle
- Lack of muscular wall results in stasis, which has pivotal role in development of complications
- **Complications: Infection, stone, neoplasm**
  - Urothelial carcinoma is most prevalent type
  - Lack of muscularis propria leads to more rapid local spread and poor prognosis

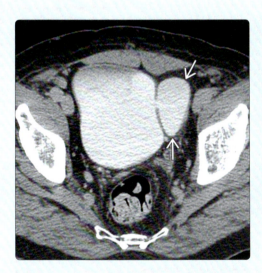
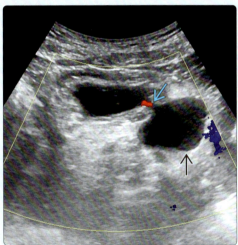

(Left) Axial CT urography in a 78-year-old male patient with history of hematuria shows a large diverticulum ➡, with a relatively narrow neck and with smooth surface, along the left lateral aspect of bladder. (Right) Axial duplex US in a 65-year-old male patient shows a large diverticulum ➡ in the left posterolateral aspect of the bladder with jet flow through its neck ➡ due to the differing specific gravity of urine within the bladder and diverticulum.

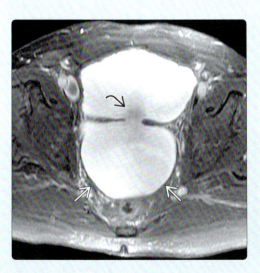
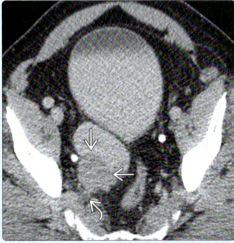

(Left) Axial T2WI MR shows a large posterior bladder diverticulum ➡ connected to the bladder via a broad neck. Signal loss in the connecting channel ➡ is due to the turbulent motion of urine and resultant dephasing. (Right) Axial CECT shows a large enhancing mass ➡ inside a diverticulum. Bulging outside the diverticulum and stranding in perivesical fat ➡ are findings highly suspicious for extramural extension. Pathology showed poorly differentiated carcinoma. The patient developed metastases to liver and lung.

Bladder

TERMINOLOGY

- Nonanatomic communication between bladder and skin or adjacent viscus

IMAGING

- Cystography and contrast enemas
  - Identify fistula in < 50% of cases
- CT: Good overall test for fistula and underlying etiology
  - Enterovesical/colovesical fistula
    - Gas in bladder (90%)
    - CT may depict tract itself, especially if it is in plane of CT section (< 50%)
  - Vesicovaginal
    - Contrast-opacified urine in vagina
- MR: High sensitivity/specificity for depiction of colovesical fistula
  - Majority (~ 70%) of cases have associated abscess
  - Focal bladder wall thickening, gas in bladder, and loss of perivesical fat plane are sensitive findings on MR

TOP DIFFERENTIAL DIAGNOSES

- Cystitis (with gas-forming bacteria)
- Emphysematous cystitis
- Presence of indwelling or recent bladder catheter

PATHOLOGY

- Colovesical fistula
  - Diverticulitis (most common cause: 80% of cases)
- Enterovesical fistula
  - Crohn disease: Most common cause
- Vesicocutaneous fistula
  - Usually due to surgical complication or trauma
- Vesicovaginal
  - Gynecologic surgery (hysterectomy) most common cause
- Colovaginal fistula
  - Diverticulitis or complication of hysterectomy

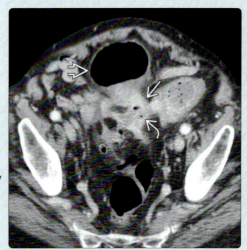
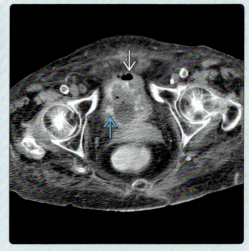

(Left) *Axial CECT in a patient with colovesical fistula from diverticulitis shows extensive sigmoid diverticulosis and inflammation of the surrounding tissues. The bladder contains a large amount of gas ➡. Note the pericolonic collection of gas and fluid ➡ tracking directly to the bladder dome. The fistula ➡ is seen as a contrast-enhancing track.* (Right) *Axial CECT in an elderly woman with history of persistent pyuria shows particulate matter, gas ➡, and enteric contrast medium ➡ within the bladder lumen.*

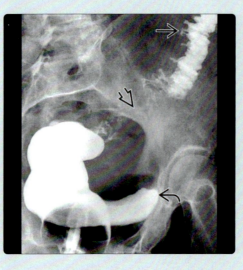
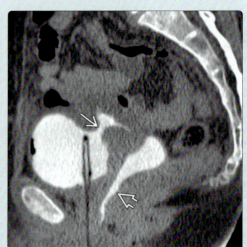

(Left) *Contrast enema in a patient with a history of colovesical fistula from diverticulitis shows several colonic diverticula ➡, spasm of the sigmoid colon ➡, and contrast filling of the bladder ➡, indicating a colovesical fistula.* (Right) *Sagittal CT cystogram in a patient with history of vesicouterine fistula following cesarean section shows a fistulous connection ➡ between the bladder, which has an indwelling catheter, and the uterus. There is subsequent filling of the vagina ➡.*

IMAGING

- **Suprapontine** (above pontine center) lesions → detrusor hyperreflexia
  - Rounding of bladder shape and serration of mucosa above trigone (detrusor contractions)
  - ± trabeculations and ↑ wall thickness
- **Suprasacral** (above S2-S4) lesions → detrusor hyperreflexia with detrusor-sphincter dyssynergia
  - Christmas tree or pine cone shape (severe): Elongated and pointed with pseudodiverticula
- **Peripheral** (below S2-S4) lesions → detrusor areflexia
  - Large atonic bladder
- **Sensory** lesions → inability to sense bladder fullness
  - Rounding of bladder shape and serration of mucosa
- Secondary bladder and upper tract abnormalities
  - Trabeculation, dilated upper tracts, pseudodiverticula, vesicoureteral reflux
- Best imaging test: Cystourethrography at rest and during voiding
- Findings on US vary depending on type and level of neurological damage

TOP DIFFERENTIAL DIAGNOSES

- Bladder outlet obstruction
- Bladder carcinoma

PATHOLOGY

- Suprapontine: Stroke, arteriosclerosis, brain tumor, multiple sclerosis
- Suprasacral: Trauma, tumor, or multiple sclerosis
- Epiconal: Myelomeningocele, tumor, or trauma
- Peripheral (pelvic ± pudendal nerve): Pelvic surgery, cauda equina
- Sensory: Diabetes mellitus, pernicious anemia, or tabes dorsalis

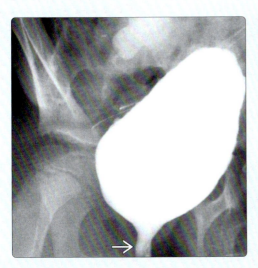

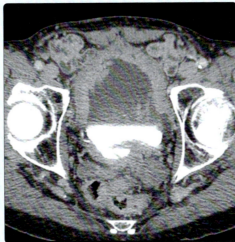

(Left) *Oblique cystogram in a young man with a history of spina bifida demonstrates an elongated, pointed, and mildly trabeculated bladder as well as a distended posterior urethra* ➡️: *Features associated with suprasacral-type (above S2) neurogenic bladder.* (Right) *Axial CECT in a young woman with a traumatic spinal cord injury shows a markedly thickened and trabeculated bladder wall compatible with neurogenic bladder.*

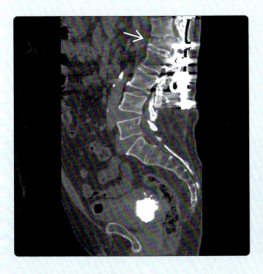

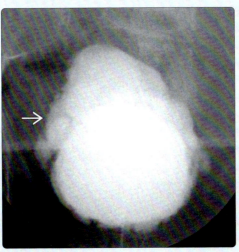

(Left) *Sagittal CECT obtained during urographic phase shows a markedly thickened and trabeculated bladder in this patient with history of a neurogenic bladder due to traumatic spine injury. Note the compression fracture of the L1 vertebral body* ➡️. (Right) *Retrograde cystogram in the same patient better delineates the trabeculae* ➡️. *This appearance can also be seen with chronic urinary outlet obstruction.*

Bladder Trauma

TERMINOLOGY

- Injury due to blunt, penetrating, or iatrogenic trauma

IMAGING

- Extravasation of contrast-opacified urine at cystography (CT or conventional): Almost 100% accuracy
- Contusion (type 1)
  - Ecchymosis of localized segment of bladder wall
- Intraperitoneal rupture (type 2)
  - Opacified urine in peritoneal spaces (pouch of Douglas), outlining bowel loops & intraperitoneal viscera
  - Requires surgical repair
- Interstitial injury (type 3)
  - Intramural tear with intact serosa
- Extraperitoneal rupture (type 4)
  - Perforation by bony spicules of pelvic fractures
  - **Molar tooth sign**: Extravasated perivesical urine assumes rounded configuration cranially & pointed contours inferolaterally

- Usually managed nonoperatively
- Complex (type 4B): Extravasation extends beyond perivesical space; thigh, scrotum, etc.
- Combined injury (type 5): Intra- & extraperitoneal rupture

TOP DIFFERENTIAL DIAGNOSES

- Male urethral injury
  - Extravasated urine can extend into perivesical spaces
- Pelvic or abdominal bleeding
  - Active hemorrhage may simulate bladder rupture
- Blood clot in bladder

PATHOLOGY

- Location of extravasation depends on anatomy
  - Anterosuperior rupture: Extravasation to intraperitoneal, Retzius space, or both
  - Injury below peritoneal reflection → extraperitoneal (paravesical, presacral spaces)

(Left) Axial CECT reveals diastasis ➡ of the pubic symphysis and fluid ➡ within the ventral soft tissues; it is difficult to determine if this is due to urine, hematoma, or a combination of both. (Right) AP view from a follow-up cystogram in the same patient shows extravasation of contrast from the urinary bladder into the extraperitoneal tissues ➡ surrounding the bladder and along the left superior thigh and scrotum. A small volume of contrast is within the urinary bladder ➡.

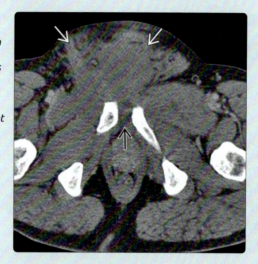
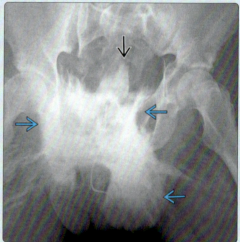

(Left) Axial CECT during the initial trauma evaluation reveals perivesical fluid ➡ for which differential considerations include urine and blood. Mild hemorrhage resides in the ventral subcutaneous tissues ➡ and presacral space ➡. (Right) Axial CT cystogram in the same patient reveals that the perivesical fluid was from extravasated contrast-opacified urine ➡ due to extraperitoneal bladder rupture. Note the molar tooth configuration of the extraperitoneal contrast in the perivesical spaces.

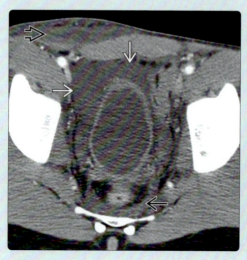
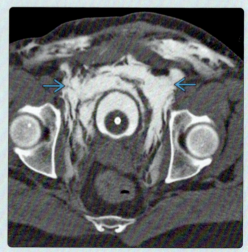

IMAGING

General Features
- Best diagnostic clue
  - Extravasation of contrast-opacified urine at cystography (CT or conventional)
- Other general features
  - Classification of bladder injury after blunt trauma
    - Type 1: Bladder contusion
    - Type 2: Intraperitoneal rupture
    - Type 3: Interstitial injury
    - Type 4A: Simple extraperitoneal rupture
    - Type 4B: Complex extraperitoneal rupture
    - Type 5: Combined injury

Radiographic Findings
- Cystography
  - Bladder contusion (type 1)
    - Pear-shaped bladder: Extrinsic compression of bladder (symmetrical extraperitoneal hematoma)
  - Intraperitoneal rupture (type 2)
    - Intraperitoneal contrast: Outlines small bowel loops & intraperitoneal viscera; layers in dependent peritoneal recesses (pouch of Douglas, Morrison pouch)
    - ± pelvic fractures
  - Interstitial injury (type 3)
    - Focal mural defect along wall of bladder
  - Extraperitoneal rupture (type 4)
    - Simple (type 4A)
      - Flame-shaped extravasation around bladder
    - Complex (type 4B)
      - Extravasation extends beyond pelvis
    - Extravasation often best seen on postdrainage films
  - Combined rupture (type 5)
    - Features of intra- & extraperitoneal ruptures
  - Penetrating injury
    - Foreign bodies (e.g., metallic fragments from bullet) along course of penetration
    - Extravasation ± foreign body (e.g., bullet) best seen on postdrainage films

CT Findings
- CT cystography
  - Bladder contusion (type 1)
    - Normal findings
  - Intraperitoneal rupture (type 2)
    - Opacified urine fills peritoneal spaces (pouch of Douglas, Morrison pouch), outlines bowel loops & intraperitoneal viscera
  - Interstitial injury (type 3)
    - Intramural & submucosal extravasation of contrast without transmural extension
  - Extraperitoneal rupture (type 4)
    - Perforation by bony spicules of pelvic fractures
    - "Knuckle" of bladder: Trapped bladder by displaced fracture of anterior pelvic arch
    - Simple (type 4A): Extravasation is confined to perivesical space

- Complex (type 4B): Extravasation extends beyond perivesical space; thigh, scrotum, penis, perineum, anterior abdominal wall, retroperitoneum (pararenal or perirenal spaces), or hip joint
    - **Molar tooth sign**: Extravasated perivesical contrast assumes rounded contour cranially & pointed contours inferolaterally
  - Combined injury (type 5)
    - Features of intra- & extraperitoneal ruptures

Ultrasonographic Findings
- Grayscale ultrasound
  - "Bladder within bladder": Fluid around bladder
  - Intravesical hematoma

Imaging Recommendations
- Best imaging tool
  - Cystography (CT or conventional): 95-100% sensitivity
    - Nearly 100% accurate if filled to 350 mL
- Protocol advice
  - Cystography
    - Exclude urethral injury in males prior to cystography; if positive, use suprapubic cystostomy tube
    - Postdrainage x-ray to check for extravasation hidden by contrast
    - CT cystography: Instill diluted contrast (10 mL contrast)
      - Multiplanar reformation aids visualization of leak

DIFFERENTIAL DIAGNOSIS

Simple Male Urethral Injury
- Contrast extravasation into base of penis or thigh may result from urethral or extraperitoneal bladder injury
- Blood in urethral meatus suggestive of urethral injury

Hemoperitoneum
- Active extravasation of enhanced blood may simulate extravesical urine from bladder rupture
  - Compare with density of blood and urine
- CT cystography usually diagnostic

Pelvic Bleeding
- Bleeding from other pelvic trauma can appear similar to contrast extravasation from bladder
- Synchronous occurrence with bladder trauma likely; complete pelvic assessment needed

Blood Clot in Bladder
- Blood from renal or bladder injury may cause irregular filling defect within bladder

DIAGNOSTIC CHECKLIST

Consider
- Cystography ± CT still procedure of choice
- Bloody urethral discharge requires urethrogram prior to catheterization of bladder

Image Interpretation Pearls
- CT only after IV contrast may miss bladder rupture
- CT cystogram best single study

(Left) AP view during cystogram reveals bladder displacement ➡ due to hematoma, fracture ➡, and intraperitoneal extravasation ➡ of urine; note that bowel loops ➡ are outlined by the extravasated urine. (Right) Axial NECT in the same patient shows opacified urine layering in the perihepatic space ➡. The density of the fluid ➡ around the spleen is mixed due to a splenic laceration with hematoma and intermixed extravasated urine.

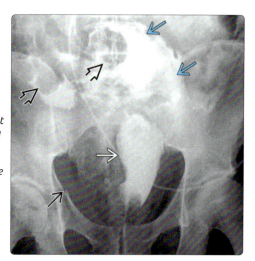

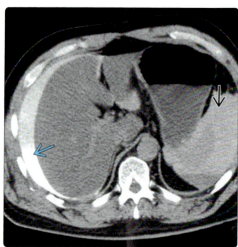

(Left) Axial NECT in the same patient shows the kidneys excreting contrast-opacified urine due to absorption of contrast from the intraperitoneal fluid. Intraperitoneal opacified urine outlines small bowel loops ➡ and distends the Morrison pouch ➡. (Right) Sagittal NECT reformation in the same patient shows the collapsed bladder due to a Foley catheter ➡ and intraperitoneal extravasation of urine ➡ surrounding bowel loops ➡.

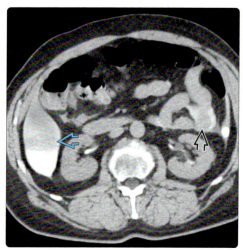

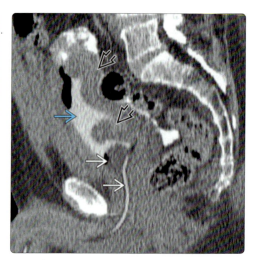

(Left) Axial CECT following a cystogram demonstrates extravasated, contrast-opacified urine ➡ surrounding the uterus ➡, ovaries ➡, and small bowel loops ➡, consistent with intraperitoneal bladder rupture. (Right) Axial CECT following cystogram shows extravasated contrast-opacified urine ➡ in the perivesical spaces due to extraperitoneal bladder rupture. A few locules of gas ➡ deep to the rectus abdominis musculature were due to traumatic soft tissue injuries and pelvic fractures.

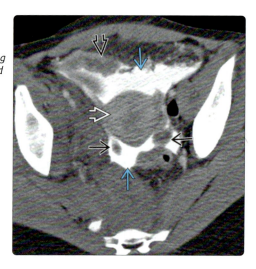

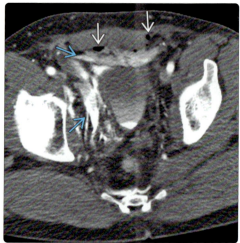

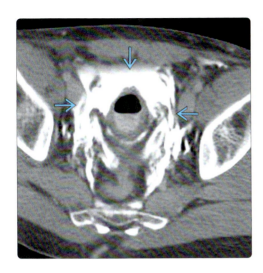

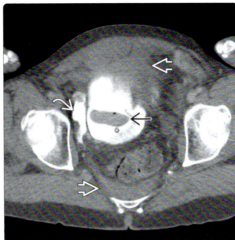

(Left) *Axial CECT following cystogram shows extraperitoneal extravasated urine* ⇨ *with a molar tooth appearance.* (Right) *Axial CT cystogram shows extravasated urine* ⇨ *from the urinary bladder due to extraperitoneal rupture. A hematoma* ⇨ *is in the space of Retzius and the presacral space. A clot* ⇨ *is within the bladder lumen.*

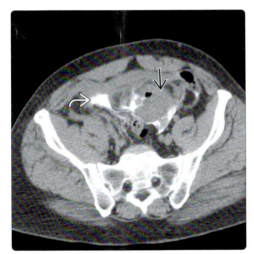

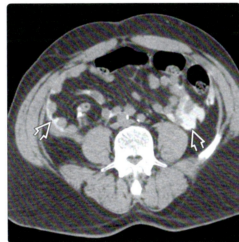

(Left) *Axial CT cystogram shows intraperitoneal extravasation of urine* ⇨ *evidenced by contrast outlining a loop of bowel* ⇨. (Right) *More superior axial image from the same patient during CT cystogram shows extravasated urinary contrast* ⇨ *outlining small bowel segments in the peritoneal cavity.*

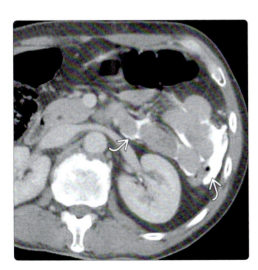

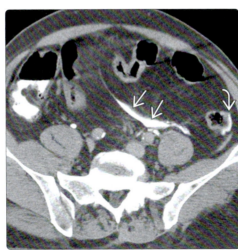

(Left) *Axial CECT following cystogram shows extravasated, opacified urine* ⇨ *outlining the small bowel segment within the peritoneal cavity.* (Right) *Axial CECT following cystogram shows combined intra- and extraperitoneal bladder rupture. Note the small volume of extravasated urine along the left paracolic gutter* ⇨ *and the smooth layering of intraperitoneal contrast* ⇨ *adjacent to the root of the mesentery.*

Postoperative State, Bladder

TERMINOLOGY

- **Segmental cystectomy**
  - Removing full-thickness portion of bladder wall
  - Used for benign and malignant lesions of bladder
- **Simple cystectomy**
  - Total resection of bladder
- **Radical cystectomy**
  - Resection of bladder with its peritoneal covering, perivesical fat, lower ureters, urachal remnant, regional lymph nodes, and adjacent structures
- **Urinary diversion techniques**
  - **Incontinent** diversion techniques
    - Cutaneous ureterostomy, ileal conduit creation
    - Usually performed in patients with poor prognosis
  - **Continent** diversion techniques
    - Cutaneous diversion, orthotopic neobladder reconstruction

- More complicated techniques; method of choice in patients with better prognosis
- **Bladder augmentation**
  - For patients who lack adequate bladder capacity or detrusor compliance
- **Psoas-hitch ureterocystostomy**
  - Technique used for ureteral reimplantation if ureter is not long enough to be sutured without tension
- **Boari flap**
  - Used in cases of ureteral injury when primary repair and primary anastomosis are not achievable due to foreshortening of the ureter
- **Complications**
  - Early complications (< 1 month): Ileus, obstruction, urinary leak, urinary obstruction, fluid collection (urinoma, hematoma, lymphocele, abscess)
  - Late complications: Ureteral stenosis, infection, parastomal herniation, lithiasis, tumor recurrence, metabolic acidosis

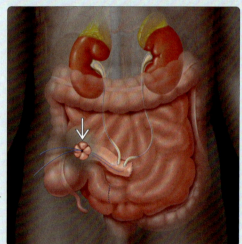
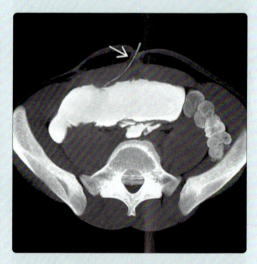

(Left) Graphic shows an ileal conduit diversion in which a segment of ileum is mobilized and serves as a reservoir and conduit for urine. The cutaneous stoma ➡ is at one end, and the ureters are anastomosed to the other end with temporary stents in place. (Right) Axial CT in a patient with a history of neurogenic bladder shows bladder augmentation utilizing ileocecal reservoir and using the appendix as the continent conduit (Mitrofanoff technique). The appendiceal conduit opens to the umbilicus for catheterization ➡.

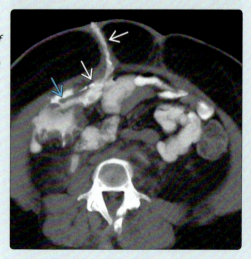
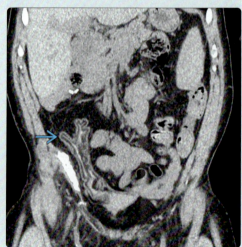

(Left) Axial CECT shows Indiana pouch continent reservoir which is composed of proximal colon and terminal ileum. The terminal ileum (➡) is brought to the skin and is used as the catheterizable stoma while the ileocecal valve (➡) creates a continent valve mechanism. (Right) Coronal CT in a patient with history of a neurogenic bladder shows bladder augmentation ➡ using a segment of ileum. Note the submucosal fat deposition in the ileal loop used for augmentation.

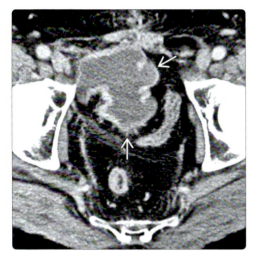
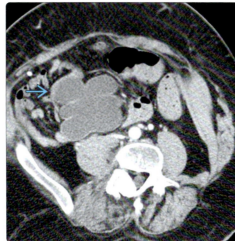

(Left) Axial CECT shows a "neobladder" ➡ constructed from an ileal segment that was anastomosed to the ureters and urethra. This is an example of orthotopic bladder replacement (Studer technique). (Right) Axial CT in a patient with a history of a neurogenic bladder, in the setting of a spine tumor, shows bladder augmentation ⇨ utilizing a segment of ileum.

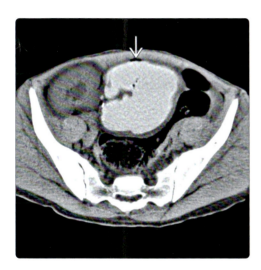
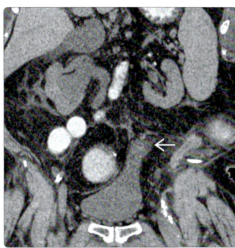

(Left) Axial NECT cystogram in a young man with renal transplant malfunction attributed to low bladder capacity and reflux shows the native bladder augmented by a segment of bowel ➡. (Right) Coronal NECT in a patient with a history of psoas-hitch ureteroneocystostomy shows the bladder mobilized and sutured to the left psoas muscle, resulting in an asymmetric appearance of the bladder dome ➡. The patient was post distal ureteral resection for retroperitoneal fibrosis.

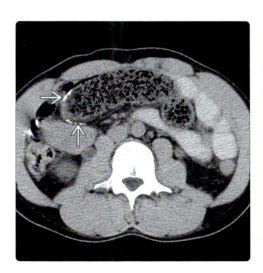
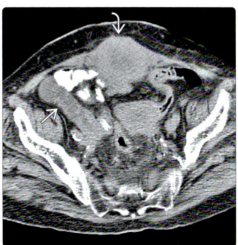

(Left) Axial NECT in patient with history of ileal conduit formation shows dilatation of the ileum and small bowel feces sign reflective of chronic bowel obstruction, presumably related to a stricture at the anastomosis site ➡. (Right) Axial NECT in a patient with history of radical cystectomy and ileal conduit diversion ➡ for bladder cancer shows a soft tissue attenuation mass ➡ that represents recurrent carcinoma.

TERMINOLOGY

- Primary neoplasms of urinary bladder deriving from nonepithelial elements
- Mesenchymal bladder tumors are rare; < 5% of tumors

IMAGING

- **Leiomyoma**
  - Most common mesenchymal tumor showing smooth muscle differentiation
  - Soft tissue-density intramural lesion with avid enhancement; larger lesions tend to be heterogeneous with nonuniform enhancement
  - Low/intermediate signal on T1WI & **low signal on T2WI**; areas of degeneration show ↑ T2 & no enhancement
  - May involved urethra & are thought to be estrogen sensitive
- **Paraganglioma**
  - Round or oval-shaped soft tissue-density mass with broad base
  - Usually have ↑ T1 & intermediate T2 signal on MR
  - Majority of reported cases are symptomatic & functional
- **Neurofibroma**
  - Nodular bladder wall thickening with low density (due to myxoid matrix) & nonuniform enhancement
  - Low to intermediate signal on T1WI MR & ↑ signal (**target sign**) on T2WI; + enhancement
    - Target sign: ↓ intensity central dot (fibrosis) surrounded by ↑ intensity myxoid stroma
- **Hemangioma/vascular malformation**
  - Solitary, small (< 3 cm), intramural mass bulging into bladder lumen
  - Highly vascular & enhancing (similar to hemangioma & vascular malformation in other parts)

TOP DIFFERENTIAL DIAGNOSES

- Bladder urothelial carcinoma
- Bladder metastasis

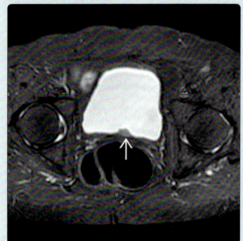
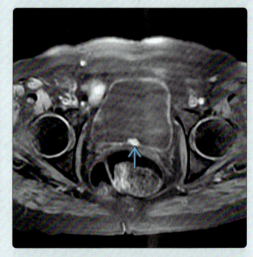

(Left) Axial fat-suppressed STIR MR in a 68-year-old woman with a history of hematuria shows a broad-base filling defect ➡ at the midline bladder trigone. The lesion has intermediate T2 signal. (Right) Axial T1WI MR in the same patient demonstrates inherent T1 hyperintensity of the lesion ➡. The patient underwent partial cystectomy, and the pathology was consistent with paraganglioma.

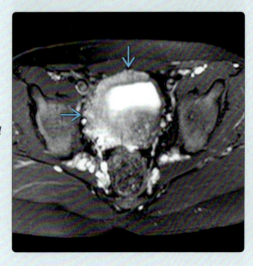
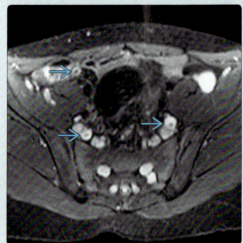

(Left) Axial T2WI MR with fat saturation shows marked nodular bladder wall thickening ➡ in this 9-year-old boy with a history of neurofibromatosis type 1. Note additional plexiform neurofibromas along the pelvic sidewalls and in the perirectal region. (Right) Axial T2WI MR with inversion recovery (a technique utilized to suppress fat) in the same patient shows the target sign in multiple neurofibromas ➡. The target sign is due to central fibrosis surrounded by T2-hyperintense myxoid stroma.

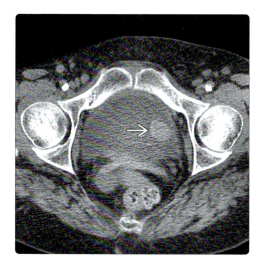

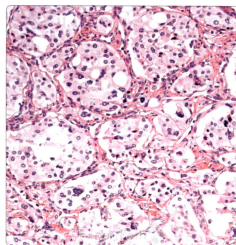

(Left) *Axial unenhanced CT in a 74-year-old man with no urinary symptoms shows an incidental pedunculated lesion ➡ along the left lateral bladder wall. The patient underwent transurethral resection of the tumor. Pathology was consistent with a paraganglioma.* (Right) *Photomicrograph with H&E staining shows classic nested, or zellballen, architecture of paraganglioma.*

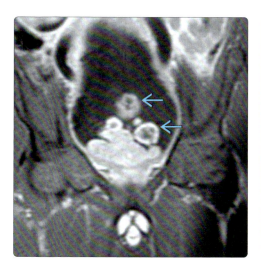

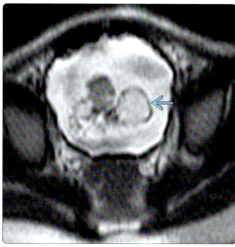

(Left) *Coronal postcontrast T1WI MR in 3 year-old boy shows a large enhancing bladder mass with polypoid intraluminal growth ➡, typical for bladder rhabdomyosarcoma (sarcoma botryoides).* (Right) *Axial T2WI MR in the same patient shows high T2 intensity of the intraluminal polypoid projections ➡, which is attributed to myxoid stroma.*

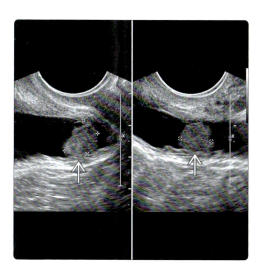

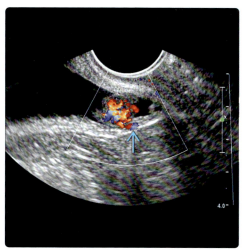

(Left) *Transverse and longitudinal US images through the bladder in a 66-year-old woman show a polypoid lesion ➡ at the inferior aspect of the bladder.* (Right) *Color Doppler shows that the lesion is vascular. Note the lesion's pedicle ➡, which arises from posterior wall. The patient underwent transurethral resection of the tumor. Pathology was compatible with a bladder paraganglioma.*

TERMINOLOGY

- Polypoid bladder mass caused by nonneoplastic proliferation of myofibroblasts and inflammatory cells
- Depending on predominant inflammatory cell in lesion, it might have different names

IMAGING

- Polypoid mass projecting into lumen of bladder
- More common in bladder dome and posterior wall
  - Tends to spare trigone
- Ring enhancement and calcified surface may be seen

TOP DIFFERENTIAL DIAGNOSES

- Bladder urothelial carcinoma
- Bladder rhabdomyosarcoma
- Bladder myxoid leiomyosarcoma

PATHOLOGY

- Unclear etiology

- May be secondary to inflammation following infection, minor trauma, surgery, or malignancy
- Immune-mediated mechanism may play role

CLINICAL ISSUES

- Presenting symptoms: Painless hematuria, dysuria, frequency, lower abdominal pain
- More common in adults; mean age: 39 years
- Locally aggressive tumor; may invade through bladder wall
  - Local recurrence after resection is unusual (< 5%)
- Treatment
  - Surgical resection (transurethral resection of bladder tumor or partial cystectomy)
  - Medical management with long-term antibiotics &/or antiinflammatory medications (steroidal and nonsteroidal)

DIAGNOSTIC CHECKLIST

- Tissue biopsy is needed to establish diagnosis

(Left) Axial NECT shows a large bladder mass with a partially calcified surface ➡ in this 76-year-old woman with gross hematuria and pelvic pain. (Right) Axial CECT in the same patient shows enhancement of the mass ➡. The perivesical fat planes adjacent to the mass are indistinct, suggesting transmural extension of this process.

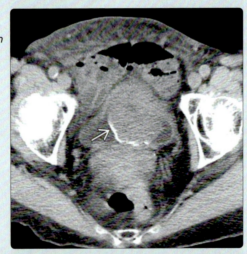
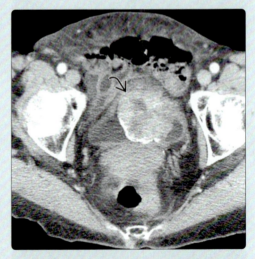

(Left) More caudal axial CECT section in the same patient shows brisk enhancement of the mass ➡ with a central zone of necrosis. (Right) Delayed-phase CECT in the same patient shows the polypoid mass as a filling defect within the contrast-opacified urine. There is a broad-base attachment to the bladder wall ➡. At surgery, the mass was very hard and difficult to extract. The frozen section diagnosis favored sarcoma, but the final diagnosis was inflammatory pseudotumor of the bladder.

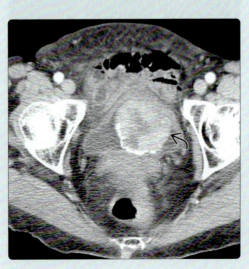
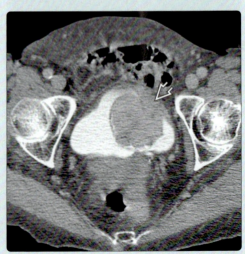

Bladder and Ureteral Intramural Masses

IMAGING

- Mass centered in bladder wall causing impression on bladder lumen; makes obtuse angles with bladder lumen
- Usually have both intravesical and extravesical growth and makes smooth interface with bladder lumen

TOP DIFFERENTIAL DIAGNOSES

- **Leiomyoma**
  - **Most common** mesenchymal tumor of bladder
  - Low signal on T1WI and T2WI MR; shows different degrees of enhancement
  - Shows T2-hyperintense areas of cystic degeneration
- **Leiomyosarcoma**
  - **Most common malignant** mesenchymal tumor of bladder
  - Imaging findings overlap with leiomyoma; usually larger and more heterogeneous containing areas of necrosis
- **Rhabdomyosarcoma**
  - Most common bladder tumor in pediatric population

- **Neurofibroma**
  - Typically low signal on T1WI MR with **target sign** on T2WI MR
- **Paraganglioma**
  - Shows high T1 signal and restricted diffusion on MR
- **Lymphoma**
  - Most often secondary involvement rather than primary
- **Endometriosis**
  - Almost always along posterior aspect of bladder (dependent) and inseparable from adjacent uterus
- **Metastasis**
  - Melanoma, breast, and gastric adenocarcinoma are most frequent primaries
- **Extrinsic masses (mimic)**
  - External compression on bladder can mimic intramural process on antegrade/retrograde cystography and on cystoscopy

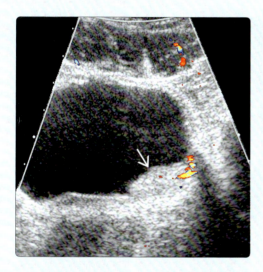

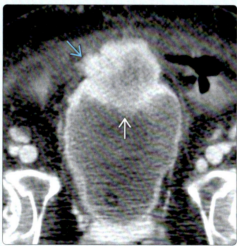

(Left) *Longitudinal color Doppler US of the bladder in a 64-year-old woman with symptoms of cystitis reveals a smooth isoechoic intramural mass* ➡ *in the bladder base without significant flow. Endoscopic biopsy proved this to be a leiomyoma.* (Right) *Axial CECT in a 48-year-old woman with pelvic pain shows a heterogeneous soft tissue mass* ➡ *infiltrating the bladder wall; note the extramural tumor invasion into surrounding perivesicular fat* ➡*. Endoscopic biopsy identified the tumor as a leiomyosarcoma.*

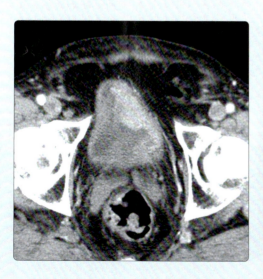

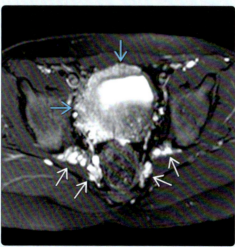

(Left) *Axial CECT of a distended urinary bladder reveals an infiltrating soft tissue mass involving the lateral wall of the bladder, identified by an endoscopic biopsy as a B-cell lymphomatous tumor.* (Right) *Axial T2WI MR with fat suppression shows marked nodular bladder wall thickening* ➡ *in this 9-year-old boy with a history of neurofibromatosis type 1. Note the additional plexiform neurofibromas along the pelvic sidewalls and in the perirectal space* ➡*.*

TERMINOLOGY

- Urothelial carcinoma accounts for 90% of bladder malignancies in USA and Europe
- Bladder is most prevalent site of urothelial carcinoma (previously known as transitional cell carcinoma)

IMAGING

- More common in bladder base (80% at initial diagnosis)
- Majority are single at time of diagnosis (~ 60%)
  - High propensity for multifocal disease and synchronous/metachronous upper tract disease
- Polypoid, sessile, or nodular
- **CT urography (CTU)** has 90% sensitivity and specificity for detection of urothelial neoplasm
  - Majority of lesions are detectable on postcontrast nonurographics set of images, seen as abnormal urothelial enhancement and wall thickening
- **MR**: More accurate than CT for local staging of tumor

- **US**: Useful for detection of bladder mass but inferior to CT/MR for local staging
  - Presence of flow helps to differentiate from clot
- Cystoscopy remains gold standard for detection of lower tract disease

TOP DIFFERENTIAL DIAGNOSES

- Extensive imaging overlap among all bladder tumors
- **Squamous cell carcinoma**
- **Adenocarcinoma**
- **Mesenchymal bladder tumors**

PATHOLOGY

- Morphological classification
  - Papillary (most common type, usually low grade and non muscle invading)
  - Sessile (infiltrating): Usually high grade
  - Mixed papillary and infiltrating
  - Carcinoma in situ

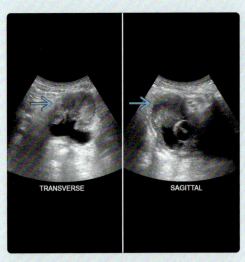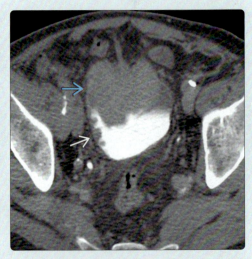

(Left) Transverse and sagittal US images of the bladder in 88-year-old male patient with a history of gross hematuria demonstrate eccentric mass-like thickening ➡ of the bladder wall. (Right) Axial image from subsequent CTU in the same patient shows a large anterior bladder wall mass ➡ as well as smaller synchronous lesions ➡ along the right lateral bladder wall. Pathology was consistent with invasive urothelial carcinoma.

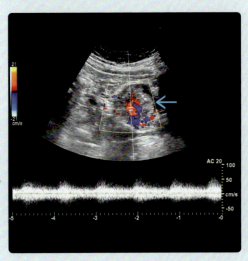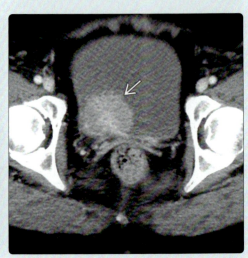

(Left) Spectral and color Doppler evaluation of an incidental bladder mass ➡ shows arterial flow within the stalk of the mass, differentiating it from blood clot. (Right) Axial CECT in the same patient shows an enhancing polypoid lesion ➡ along the right bladder trigone. Pathology was consistent with high-grade papillary urothelial cancer without invasion to the lamina propria.

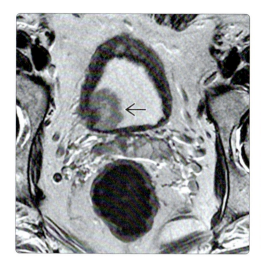
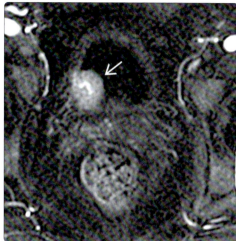

(Left) *Axial T2WI in 68-old-year male patient, who was being evaluated for elevated PSA, shows an incidental polypoid bladder mass* ➡. (Right) *Axial arterial-phase postcontrast T1WI MR from a dynamic perfusion study shows avid enhancement of the tumor* ➡.

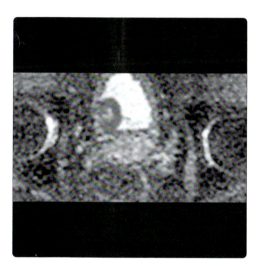
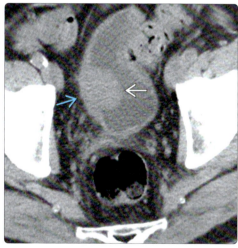

(Left) *ADC map through the incidental bladder mass shows marked hypointensity due to significant restricted diffusion.* (Right) *Axial NECT in this patient with a history of colonic diverticular disease shows an incidental polypoid bladder mass* ➡. *Note broad thickening of the right lateral bladder wall as well as mild perivesical fat stranding* ➡ *adjacent to the tumor suspicious for invasion through the detrussor muscle. Pathology showed urothelial carcinoma with invasion to perivesical fat.*

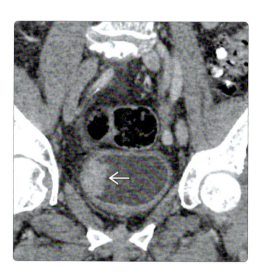
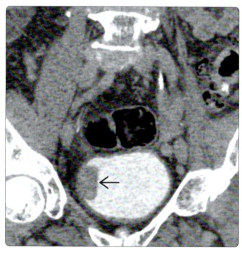

(Left) *Coronal CECT in 88-year-old male patient with a history of gross hematuria shows a broad-based enhancing polypoid mass* ➡, *which was proven to be urothelial carcinoma. The mass extends into the detrusor muscle (T2).* (Right) *Coronal image from a CTU in the same patient again shows the broad-based polypoid mass* ➡. *While CTU offers better contrast resolution for detection of small lesions, venous-phase CECT provides more information regarding the local extent of tumor.*

T | Definition of Primary Tumor (T)

T Category	T Criteria
TX	Primary tumor cannot be assessed
T0	No evidence of primary tumor
Ta	Noninvasive papillary carcinoma
Tis	Urothelial carcinoma in situ: "flat tumor"
T1	Tumor invades lamina propria (subepithelial connective tissue)
T2	Tumor invades muscularis propria
pT2a	Tumor invades superficial muscularis propria (inner half)
pT2b	Tumor invades deep muscularis propria (outer half)
T3	Tumor invades perivesical soft tissue
pT3a	Microscopically
pT3b	Macroscopically (extravesical mass)
T4	Extravesical tumor directly invades any of the following: Prostatic stroma, seminal vesicles, uterus, vagina, pelvic wall, abdominal wall
T4a	Extravesical tumor invades directly into prostatic stroma, uterus, vagina
T4b	Extravesical tumor invades pelvic wall, abdominal wall

Adapted with permission from AJCC Cancer Staging Manual 8th ed., 2017.

N | Definition of Regional Lymph Node (N)

N Category	N Criteria
NX	Lymph nodes cannot be assessed
N0	No lymph node metastasis
N1	Single regional lymph node metastasis in the true pelvis (perivesical, obturator, internal and external iliac, or sacral lymph node)
N2	Multiple regional lymph node metastasis in the true pelvis (perivesical, obturator, internal and external iliac, or sacral lymph node metastasis)
N3	Lymph node metastasis to the common iliac lymph nodes

Adapted with permission from AJCC Cancer Staging Manual 8th ed., 2017.

M | Definition of Distant Metastasis (M)

M Category	M Criteria
M0	No distant metastasis
M1	Distant metastasis
M1a	Distant metastasis limited to lymph nodes beyond the common iliacs
M1b	Non-lymph-node distant metastases

Adapted with permission from AJCC Cancer Staging Manual 8th ed., 2017.

Bladder

AJCC Prognostic Stage Groups

When T is...	And N is...	And M is...	Then the stage group is...
Ta	N0	M0	0a
Tis	N0	M0	0is
T1	N0	M0	I
T2a	N0	M0	II
T2b	N0	M0	II
T3a, T3b, T4a	N0	M0	IIIA
T1-T4a	N1	M0	IIIA
T1-T4a	N2, N3	M0	IIIB
T4b	N0	M0	IVA
Any T	Any N	M1a	IVA
Any T	Any N	M1b	IVB

Adapted with permission from AJCC Cancer Staging Manual 8th ed., 2017.

T Staging of Urinary Bladder Carcinoma

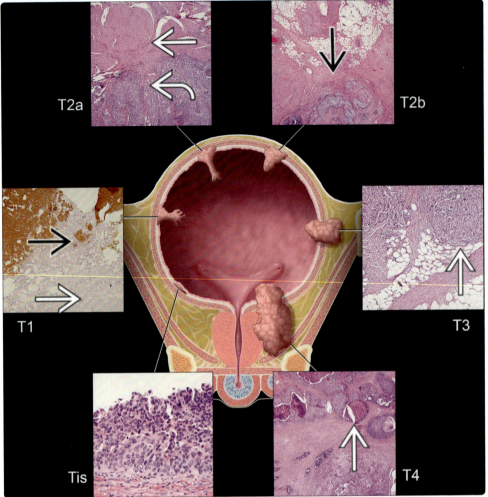

Graphics show T stages of urinary bladder carcinoma with histologic correlation. Tis or carcinoma in situ refers to nonpapillary (flat) mucosa in which the normal urothelium has been replaced by cancer cells that have not invaded through the basement membrane. Carcinoma in situ is a high-grade lesion and essentially recognized because of cytologic abnormalities similar to those noted in high-grade papillary tumors. Neoplastic cells are pleomorphic, hyperchromatic, and occupy a portion of the thickness of the urothelium. They lack polarity in relation to the basement membrane. (Original magnification 400x.) T1 describes urothelial tumor invasion through the basement membrane into the subepithelial connective tissue. In this photomicrograph, cytokeratin immunohistochemical stain is used to highlight the tumor ➡ invading into subepithelial connective tissue but not to muscularis propria ➡. (Original magnification 200x.) T2 designates a tumor that invades muscularis propria. T2a: H&E stain shows tumor cell invading the superficial/inner 1/2 of muscularis propria ➡. Note that outer 1/2 of muscularis propria ➡ is not involved. (Original magnification 100x.) T2b: H&E stain shows tumor cells ➡ invading the outer 1/2 of the muscularis propria. (Original magnification 100x.) T3 applies to a tumor invading perivesical tissue. H&E stain shows tumor cells ➡ invading perivesical fat tissue. (Original magnification 200x.) Tumor is considered T3a if perivesical fat involvement is microscopic (not evident by imaging) and T3b if macroscopic (potentially detected by imaging). T4 describes a tumor invading any of the following: Prostate, uterus, vagina, pelvic wall, or abdominal wall. It is T4a when the tumor invades prostate, uterus, and vagina; tumor is T4b when it invades pelvic wall and abdominal wall. H&E stain demonstrates neoplastic transitional cell carcinoma cells ➡ invading prostate. (Original magnification 100x.)

T4a: Male

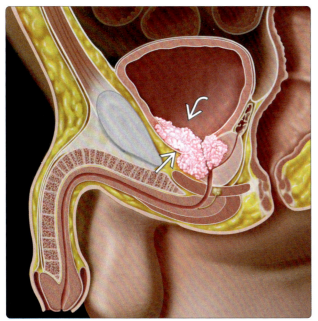

Graphic shows a bladder neck tumor ⬊ in a male patient; the tumor invades the prostate ⬈, constituting stage T4a. To be considered T4a disease, the tumor should have prostatic stromal invasion directly from the bladder tumor. Subepithelial invasion of prostatic urethra will not constitute T4 staging status.

T4a: Female

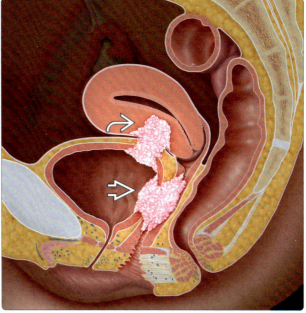

Graphic shows posterior wall bladder tumors in a female patient invading the uterus ⬈ and vagina ⬊. Invasion of the uterus &/or vagina constitutes stage T4a.

T4b: Male

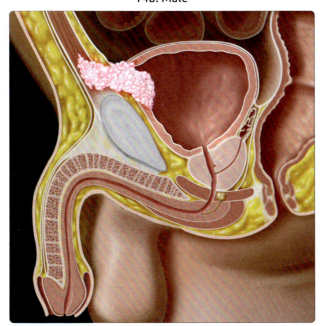

Graphic shows a tumor of the anterior wall of the urinary bladder that invades into the extraperitoneal prevesical fat (space of Retzius) and eventually the muscles of the anterior abdominal wall, constituting stage T4b.

T4b: Female

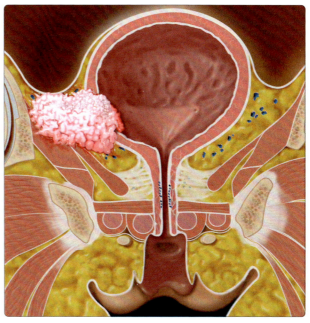

Graphic shows a lateral wall bladder tumor invading the muscles of the lateral pelvic wall, constituting stage T4b.

N1 and N2

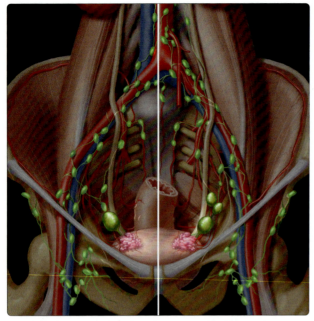

N3 and Distant Nodal Metastases

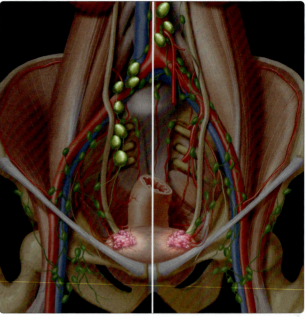

Graphics show N1 and N2 disease in urinary bladder carcinoma. Both classifications describe nodal metastases confined to the true pelvis. N1 (left) is a single metastatic pelvic lymph node, whereas N2 (right) is defined as multiple metastatic pelvic lymph nodes.

The graphic on the left shows N3 disease, which describes involvement of the common iliac lymph nodes. The graphic on the right shows involvement of paraaortic lymph nodes, which constitute distant metastases and M1 staging in the 7th edition of the AJCC Cancer Staging Manual.

Metastases, Organ Frequency

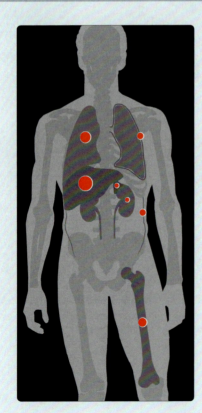

Liver	47%
Lung	45%
Bone	32%
Peritoneum	19%
Pleura	16%
Kidney	14%
Adrenal gland	14%

Adapted from Wallmeroth A et al: Patterns of metastasis in muscle-invasive bladder cancer (pT2-4): an autopsy study on 367 patients. Urol Int. 62:69-75, 1999.

Stage 0a (Ta N0 M0)

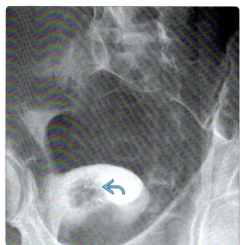

Stage 0a (Ta N0 M0)

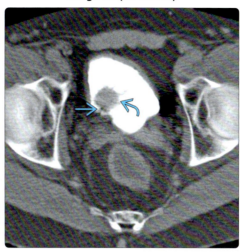

(Left) Right posterior oblique intravenous pyelography in a patient who presented with gross hematuria shows a papillary mass ⊿ projecting into the contrast-filled lumen of the urinary bladder. (Right) Axial CECT in the same patient shows a pedunculated papillary mass ⊿ with a narrow stalk ⊿ attached to the right posterolateral aspect of the urinary bladder. The tumor was found to be a noninvasive papillary carcinoma.

Stage I (T1 N0 M0)

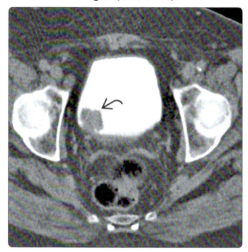

Stage I (T1 N0 M0)

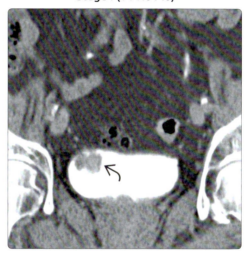

(Left) Axial CECT shows a polypoid mass ⊿ involving the right side of the posterior wall of the bladder lateral to the ureteric orifice. The tumor was found to invade into the subepithelial connective tissue without extension into the muscle layer. (Right) Coronal CECT in the same patient shows the polypoid tumor ⊿ attached to the superior aspect of the right posterior bladder wall.

Stage II (T2a N0 M0)

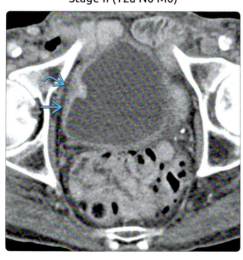

Stage II (T2a N0 M0)

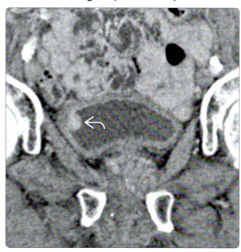

(Left) Axial CECT shows an enhancing polypoid mass arising from the right lateral wall of the urinary bladder ⊿. There is associated thickening of the adjacent bladder wall ⊿. (Right) Coronal CECT in the same patient shows the enhancing urinary bladder mass ⊿. Enhancement is limited to the mass without involvement of the underlying wall, suggesting the absence of muscle invasion, although CT is not adequate to definitely make this distinction. This was found to be a T2a tumor.

(Left) *Axial CECT in a 38-year-old woman who presented with repeated urinary tract infection and gross hematuria shows a heterogeneous mass ➦ in the anterior aspect of the dome of the urinary bladder with focal calcifications ➥. There is no evidence of extravesical extension.* **(Right)** *Axial CECT in the same patient shows the bladder dome mass ➦ with peripheral curvilinear calcifications ➥, which is pathognomonic for urachal adenocarcinoma.*

Stage II (T2a N0 M0)

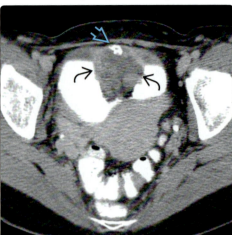

Stage II (T2a N0 M0)

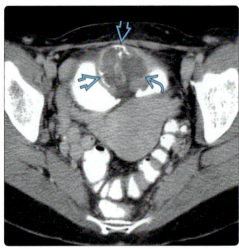

(Left) *Transverse ultrasound image of the urinary bladder shows an echogenic mass ➦ centered on and obstructing the left ureteric orifice ➥. Note the normal right side ureteric jet ➦. Ultrasound is not useful for staging bladder carcinoma but can help in tumor detection and evaluation of ureteric orifice.* **(Right)** *Longitudinal duplex Doppler ultrasound in the same patient shows blood flow in the mass, which helps differentiate a solid mass from blood clot.*

Stage II (T2b N0 M0)

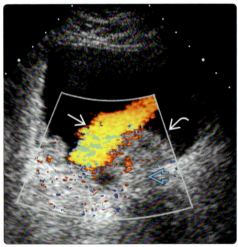

Stage II (T2b N0 M0)

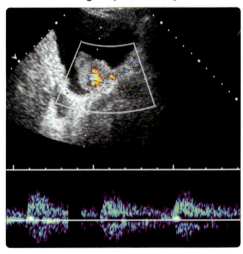

(Left) *Axial CECT shows a large mass filling the bladder ➦ without evidence of perivesical infiltration. Calcifications ➥ are seen on the surface of the mass.* **(Right)** *Coronal CECT in the same patient shows that the mass ➦ is attached to the superior wall of the bladder. Note the smooth outer contour of the bladder at the site of tumor attachment ➦, indicating the absence of perivesical infiltration despite the large tumor size.*

Stage II (T2b N0 M0)

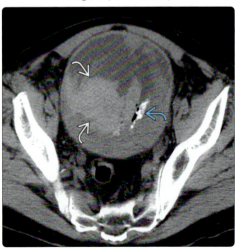

Stage II (T2b N0 M0)

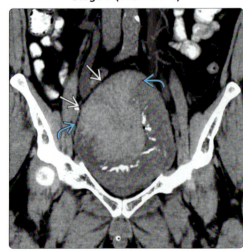

Stage II (T2b N0 M0)

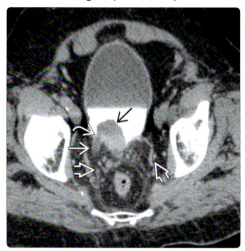

Stage II (T2b N0 M0)

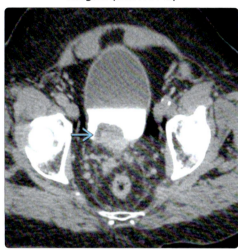

(Left) *Axial CECT in a patient who presented with hematuria shows a posterior wall bladder mass* ➡️ *that involves the ureteric orifice* ➡️*. The right ureter is slightly dilated* ➡️*. No regional adenopathy is present. Small nodular densities in the perivesical fat represent dilated veins* ➡️*.* (Right) *Axial CECT in the same patient shows involvement of the right ureteric orifice* ➡️*. Ureteric involvement is a strong indication of muscle-invasive (T2) disease.*

Stage II (T2b N0 M0)

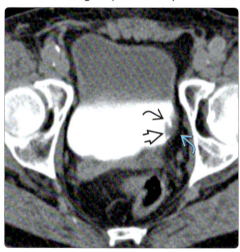

Stage III (T3b N0 M0)

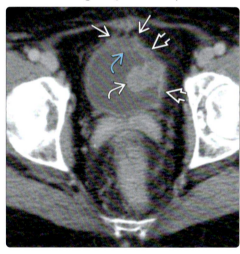

(Left) *Axial CECT shows a polypoid lesion arising from the left lateral wall of the urinary bladder* ➡️*. Contrast is extending into a superficial ulcer* ➡️*. There is no perivesical tumor extension* ➡️*.* (Right) *Axial CECT shows thickening of the anterior* ➡️ *and left lateral wall of the urinary bladder* ➡️ *with a large polypoid mass projecting into the bladder lumen* ➡️*. There is stranding of the perivesical fat almost reaching to the anterior abdominal wall* ➡️*.*

Stage III (T3b N0 M0)

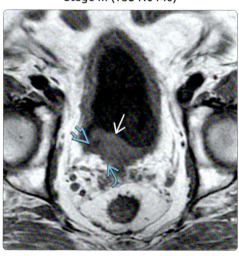

Stage III (T3b N0 M0)

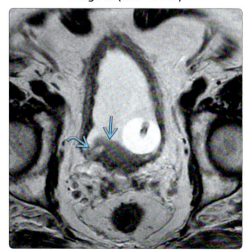

(Left) *Axial T1WI MR shows an intermediate signal intensity posterior wall bladder mass* ➡️ *that is hyperintense to urine, hypointense to fat, and isointense to muscle. Tumor nodules extend into high signal perivesical fat* ➡️*. The ureteric orifice is embedded in the mass* ➡️*.* (Right) *Axial T2WI MR in the same patient shows an intermediate signal bladder mass* ➡️ *that is hypointense to the urine and perivesical fat. Note also involvement of the ureteric orifice* ➡️*.*

(Left) *Axial T1WI MR shows a right posterolateral urinary bladder mass ➡ that has a large extravesical component ➡. The mass is isointense to the bladder wall on T1WI MR. **(Right)** Axial T2WI MR shows a bladder mass ➡ that is hyperintense relative to the dark urinary bladder wall and hypointense relative to urine and perivesical fat. Note the interruption of the dark urinary bladder wall signal where the mass extends into the perivesical fat ➡.*

Stage III (T3b N0 M0)

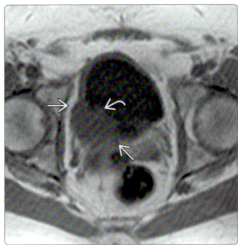

Stage III (T3b N0 M0)

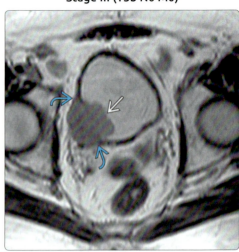

(Left) *Axial T1WI MR shows diffuse thickening of the left lateral urinary bladder wall ➡. Note focal disruption of the smooth outer contour of the bladder ➡ and tumor extension into the high signal perivesical fat. The left ureter ➡ is dilated, which suggests muscle-invasive disease. **(Right)** Axial T1WI C+ FS MR in the same patient shows tumor enhancement ➡ and confirms the extension of enhancing tumor tissue into the low signal perivesical fat ➡.*

Stage III (T3b N0 M0)

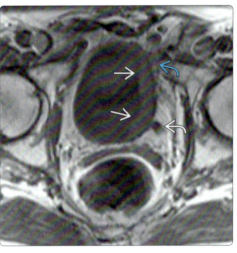

Stage III (T3b N0 M0)

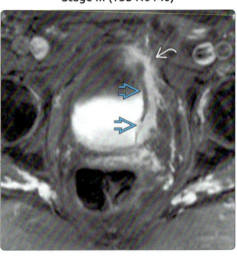

(Left) *Coronal T1WI C+ FS MR in the same patient shows a polypoid bladder mass ➡ that infiltrates into the prostate ➡. **(Right)** Coronal T1WI C+ FS MR in the same patient again shows the bladder mass ➡ invading into the prostate ➡ and displacing the Foley catheter ➡ toward the left side. It can be difficult to differentiate primary bladder masses invading the prostate from prostate carcinoma invading the neck of the urinary bladder.*

Stage III (T4a N0 M0)

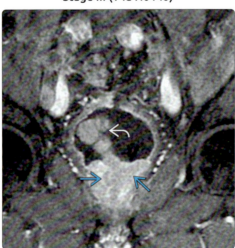

Stage III (T4a N0 M0)

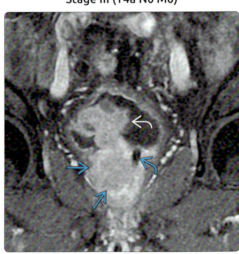

Stage III (T4a N0 M0)

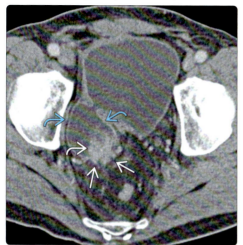

Stage III (T4a N0 M0)

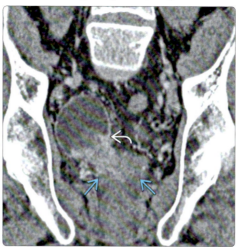

(Left) *Axial CECT shows a right posterolateral bladder diverticulum ⇨ with a polypoid mass ⇨ arising within the diverticulum and infiltrating into the perivesical fat ⇨. Pathology confirmed the diagnosis of squamous cell carcinoma.* (Right) *Coronal CECT in the same patient shows that the mass ⇨ within the diverticulum invades into the prostate ⇨. Because bladder diverticula lack a muscle layer, tumors arising within a diverticulum and invading the wall are at least T3.*

Stage III (T4a N0 M0)

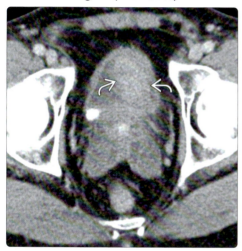

Stage III (T4a N0 M0)

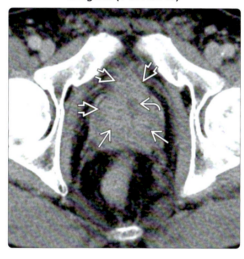

(Left) *Axial CECT shows an enhancing mass in the region of the neck of the urinary bladder ⇨.* (Right) *Axial CECT in the same patient at the level of the prostate shows tumor ⇨ surrounding the urethra ⇨ and invading into the prostate ⇨. It can be difficult to differentiate prostatic tumor invading the bladder neck from bladder tumors invading the prostate. The presence of prostate invasion makes this T4a disease.*

Stage IV (T4b N0 M0)

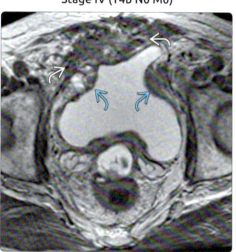

Stage IV (T4b N0 M0)

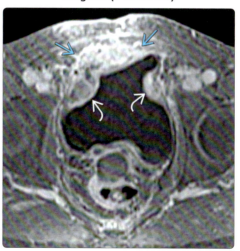

(Left) *Axial T2WI MR shows extensive infiltrative tumor ⇨ involving mainly the anterior bladder wall with focal invasion of the rectus abdominus muscle ⇨. The tumor shows heterogeneous T2 signal intensity.* (Right) *Axial T1WI C+ FS MR in the same patient shows heterogeneously enhancing tumor of the anterior wall of the bladder ⇨. Enhancing tumor fills the prevesical space and invades the rectus muscles ⇨.*

(Left) *Sagittal T2WI MR in the same patient shows marked circumferential thickening of the wall of the urinary bladder ➡️, as well as invasion of the rectus muscles anteriorly ⇨.* (Right) *Sagittal T1WI C+ FS MR in the same patient shows diffuse enhancement of the bladder wall with tumor extension into the wall of the rectum ➡️ and the anterior abdominal wall muscles ⇨.*

Stage IV (T4b N0 M0)

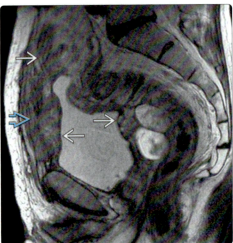

Stage IV (T4b N0 M0)

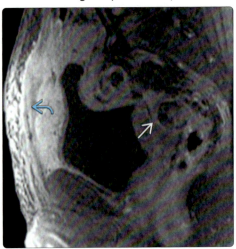

(Left) *Axial CECT shows a large dumbbell-shaped polypoid mass that has a large intraluminal component ➡️ and a large extraluminal component ⇨. The extraluminal component invades into the anterior abdominal wall ➡️.* (Right) *Coronal CECT in the same patient shows the intraluminal ⇨ and large extraluminal ➡️ components. This lesion was initially thought to be a mesenchymal mural tumor but was found at surgery to be transitional cell carcinoma.*

Stage IV (T4b N0 M0)

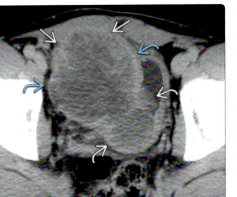

Stage IV (T4b N0 M0)

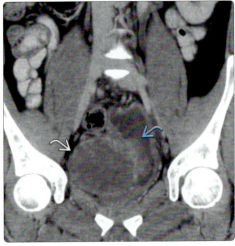

(Left) *Axial T2WI MR shows 2 urinary bladder masses. The 1st mass ⇨ is superficial and does not invade through the muscle layer (uniform low signal intensity muscle layer at the base of the lesion ⇨). The 2nd lesion invades and interrupts the muscle layer ⇨. A perivesical lymph node is present ⇨.* (Right) *Axial T1WI C+ FS MR in the same patient shows enhancement of both lesions ➡️, as well as similar enhancement of the perivesical lymph node ➡️.*

Stage IV (T2b N1 M0)

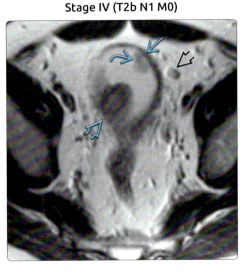

Stage IV (T2b N1 M0)

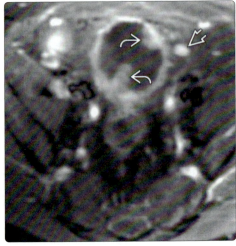

Stage IV (T2b N1 M0)

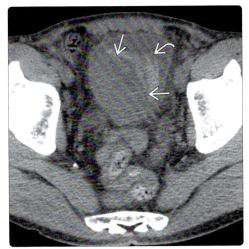

Stage IV (T2b N1 M0)

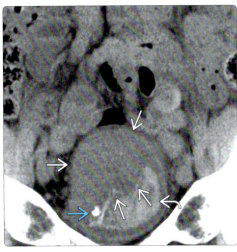

(Left) *Axial NECT in a patient who presented with gross hematuria shows high-density blood within the urinary bladder* ➡️. *The intraluminal blood outlines a large urinary bladder tumor* ➡️ *that is otherwise isodense to urine.* (Right) *Coronal NECT in the same patient shows intravesical blood* ➡️ *outlining the bladder tumor* ➡️. *There are focal tumoral calcifications* ➡️. *The bladder has a smooth outer contour, indicating the absence of perivesical invasion.*

Stage IV (T2b N1 M0)

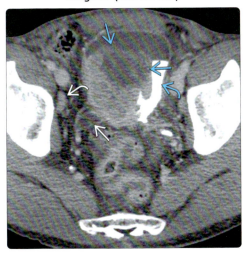

Stage IV (T2b N1 M0)

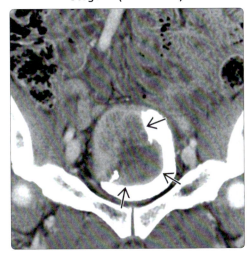

(Left) *Axial CECT in the same patient shows contrast material* ➡️ *within the urinary bladder outlining the large necrotic bladder mass* ➡️. *Note involvement of the ureteric orifice and mild ureteric dilatation* ➡️. *There is a single obturator lymph node* ➡️, *which constitutes N1 disease (stage IV).* (Right) *Coronal CECT in the same patient shows the tumor outlined by intravesical contrast* ➡️.

Stage IV (T2b N2 M0)

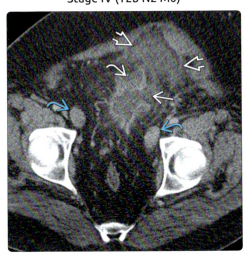

Stage IV (T2b N2 M0)

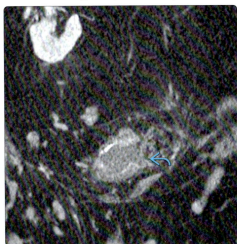

(Left) *Axial CECT in a morbidly obese patient with pathologically proven T2b disease, who presented with severe lower abdominal pain, shows focal thickening of the anterior wall of the urinary bladder* ➡️ *with a large defect of the bladder wall* ➡️ *and fluid collection in the prevesical space* ➡️ *due to bladder rupture. Bilateral enlarged external iliac nodes are seen* ➡️. (Right) *Coronal CECT in the same patient shows the bladder defect* ➡️.

Stage IV (T3b N2 M0)

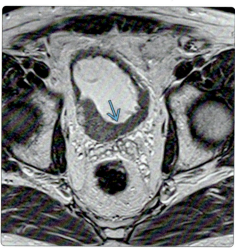

Stage IV (T3b N2 M0)

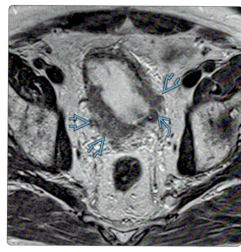

(Left) *Axial T2WI MR in a 72-year-old man who presented with painless hematuria shows posterior urinary bladder wall thickening ➡ with loss of the low signal bladder wall indicating muscle invasion.* (Right) *Axial T2WI MR in the same patient shows thickening of the wall of the distal left ureter due to tumor invasion ➡. Irregular outer contour of the urinary bladder ➡ due to gross invasion of the perivesical fat, constituting T3b disease, is also shown.*

Stage IV (T3b N2 M0)

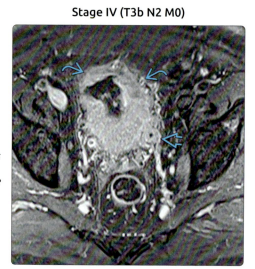

Stage IV (T3b N2 M0)

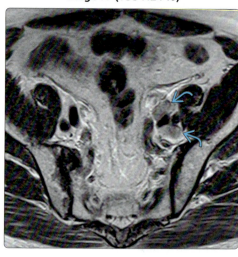

(Left) *Axial T1WI C+ FS MR obtained at a higher level in the same patient shows diffuse enhancing wall thickening ➡ involving the dome of the urinary bladder with circumferential thickening of the distal left ureter ➡ due to tumor invasion.* (Right) *Axial T2WI MR in the same patient shows 2 enlarged left external iliac lymph nodes ➡. The presence of multiple lymph nodes metastases within the true pelvis constitutes N2 disease.*

Stage IV (T4a N2 M0)

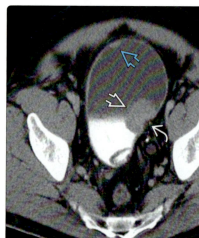

Stage IV (T4a N2 M0)

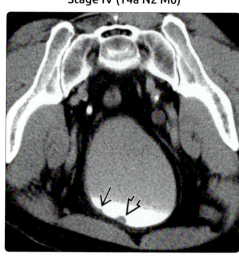

(Left) *Axial CECT in a 54-year-old man shows a large polypoid lesion ➡ with indentation of the urinary bladder wall ➡ at the site of tumor attachment indicating muscle invasion. Note the subtle nodular lesion ➡ of the anterior bladder wall.* (Right) *Axial CECT in the same patient obtained in the prone position confirms the presence of the anterior wall polypoid lesion ➡ and shows another subtle flat lesion ➡, which was pathologically proven to be carcinoma in situ.*

Stage IV (T4a N2 M0)

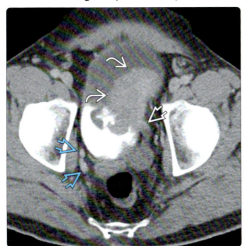

Stage IV (T4a N2 M0)

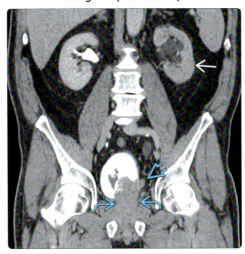

(Left) *Axial CECT in the same patient shows the large polypoid mass ⬈ invading the left ureter ⬈. Two metastatic obturator lymph nodes ⬈ are present. The presence of multiple metastatic lymph nodes within the true pelvis constitute N2 disease.* (Right) *Coronal CECT in the same patient shows invasion of the prostate ⬈ and the left ureteric orifice ⬈. The left kidney ⬈ shows delayed nephrogram due to left ureteric obstruction.*

Stage IV (T2b N0 M1)

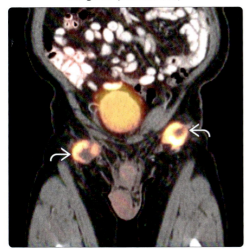

Stage IV (T2b N0 M1)

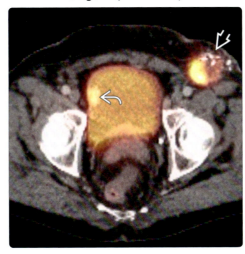

(Left) *Coronal PET/CT was obtained after forced diuresis in a patient who presented with bilateral inguinal lymphadenopathy that was pathologically proven to be metastatic transitional cell carcinoma. Bilateral FDG-avid inguinal lymph nodes ⬈ are seen.* (Right) *Axial PET/CT in the same patient shows inguinal lymphadenopathy ⬈. A polypoid bladder mass is seen ⬈, representing the primary tumor that was found to be T2b tumor at surgery.*

Stage IV (T3b N0 M1)

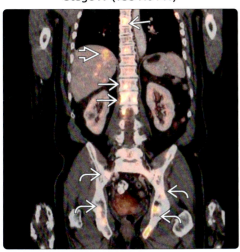

Stage IV (T3b N0 M1)

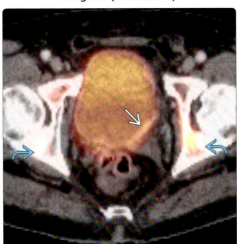

(Left) *Coronal PET/CT shows liver metastases ⬈, multiple spine metastases ⬈, as well as multiple pelvic bony metastases ⬈. Spine and bony pelvic metastases are common due to tumor spread through the Batson venous plexus.* (Right) *Axial PET/CT in the same patient shows uptake ⬈ along the left posterolateral wall of the urinary bladder following resection of a muscle-invasive tumor and bilateral acetabular uptake ⬈ due to pelvic bony metastases.*

TERMINOLOGY

- Malignant epithelial neoplasm with pure squamous cell phenotype

IMAGING

- CT with delayed-phase imaging (CT urography) is modality of choice
- Enhancing plaque-like or sessile polypoid lesion
- Tumor has predilection for trigone and lateral walls
  - May occur in bladder diverticula
- Invasion through serosal layer (T3b) is manifested by soft tissue and stranding in perivesical fat
- Differentiation between malignant and reactive nodes can be very difficult
- Tumor has intermediate T1 and T2 signal intensity on MR imaging and shows early enhancement

TOP DIFFERENTIAL DIAGNOSES

- Invasive urothelial carcinoma

  - Differentiation between urothelial carcinoma and SCC is almost impossible based on imaging alone
- Mesenchymal bladder neoplasms (such as leiomyoma)
- Chronic granulomatous cystitis

PATHOLOGY

- Chronic mucosal irritation and inflammation play major role
  - Chronic/repetitive injury → squamous metaplasia → dysplasia → carcinoma
- Staging of bladder SCC follows same TNM staging scheme used for urothelial bladder carcinoma

CLINICAL ISSUES

- Common symptoms: Painless, microscopic hematuria
- Nonschistosomal forms usually present in advanced stage (80% have detrusor muscle invasion, and up to 10% are metastatic at presentation)
  - Schistosomiasis-related forms, on other hand, have relatively low prevalence of nodal and distant metastasis
- Radical cystectomy is treatment of choice

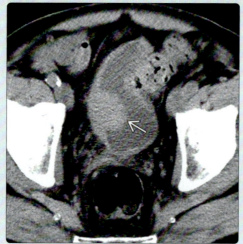
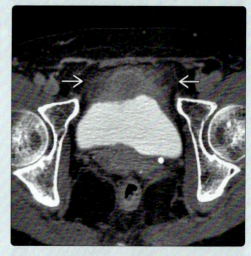

(Left) Axial NECT in a patient with a history of hematuria shows a soft tissue-attenuation polypoid mass ➡ along the lateral bladder wall. Patient underwent transurethral resection of bladder tumor. Pathology was compatible with squamous cell carcinoma. (Right) CECT shows marked, irregular wall thickening of anterior bladder wall. Note perivesical fat stranding ➡, suggestive of tumor extension into serosa (T3 disease). Patient underwent radical cystectomy; pathology was compatible with T3N1 SCC.

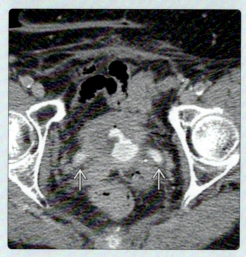
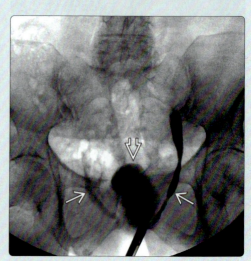

(Left) Axial delayed-phase CECT in patient with a history of remote radiation for anal cancers shows marked, irregular, circumferential bladder wall thickening. There was extension of infiltrative tumor to the ureterovesical junctions resulting in bilateral hydroureteronephrosis ➡. (Right) Frontal retrograde cystogram in the same patient shows irregular contour and decreased distensibility of the urinary bladder ➡. Note bilateral hydroureter ➡.

Rhabdomyosarcoma, Genitourinary

TERMINOLOGY

- Malignant tumor of mesenchymal origin arising from any pelvic organ (paratesticular discussed separately)

IMAGING

- Best clue: Large, heterogeneous, predominantly solid pelvic mass in child with symptoms of urinary tract obstruction &/or constipation
  - Variable cystic components
  - Botryoid variety resembles bunch of grapes with cysts protruding into lumen of vagina or urinary bladder
- May originate from bladder, vagina, cervix, uterus, pelvic side walls, prostate, & paratesticular tissues
  - May also occur in adjacent non-genitourinary soft tissues
- Tumors spread by local extension as well as lymphatic & hematogenous routes with metastases to lungs, liver, & bone
  - 15-20% have metastases at diagnosis
- Work-up typically includes
  - US for initial investigation of urinary tract symptoms or palpable mass
  - CECT or MR for further tumor characterization & localization
  - Staging with chest CT & PET/CT

PATHOLOGY

- Small round blue cell tumor of primitive muscle cells
- Major histologic types: Embryonal (majority, especially in genitourinary sites), alveolar, & undifferentiated (adults)
- Bladder & prostate sites unfavorable, automatically at least stage II

CLINICAL ISSUES

- Peak incidence: 2-6 years old
  - 75% < 5 years old at diagnosis
- Surgery, chemotherapy, & radiation therapy combined
- 5-year survival: Stage I (93%) vs. stage IV (~ 30%)
  - Embryonal type has better prognosis than alveolar

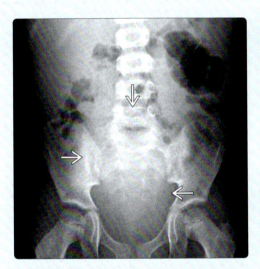
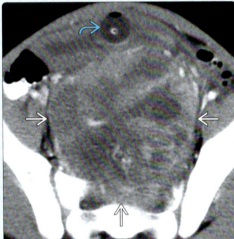

(Left) AP radiograph of a 6-year-old boy shows displacement of bowel by a soft tissue mass ➡ in the pelvis, initially suspected to be due to urinary retention but not relieved by bladder catheterization. (Right) Axial CECT in the same patient with urinary retention shows a large, heterogeneously enhancing presacral mass ➡ displacing the urinary bladder (with Foley balloon in place ➡) anteriorly.

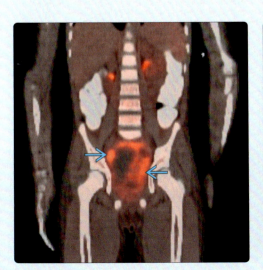
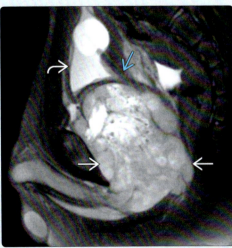

(Left) Coronal FDG PET/CT in the same patient shows predominantly peripheral uptake in the pelvic tumor ➡ but no evidence of metastatic disease. Biopsy confirmed a rhabdomyosarcoma originating from the bladder base/prostate. (Right) Sagittal T2 MR in a 7-year-old boy shows a large, heterogeneous, intermediate to high signal intensity rhabdomyosarcoma ➡ arising from the prostate. Note the superior displacement of the bladder ➡ and the altered course of the Foley catheter ➡ caused by the mass.

TERMINOLOGY

- Primary gland-forming carcinoma of urinary bladder
- 1/3 are associated with urachal remnant (urachal type)

IMAGING

- Predilection for bladder base and urachus (urachal remnant)
- Tumor may present as heterogeneous mass or irregular focal or diffuse bladder wall thickening
- Most tumors are **mixed solid and cystic**
  - Cystic component is due to mucin (which is T2 hyperintense on MR)
- ~ 70% of cases have **calcification**
- Extravesical extension is common
- Bulk of tumor in urachal adenocarcinoma is extravesical
- Urachal adenocarcinomas are usually large at time of presentation (mean size: 6 cm)

TOP DIFFERENTIAL DIAGNOSES

- Urothelial carcinoma
  - Urothelial carcinoma usually shows papillary intravesical growth, which is unusual in adenocarcinoma
  - Presence of cystic spaced (mucin) and calcification are clues for adenocarcinoma
- Other uncommon bladder neoplasms
- Cystitis

PATHOLOGY

- Proposed pathogenesis: Chronic mucosal irritation → intestinal metaplasia → adenocarcinoma
- Risk factors: Bladder exstrophy, **urachal remnant**, chronic mucosal irritation/inflammation, cystitis glandularis (such as with pelvic lipomatosis), endometriosis

CLINICAL ISSUES

- Rare; < 2% of bladder malignancies
- Usually in advanced stage at time of presentation

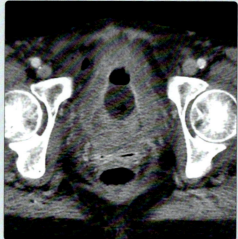
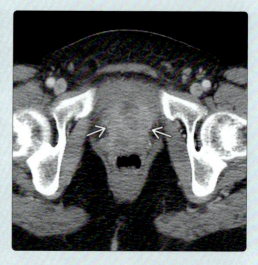

(Left) Axial CECT in a 63-year-old female patient shows marked circumferential bladder wall thickening. Tissue biopsy was compatible with clear cell adenocarcinoma. Tumor extended into the urethra and invaded the anterior vaginal wall (T4a lesion). The patient underwent pelvic exenteration. (Right) Axial CECT shows a heterogeneously enhancing mass at the bladder base ➡, which was shown to be bladder adenocarcinoma (nonurachal type). The patient underwent radical cystectomy.

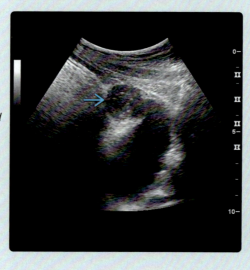
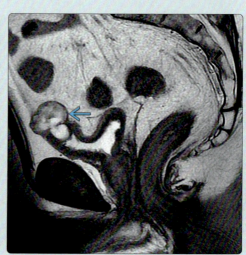

(Left) Longitudinal US of the bladder shows an incidental complex mass ➡ superior to the bladder dome. (Right) Sagittal T2WI MR in the same patient shows a complex solid/cystic mass ➡ attached to the bladder dome. The T2-hyperintense areas are related to mucin content. The patient underwent partial cystectomy and pathology was consistent with urachal adenocarcinoma.

Adenocarcinoma

TERMINOLOGY

Definitions
- Primary gland-forming carcinoma of urinary bladder
- 1/3 are associated with urachal remnant (urachal type)

IMAGING

General Features
- Location
  - Predilection for bladder base and urachus (urachal remnant)
- Size
  - Urachal adenocarcinomas are usually large at time of presentation (mean size: 6 cm)
- Morphology
  - Urachal: Large midline supravesical/infraumbilical mass with calcification
  - Nonurachal: Could present as mass or marked bladder wall thickening

Radiographic Findings
- Antegrade/retrograde cystography
  - Filling defect in bladder base
  - Contour deformity and external compression in bladder dome (urachal form)

CT Findings
- Irregular focal or diffuse bladder wall thickening
- Most tumors are mixed solid and cystic
  - Cystic component due to mucin
- ~ 70% of cases have calcification
  - Usually peripheral
- Extravesical extension is common
  - Perivesical fat stranding
  - Regional or distant lymphadenopathy
  - Peritoneal carcinomatosis
- Bulk of tumor in urachal adenocarcinoma is extravesical
  - May also have intraluminal component

MR Findings
- Enhancing mass with heterogeneous signal on T1WI and T2WI
- Contains areas of high T2 signal intensity corresponding to mucin
- Extravesical extension (T3 tumor) manifests as perivesical fat stranding and enhancement
- Multiplanar imaging allows better assessment for invasion to adjacent organs (T4 tumor)

Ultrasonographic Findings
- Heterogeneous intravesical mass
  - Shadowing calcification
- Complex solid/cystic mass superior to bladder dome (urachal type)
- ± vascularity on Doppler

DIFFERENTIAL DIAGNOSIS

Urothelial Carcinoma
- Urothelial carcinoma usually shows papillary intravesical growth, which is unusual in adenocarcinoma

- Presence of cystic spaces (mucin) and calcification are clues for adenocarcinoma
- Adenocarcinoma is most common urachal neoplasm
- Differentiation between the 2 can be very difficult based on imaging and tissue sampling is required

Other Uncommon Bladder Neoplasms
- Such as squamous cell carcinoma, small cell tumor, carcinoid, etc.
- Differentiation between these conditions based on imaging alone is difficult

Cystitis
- Adenocarcinoma can present as diffuse bladder wall thickening and mimic cystitis

PATHOLOGY

General Features
- Etiology
  - Proposed pathogenesis: Chronic mucosal irritation → intestinal metaplasia → adenocarcinoma
  - Risk factors: Bladder exstrophy, urachal remnant, chronic mucosal irritation/inflammation, cystitis glandularis (such as with pelvic lipomatosis), endometriosis
  - 80% of urachal carcinomas are adenocarcinoma
    - Urachal adenocarcinoma is thought to arise from rests of embryonic hindgut epithelium

Microscopic Features
- Important to differentiate primary from secondary adenocarcinoma (invasion from adjacent organs or distant metastasis)
- Gland-forming with vacuolated cytoplasm

CLINICAL ISSUES

Presentation
- Most common signs/symptoms
  - Hematuria
  - Irritative symptoms (dysuria, frequency)

Demographics
- Age
  - Peak incidence in 6th decade
  - Patients with urachal type present ~ 10 years earlier
- Gender
  - More common in male (M:F = 2.6:1.0)
  - No gender predilection in urachal type
- Epidemiology
  - Rare; < 2% of bladder malignancies

Natural History & Prognosis
- Usually in advanced stage at time of presentation
  - > 90% of cases show invasion into detrusor muscle (T2)
  - ~ 50% of cases have distant metastasis at time of presentation
- Poor prognosis; 5-year survival: 18-47%

Treatment
- Radical cystectomy ± adjuvant chemoradiation
- En bloc resection of urachal tumor and adjacent abd wall in cases of advanced urachal adenocarcinom

SECTION 7
Urethra/Penis

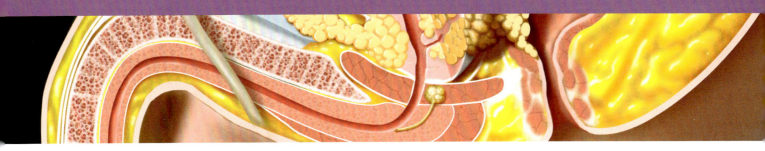

Anatomy

Female Urethra

The female urethra is ~ 4 cm in length and follows an oblique course anteroinferiorly from the internal urethral meatus at the bladder neck to the external urethral meatus anterior to the vaginal opening. The urethra passes through the pelvic diaphragm, which is formed by the levator ani and coccygeus muscles and fascia. The levator ani separates the pelvic cavity from the perineum. Inferior to the levator ani, the urethra is surrounded by the urogenital diaphragm, which is formed by the sphincter urethrae and deep transverse peroneus muscles and their fascia. Due to its short course, traumatic injury isolated to the female urethra is extremely rare.

Male Urethra

The male urethra is ~ 18-20 cm in length and has 2 major divisions: The **anterior** and **posterior urethra**, each of which can be further subdivided into 2 parts. The posterior urethra is composed of the prostatic and membranous portions, and the anterior urethra is composed of the bulbous and penile portions.

The **prostatic urethra** begins at the bladder neck and extends to the apex of the prostate gland. The **membranous urethra** traverses the urogenital diaphragm. It is the shortest portion (~ 1 cm) of the urethra but the area most vulnerable to injury in the setting of lower abdominal blunt trauma that results in pelvic fractures. The **bulbous urethra** extends from the inferior border of the urogenital diaphragm to the penoscrotal junction. The bulbous urethra passes beneath the inferior margin of the symphysis pubis and may be disrupted with a straddle injury. The **penile urethra** is distal to the penoscrotal junction and travels through the pendulous portion of the penis within the corpus spongiosum. It widens into the fossa navicularis at the distal glans. Both the penile and bulbous urethra are most prone to either iatrogenic or straddle injuries.

The **verumontanum** is a 1-cm ovoid mound of smooth muscle along the posterior wall of the prostatic urethra. The prostatic utricle (an embryologic remnant of the müllerian system) enters in the center of the verumontanum, along with the ejaculatory ducts, which are just distal on either side.

Cowper glands are located within the urogenital diaphragm, but their ducts course distally ~ 2 cm to enter the bulbous urethra. Multiple small mucosal glands (glands of Littré) line the mucosa of the anterior urethra.

Imaging Techniques and Indications

Retrograde Urethrogram

A retrograde urethrogram (RUG) is the study of choice for evaluating the male urethra and is most often used in the setting of acute trauma. It is also the study of choice for evaluating for the sequelae of trauma, including strictures and fistulae formation.

Proper positioning is very important when performing a RUG. The penis should be imaged in an oblique position to visualize the full length of the urethra, avoid overlapping structures, and optimize evaluation of the membranous urethra (the most common site of urethral injury in the setting of blunt abdominal trauma). If the clinical history is a straddle injury, the examination should be focused on the bulbous portion of the urethra.

It is also imperative to get adequate distention of the urethra. Inadequate distention may result in the failure to diagnose a urethral tear. This is particularly true when a partial tear is present.

Voiding Cystourethrogram

The urethra can also be evaluated with a voiding cystourethrogram. This is most often used to evaluate for diverticula of the female urethra and obstructing valves in the male urethra.

If a patient has a suprapubic catheter placed for trauma, a combined cystogram and RUG can be performed prior to reparative surgery to determine the length of injured urethra.

MR

T2WI MR sequences provide the best images of the urethra and are particularly helpful for demonstrating the female urethra, as it is poorly evaluated on other imaging studies. T2WI with fat saturation is the best technique when evaluating for urethral diverticula. T2WI and postcontrast T1WI with fat suppression are key sequences for evaluating local invasion of urethral carcinoma.

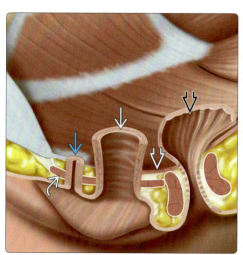
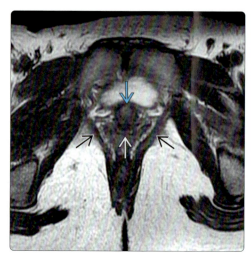

(Left) Sagittal graphic of the female pelvis shows the urethra ➡, vagina ➡, and rectum ➡ passing through the pelvic diaphragm ➡, which separates the pelvic cavity from the perineum. The urethra and vagina then pass through the muscular urogenital diaphragm ➡. (Right) Axial T2WI MR shows the female urethra ➡ as a round, intermediate signal intensity structure anterior to the vagina ➡. The levator muscles ➡ are shown well laterally.

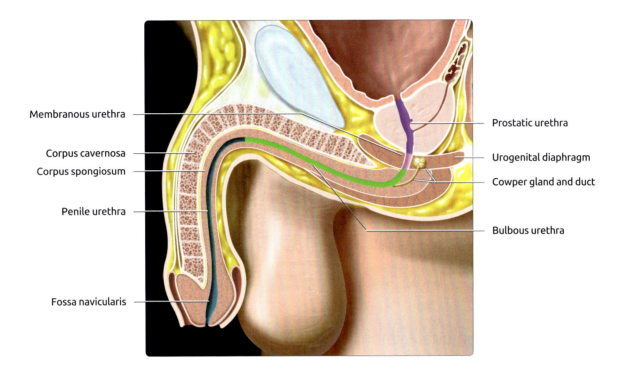

Membranous urethra

Corpus cavernosa

Corpus spongiosum

Penile urethra

Fossa navicularis

Prostatic urethra

Urogenital diaphragm

Cowper gland and duct

Bulbous urethra

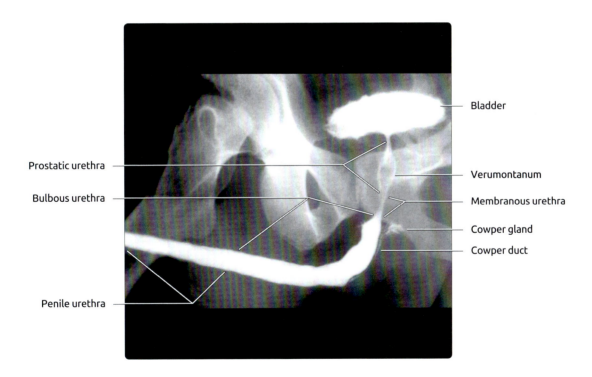

Prostatic urethra

Bulbous urethra

Penile urethra

Bladder

Verumontanum

Membranous urethra

Cowper gland

Cowper duct

(Top) *The male urethra is divided into 2 large segments: The posterior urethra, which is composed of the prostatic (purple) and membranous (pink) portions, and the anterior urethra, which is composed of the bulbous (green) and penile (blue) portions. The membranous urethra is the shortest segment; it passes through the urogenital diaphragm and is a vulnerable site for injury.* **(Bottom)** *Retrograde urethrogram shows the segments of the urethra. The verumontanum is seen as a smooth filling defect along the posterior wall of the prostatic urethra. The paired Cowper glands lie within the urogenital diaphragm, but their ducts extend ~ 2 cm distal to enter the bulbous urethra.*

T | Definition of Primary Tumor (T)

T Category	T Criteria
Male Penile Urethra and Female Urethra	
TX	Primary tumor cannot be assessed
T0	No evidence of primary tumor
Ta	Noninvasive papillary carcinoma
Tis	Carcinoma in situ
T1	Tumor invades subepithelial connective tissue
T2	Tumor invades any of the following: Corpus spongiosum, periurethral muscle
T3	Tumor invades any of the following: Corpus cavernosum, anterior vagina
T4	Tumor invades other adjacent organs (e.g., invasion of the bladder wall)
Prostatic Urethra	
Tis	Carcinoma in situ involving the prostatic urethra or periurethral or prostatic ducts without stromal invastion
T1	Tumor invades urethral subepithelial connective tissue immediately underlying the urothelium
T2	Tumor invades the prostatic stroma surrounding ducts either by direct extension from the T3 surface or by invasion from prostatic ducts
T3	Tumor invades the preprostatic fat
T4	Tumor invades other adjacent organs (e.g., extraprostatic invasion of the bladder wall, rectal wall)

Adapted with permission from AJCC Cancer Staging Manual 8th ed., 2017.

N | Definition of Regional Lymph Node (N)

N Category	N Criteria
NX	Regional lymph nodes cannot be assessed
N0	No regional lymph node metastasis
N1	Single regional lymph node metastasis in the inguinal region or true pelvis [perivesical, obturator, internal (hypogastric) and external iliac], or presacral lymph node
N2	Multiple regional lymph node metastasis in the inguinal region or true pelvis [perivesical, obturator, internal (hypogastric) and external iliac], or presacral lymph node

Adapted with permission from AJCC Cancer Staging Manual 8th ed., 2017.

M | Definition of Distant Metastasis (M)

M Category	M Criteria
M0	No distant metastasis
M1	Distant metastasis

Adapted with permission from AJCC Cancer Staging Manual 8th ed., 2017.

AJCC Prognostic Stage Groups

When T is...	And N is...	And M is...		Then the stage group is...
Tis	N0	M0		0is
Ta	N0	M0		0a
T1	N0	M0		I
T1	N1	M0		III
T2	N0	M0		II
T2	N1	M0		III
T3	N0	M0		III
T3	N1	M0		III
T4	N0	M0		IV
T4	N1	M0		IV
Any T	N2	M0		IV
Any T	Any N	M1		IV

Adapted with permission from AJCC Cancer Staging Manual 8th ed., 2017.

G Histologic Grade (G)

G Category	G Definition
Urolthelial Carcinoma	
LG	Low grade
HG	High grade
Squamous Cell Carcinoma and Adenocarcinoma	
GX	Grade cannot be assessed
G1	Well differentiated
G2	Moderately differentiated
G3	Poorly differentiated

Adapted with permission from AJCC Cancer Staging Manual 8th ed., 2017.

Incidence of Primary Urethral Carcinoma

Histologic Subtype	Incidence in Males	Incidence in Females
Transitional cell carcinoma	70.2%	33.9%
Squamous cell carcinoma	18.4%	31.1%
Adenocarcinoma	11.4%	35.0%

Observed and Overall 1- and 5-Year Survival Rates

Stage	1-Year Survival	5-Year Survival
0a	97%	79%
0is	93%	62%
I	90%	59%
II	82%	51%
III	79%	28%
IV	59%	22%

Adapted with permission from AJCC Cancer Staging Manual 8th ed., 2017.

T1: Female

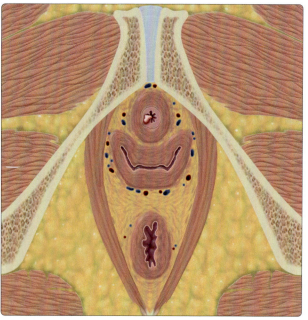

Axial illustration demonstrates T1 disease, which is limited to focal tumor with submucosal invasion. Periurethral tissue is not involved. It is unlikely that this minimal disease burden would be visible on imaging.

T2: Female

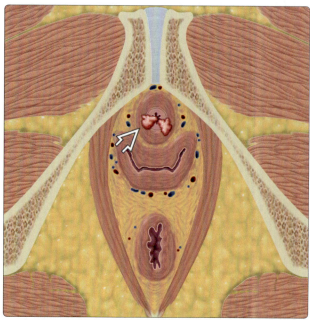

Axial illustration demonstrates T2 disease, which is centered in the urethra and extends through the subepithelial tissue into the periurethral muscle ➡ layer.

T3: Female

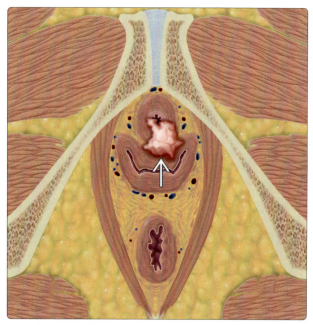

Axial illustration demonstrates T3 disease, which extends through the periurethral muscle into the adjacent anterior vagina ➡.

T4: Female

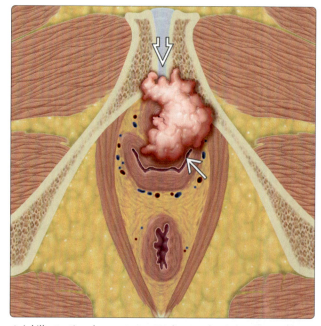

Axial illustration demonstrates T4 disease that is locally advanced and involves both the anterior vagina ➡ and the pubic symphysis ➡.

T1 and T2: Female

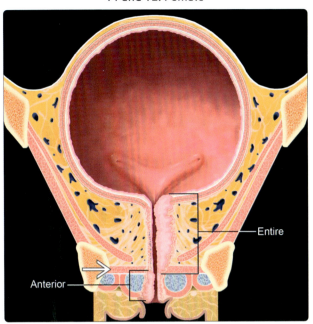

Coronal illustration of the bladder shows primary urethral cancer. The distribution of disease is divided into the anterior and entire urethra. Anterior urethral cancer is limited to the distal 1/3 of the urethra, external to the urogenital diaphragm ➡. Entire urethral cancer is usually high grade and locally advanced.

T3 and T4: Female

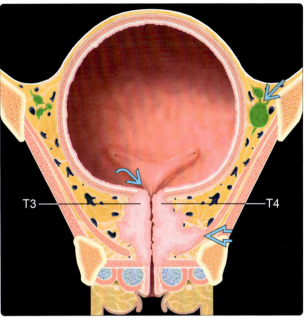

Coronal illustration of the bladder shows T3 disease on the left. It extends into the periurethral soft tissues and may involve the bladder neck ➡. T4 disease (right) involves the entire urethra and periurethral muscles ➡. N1 disease is illustrated by the enlarged regional lymph node ➡, which measures < 2 cm.

Tis and T1: Male

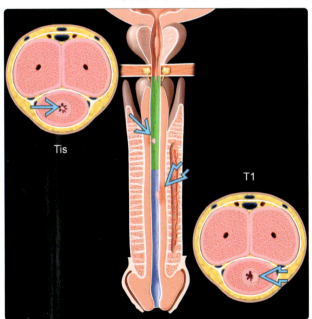

Primary urethral cancer in a male is divided into anterior (penile urethra in blue) and posterior (bulbomembranous urethra in green) distributions. On the left, Tis disease ➡ is papillary and localized, without submucosal invasion. On the right, T1 disease ➡ extends into the submucosal layer.

T2 and T3: Male

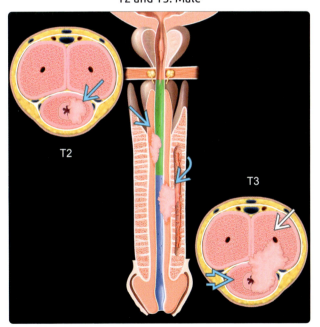

On the left, T2 disease extends into the corpus spongiosum ➡. On the right, T3 disease ➡ extends beyond the corpus spongiosum ➡ into the corpus cavernosum ➡. If prostatic urethra is involved, the etiology is more often prostatic or bladder cancer extending into prostatic urethra.

T2: Male

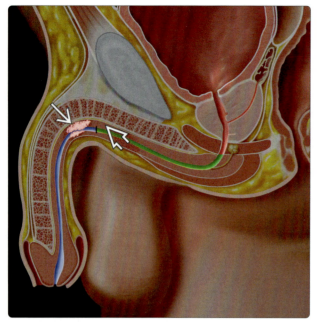

Sagittal illustration through the bladder and penis demonstrates anterior disease ➔ in the penile urethra (blue). Disease extends into the corpus spongiosum ➔, making this at least T2/stage II disease.

T2: Male

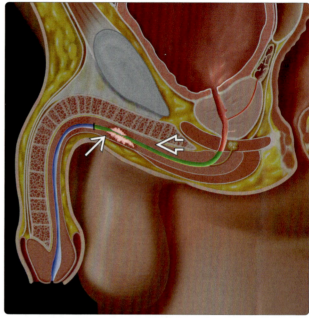

Sagittal illustration through the bladder and penis demonstrates posterior disease ➔ centered in the bulbous urethra (green). Again, there is disease demonstrated that extends into the corpus spongiosum ➔, resulting in at least T2/stage II classification.

T3: Male

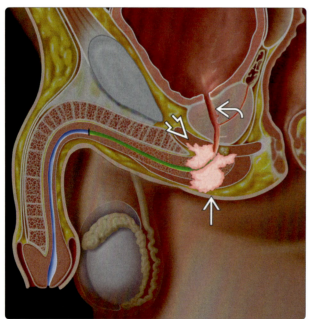

Locally advanced disease in the bulbomembranous urethra (green) is shown. Tumor invades periurethral muscle, urogenital diaphragm ➔, and perineal tissues ➔. Note the normal prostatic urethra ➔, which is consistent with the tumor arising primarily from the urethra rather than from bladder or prostate.

T4: Male

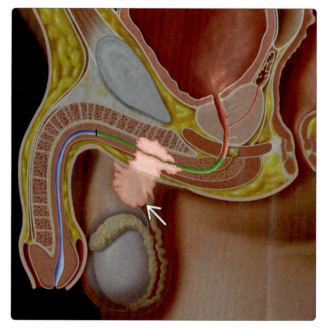

Sagittal illustration through the bladder and perineum demonstrates locally advanced posterior disease in the bulbomembranous urethra (green). This lesion extends beyond the corpus spongiosum to the scrotum ➔. A patient may present with a nonhealing scrotal ulcer in such cases.

Urethral Carcinoma Staging

N1

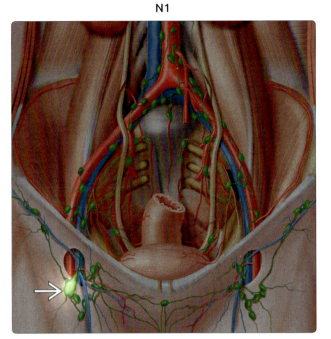

A single enlarged superficial inguinal node ➡ is present that measures ≤ 2 cm. The presence of N1 disease upgrades disease severity to stage III.

N2

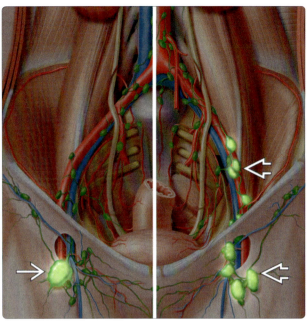

On the left, a single enlarged superficial inguinal node ➡ measures more than 2 cm. On the right, multiple nodes and multiple nodal stations are involved ➡. These are both examples of N2 disease. The presence of N2 disease upgrades disease severity to stage IV.

Metastases, Organ Frequency

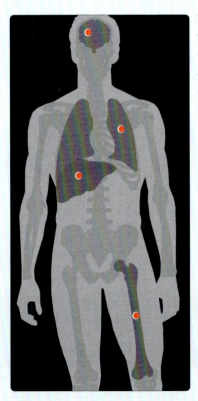

Liver	Unknown
Lung	Unknown
Bone	Unknown
Brain	Unknown

Urethral carcinoma is so uncommon that the frequency distribution of metastases is unknown. Most metastatic disease is to local lymph nodes.

Stage I (T1 N0 M0)

Stage I (T1 N0 M0)

(Left) *Axial PET/CT demonstrates minimal increased activity in the urethra ➡. Although this finding can be seen in normal mucosa, this patient had a < 1 cm anterior urethral mass, which was easily removed by local excision.* (Right) *Coronal PET/CT demonstrates minimally increased activity in the urethra ➡, corresponding to the known site of disease. No discrete lesion was identified on imaging, nor were additional sites of disease identified.*

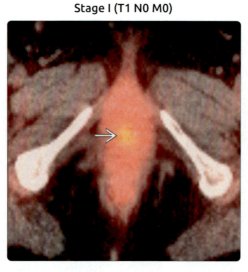

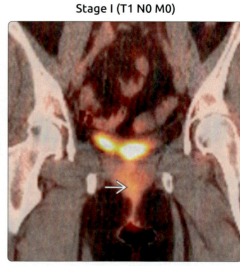

Stage I (T1 N0 M0)

Stage II (T2 N0 M0)

(Left) *Axial T2WI MR demonstrates a soft tissue nodule ➡ within a urethral diverticulum ➡. The depth of invasion is difficult to assess. On resection the lesion depth was limited to the subepithelial connective tissue layer.* (Right) *Sagittal T2WI FS MR in a male patient demonstrates a low T2 SI expansile ureteral mass ➡ in the bulbous portion of the urethra. It involves the corpus spongiosum ➡, but the corpus cavernosum ➡ is spared. (Courtesy M. Lockhart, MD, MPH.)*

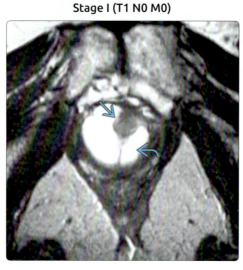

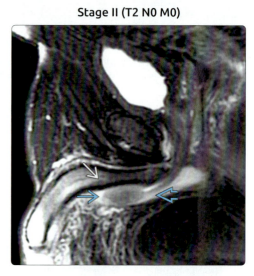

Stage II (T2 N0 M0)

Stage II (T2 N0 M0)

(Left) *Axial T2WI FS MR in the same patient demonstrates a hypointense mass ➡ centered in the bulbous urethra with expansion into the surrounding corpus spongiosum ➡. (Courtesy M. Lockhart, MD, MPH.)* (Right) *Axial T1WI C+ FS MR demonstrates relatively poor enhancement of the tumor ➡ compared to the adjacent highly vascularized corpus spongiosum ➡. (Courtesy M. Lockhart, MD, MPH.)*

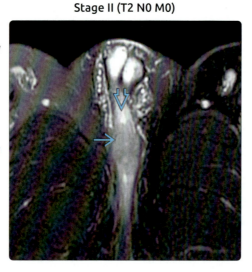

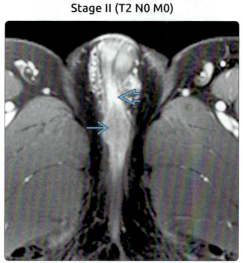

Stage II (T2 N0 M0)

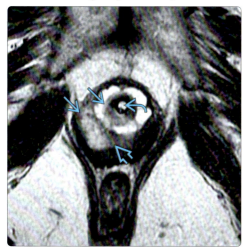

Stage II (T2 N0 M0)

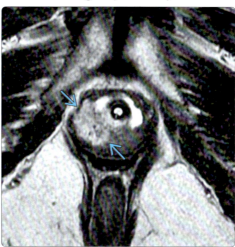

(Left) *Axial T2WI MR demonstrates a relatively low T2 signal intensity mass ➡ arising in a female urethral diverticulum, extending from the urethra into the periurethral tissues ➡. A Foley catheter is in place ➡.* **(Right)** *More caudal image in the same patient better demonstrates the extent of the relatively low T2 signal intensity mass ➡ in the diverticulum.*

Stage II (T2 N0 M0)

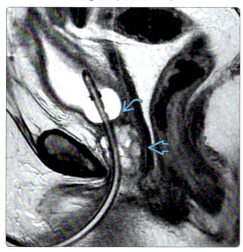

Stage II (T2 N0 M0)

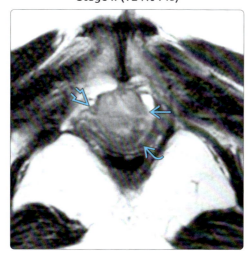

(Left) *Sagittal T2 MR in the same patient demonstrates the confinement of the mass to the urethral tissues with sparing of the bladder base ➡ and anterior vagina ➡.* **(Right)** *Axial T2WI MR in a different woman with urethral carcinoma shows a heterogeneously hypointense urethral mass ➡ with periurethral extension on the right ➡. The normally low T2 signal intensity urethral wall ➡ appears to be intact adjacent to the vagina.*

Stage III (T3 N0 M0)

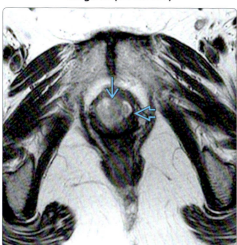

Stage III (T3 N0 M0)

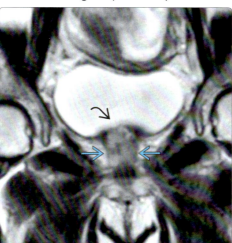

(Left) *Axial T2WI MR shows an intermediate signal intensity urethral mass ➡ that expands the urethra. The low T2 signal intensity urethral muscular wall ➡ remains intact.* **(Right)** *Coronal T2 MR shows that the entire urethra is expanded by the mass ➡. Superior extension of the mass into the bladder neck ➡ upstages this to T3 disease.*

Stage III (T3 N0 M0)

Stage III (T3 N0 M0)

(Left) Sagittal T2WI MR in the same patient shows an intermediate signal intensity urethral mass ➡ that expands the urethra. The superior extension into the bladder neck is well depicted ➡.
(Right) Postcontrast sagittal T1WI FS MR demonstrates a heterogeneously enhancing urethral mass ➡, with increased concern for involvement of the anterior vagina ➡.

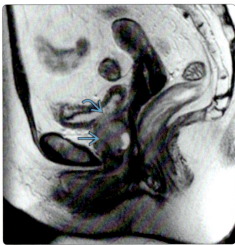

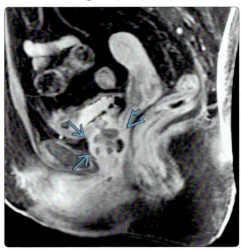

Stage III (T2 N1 M0)

Stage III (T2 N1 M0)

(Left) Axial T2WI MR demonstrates an intermediate signal intensity urethral mass ➡ expanding the female urethra. Periurethral muscle is thinned on the left ➡. Deep periurethral muscle invasion is not seen. An enlarged right inguinal node is present ➡.
(Right) Axial T1WI C+ FS MR shows the heterogeneously enhancing tumor contacting, but not involving, the left periurethral muscle ➡. Metastatic right inguinal adenopathy ➡ upstages the disease from stage II to stage III.

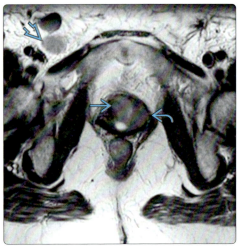

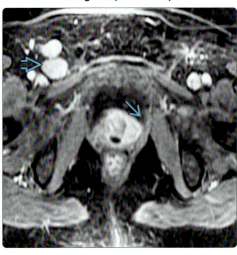

Stage IV (T2 N0 M1)

Stage IV (T2 N0 M1)

(Left) Axial CECT shows a heterogeneously enhancing urethral mass ➡; however, the integrity of periurethral tissue planes cannot be determined. Indeed, CT is of limited utility in assessing urethral T stage. (Right) Axial thoracic CECT in the same patient demonstrates an enlarged enhancing precarinal node ➡, a left pleural nodule ➡, and a right pleural effusion ➡. The extensive thoracic metastatic disease is best demonstrated on CT.

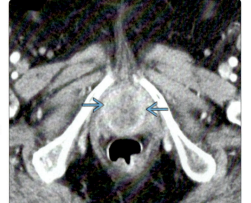

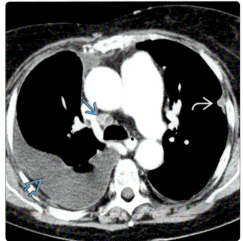

Stage IV (T4 N0 M0)

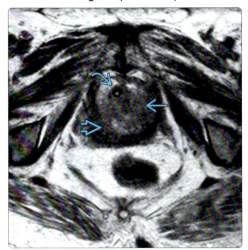

Stage IV (T4 N0 M0)

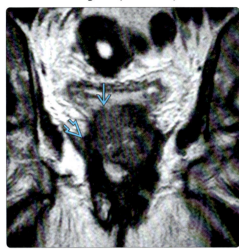

(Left) Axial T2WI MR demonstrates a heterogeneously hypointense mass ➡ expanding a female urethra with loss of a distinct high T2 signal intensity plane in the vesicovaginal space ➡. A Foley catheter is in place ➡. (Right) Coronal T2WI MR in the same patient demonstrates infiltration beyond the periurethral tissue into the adjacent levator ani muscle complex on the right ➡. Additionally, the mass is seen invading the bladder base ➡.

Stage IV (T4 N0 M0)

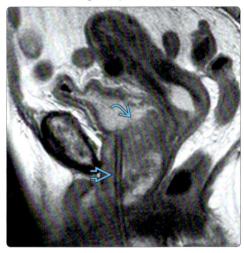

Stage IV (T4 N0 M0)

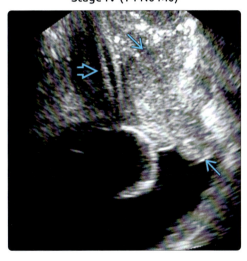

(Left) Sagittal T2WI MR in the same patient better demonstrates the heterogeneous low T2 signal intensity mass involving the entire urethra and extending cranially to invade the bladder base ➡. A Foley catheter ➡ is present. (Right) Transperineal ultrasound in the same patient demonstrates the polypoid urethral mass ➡ extending into the bladder. A Foley catheter is well demonstrated within the urethra ➡, with the catheter balloon expanded in the bladder.

Postoperative Appearance

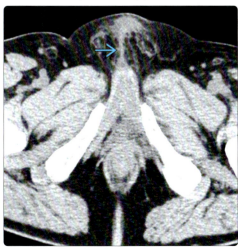

Postoperative Recurrence

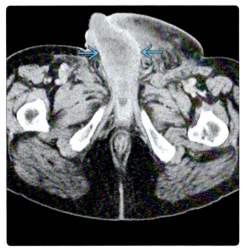

(Left) Axial CECT shows the postoperative appearance of a partial penectomy ➡ for anterior stage II disease. At this time, no local recurrence is present. Long-term survival has been reported in subjects who undergo this therapy. (Right) Axial NECT in a different patient demonstrates a local recurrence ➡ after partial penectomy. Recurrence developed along the bulbomembranous urethra.

Urethral Stricture

TERMINOLOGY

- Narrowing of urethra due to scar tissue or tumor

IMAGING

- Strictures have variable appearance
  - Focal, asymmetric indentations
  - Long segmental, tubular, or beaded constrictions
  - Proximal urethral dilatation on urethrography in chronic phase
- Filling of glands of Littre (mucous-secreting glands of urethra)
  - Highly associated with infection or inflammation
- Iatrogenic trauma
  - Located in penoscrotal junction and membranous portion of urethra (most common)
  - Other sites: Meatus and junction with bladder neck
- Retrograde urethrogram and voiding urethrography combined to evaluate proximal and distal stricture

TOP DIFFERENTIAL DIAGNOSES

- Urethral trauma
  - Stretch injury with similar appearance to stricture but in acute setting
- Urethral carcinoma

PATHOLOGY

- Etiology: Trauma (most common etiology)
  - Iatrogenic trauma (most common traumatic cause)
  - Infection: Gonorrhea, syphilis (2nd most common), tuberculosis

CLINICAL ISSUES

- Treatment: Use 1 or more procedures
  - Dilatation with catheters or balloons
  - Urethrotomy, surgical reconstruction
- US and RUG/VCUG ("up-downogram") can be used to measure stricture

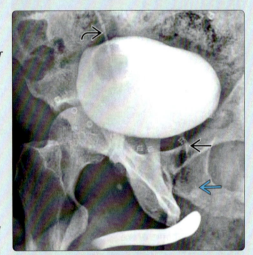
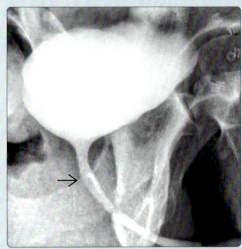

(Left) Combined retrograde urethrogram (RUG) and voiding cystourethrogram through a suprapubic catheter ➡ was performed 1 month after the patient sustained pelvic trauma. There is filling of the proximal aspect of the prostatic portion ➡ of the urethra followed by a severe stricture ➡ of the remainder of the posterior urethra. (Right) Postoperative RUG in the same patient, following the repair of the severe stricture, shows a normal urethra ➡. Trauma is one of the leading causes of urethral strictures.

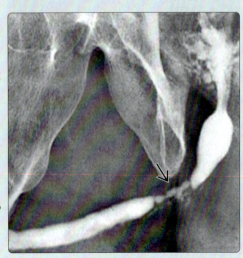
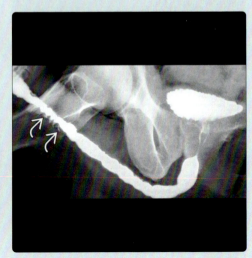

(Left) RUG shows an irregular segment of stricture ➡ in the bulbous portion of the urethra due to urothelial carcinoma. Unlike most iatrogenic strictures, malignant strictures have an irregular appearance. (Right) RUG in a patient with gonococcal urethritis shows irregularity of the penile and bulbous urethra with filling of the periurethral glands of Littre ➡. This sign is highly associated with an infectious or inflammatory etiology, which frequently progresses to stricture formation.

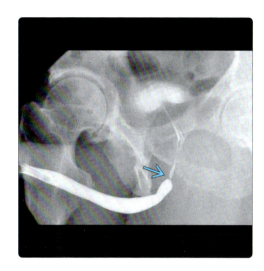
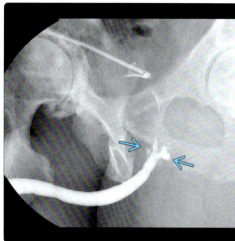

(Left) *Anterior oblique image during RUG shows a high-grade stricture ➡ in the bulbar urethra. (Courtesy P. Ramchandani, MD, FACR.)* (Right) *RUG in the same patient following urethroplasty shows a leak ➡ at the site of a previous stricture. (Courtesy P. Ramchandani, MD, FACR.)*

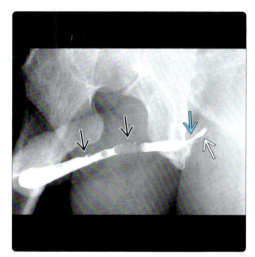
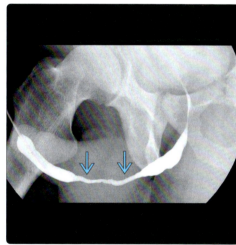

(Left) *Anterior oblique image during RUQ shows a stricture ➡ of the bulbar urethra, filling of the glands of Littre ➡ and filling of Cowper duct ➡. (Courtesy P. Ramchandani, MD, FACR.)* (Right) *Anterior oblique image during RUG shows a long-segment stricture ➡ of the distal bulbar and proximal pendulous urethra. (Courtesy P. Ramchandani, MD, FACR.)*

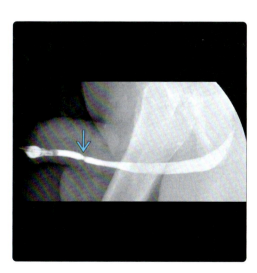
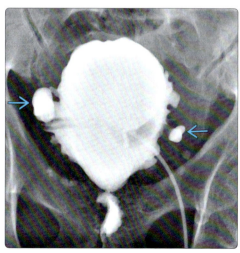

(Left) *Lateral image during RUG shows a focal stricture ➡ in the proximal aspect of the pendulous urethra. (Courtesy P. Ramchandani, MD, FACR.)* (Right) *AP image during RUG shows trabeculation ➡ of the urinary bladder, a finding which can be seen with chronic outlet obstruction due to stricture. (Courtesy P. Ramchandani, MD, FACR.)*

TERMINOLOGY

- Focal outpouching of urethra into adjacent fascia
  - Most arise from posterolateral wall of middle 1/3 of urethra

IMAGING

- MR
  - Periurethral cystic lesion that may abut or surround urethra
  - T1WI: Typically low signal intensity (SI)
    - ↑ SI with proteinaceous or hemorrhagic contents
  - T2WI: Typically ↑ SI
    - ↓ SI with proteinaceous or inflammatory debris
  - T1WI post contrast
    - Inflammation/infection: Enhancement of diverticular wall and periurethral tissues
    - Neoplasm: Enhancement of mural nodule or mass
- Voiding cystourethrogram
  - Opacification of diverticulum during voiding of contrast instilled into bladder

TOP DIFFERENTIAL DIAGNOSES

- Bartholin gland cyst
- Gartner cyst
- Skene duct cyst
- Urethral caruncle

CLINICAL ISSUES

- Etiologies: Congenital, recurrent infection of periurethral glands, traumatic delivery
- Nonspecific signs/symptoms: Recurrent/chronic urinary tract infection, dysuria, incontinence
- Classic triad of dysuria, dyspareunia, and postvoid dribbling
- Intraluminal calculi and neoplasms are rare

DIAGNOSTIC CHECKLIST

- Describe location, size, number, complexity (septa, mural nodules, calculi)

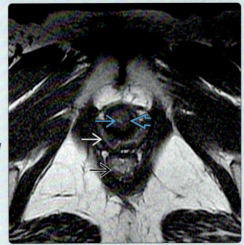
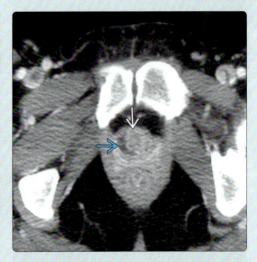

(Left) Axial single-shot fast spin-echo T2WI at the level of the pubic symphysis demonstrates the normal appearance of the female urethra; the central high signal intensity is due to the mucosa ➡, while the surrounding intermediate signal intensity is due to the muscular wall ➡. More posteriorly, the vaginal ➡ and anal ➡ canals are evident. (Right) Axial CECT reveals a crescentic, fluid-attenuation structure ➡ along the right lateral aspect of the urethra ➡ that is due to urethral diverticulum.

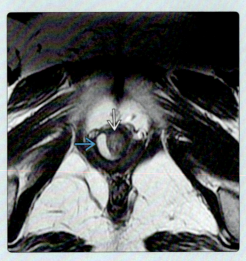
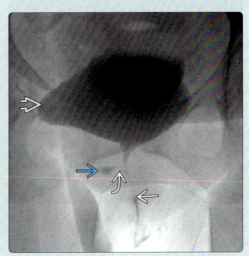

(Left) Axial single-shot fast spin-echo T2WI in the same patient demonstrates homogeneous, high signal intensity within the diverticulum ➡ that extends along the right lateral aspect of the urethra ➡. (Right) AP view during a voiding cystourethrogram in the same patient shows that the orifice ➡ of the diverticulum ➡ arises from the right posterolateral wall of the urethra ➡. The catheter used to instill contrast material into the urinary bladder ➡ had been removed prior to voiding.

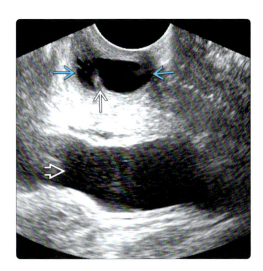
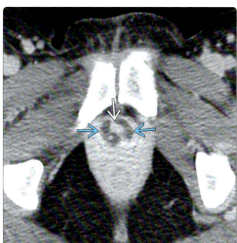

(Left) Coronal, angled endovaginal US shows an ovoid, cystic structure ➡ surrounding the urethra ➡. The cystic structure is anechoic and shows posterior acoustic enhancement. More superoposterior, the urinary bladder ➡ is shown. (Right) Axial CECT at the level of the pubic symphysis in the same patient shows a rounded, cystic structure ➡ encircling the urethra due to a urethral diverticulum. The enhancement of the urethra and adjacent tissues ➡ is normal. The patient had a history of postvoid dribbling.

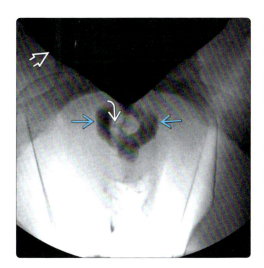
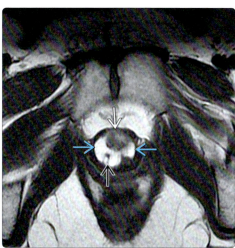

(Left) AP view during voiding cystourethrogram in the same patient demonstrates contrast material filling circumferential urethral diverticulum ➡. The orifice ➡ of the diverticulum is shown to arise posterolaterally on right side. Contrast material is within the urinary bladder ➡. (Right) Axial single-shot fast spin-echo T2WI in the same patient reveals high signal intensity in the diverticulum ➡ that surrounds the urethra ➡. A thin, partial septum ➡ is shown along the right posterolateral aspect of the diverticulum.

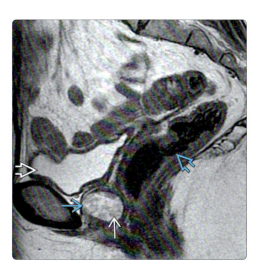
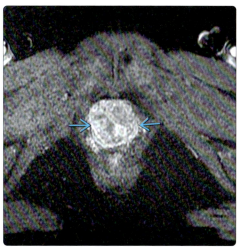

(Left) Sagittal single-shot fast spin-echo T2WI reveals an ovoid diverticulum ➡ arising from midurethra. Diverticulum has a heterogeneous appearance due to high signal intensity from fluid and intermediate signal intensity from numerous soft tissue nodules ➡. The urinary bladder ➡ and rectum ➡ are shown. (Right) Axial T1WI with fat saturation after contrast injection in the same patient shows heterogeneous enhancement throughout the diverticulum ➡ due to adenocarcinoma within the diverticular lumen.

IMAGING

- Goldman classification for retrograde urethrogram
  - Type 1: Stretched posterior urethra but no extravasation
  - Type 2: Contrast extravasation superior to level of urogenital diaphragm
    - Urogenital diaphragm remains intact
  - Type 3: Contrast extravasation surrounding membranous and proximal bulbous urethra into perineum
    - Disruption of urogenital diaphragm
  - Type 4: Bladder neck injury extending into proximal urethra
    - Type 4a: Injury at base of bladder (not involving bladder neck) with periurethral extravasation simulating true type 4 urethral injury
    - Types 4 and 4a indistinguishable on urethrogram
  - Type 5: Contrast extravasation from anterior urethra
    - Injury is isolated to anterior urethra
  - In partial ruptures, contrast fills bladder
    - In complete ruptures, contrast fails to fill bladder
- Alternative classification from American Association for Surgery of Trauma
  - Class 1: Contusion
  - Class 2: Stretch injury (intact lumen)
  - Class 3: Partial disruption
  - Class 4: Complete disruption (< 2 cm separation)
  - Class 5: Complete disruption (> 2 cm separation)

CLINICAL ISSUES

- Urethral injury is seen in 24% of men with pelvic fracture (6% in women)
- Type 3 injury (disruption of urogenital diaphragm) is most common form
- Urogenital diaphragm can be identified on retrograde urethrogram immediately superior to symmetrical, cone-shaped tip of bulbar urethra

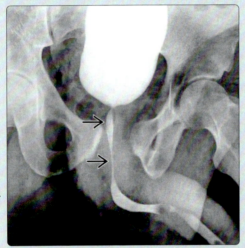
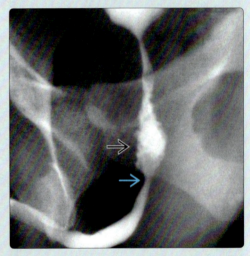

(Left) Retrograde urethrogram (RUG) shows a stretched, but intact, posterior urethra ⊅, consistent with a type 1 injury in the Goldman classification. According to the American Association for Surgery of Trauma classification, this is a type 2 injury. Note the diastasis of the pubic symphysis. (Right) RUG shows extravasation of contrast material ⊅ from the posterior urethra; note that the extravasated contrast is located superior to the level of the urogenital diaphragm ⊅, consistent with a type 2 injury in the Goldman classification.

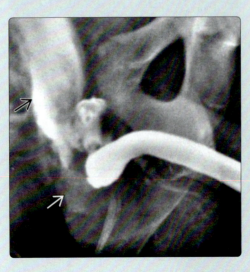
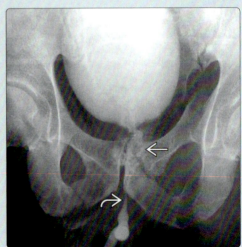

(Left) RUG shows a Goldman classification type 3 injury with extravasated contrast superior ⊅ and inferior ⊅ to the level of the urogenital diaphragm. (Right) RUG shows contrast extravasation from a bladder neck laceration that extended into the proximal urethra ⊅ (Goldman type 4 injury). Note the symmetrical, coned appearance of the proximal bulbar urethra ⊅ demarcating the approximate junction of the anterior and posterior aspects of the urethra and the level of the urogenital diaphragm.

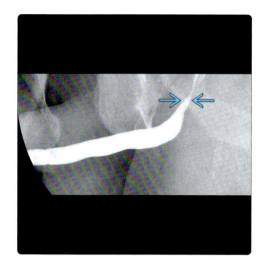

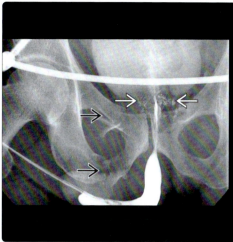

(Left) *Anterior oblique image from a RUG shows a normal male urethra. Note the normal smooth funneling* ⇨ *at the bulbomembranous junction between the anterior and posterior segments of the urethra. (Courtesy P. Ramchadani, MD, FACR.)* (Right) *Anterior image from a RUG shows contrast extravasation* ⇨ *due to injury at the junction of the bladder base and proximal prostatic urethra. Note fractures* ⇨ *of the right pubic rami. (Courtesy P. Ramchadani, MD, FACR.)*

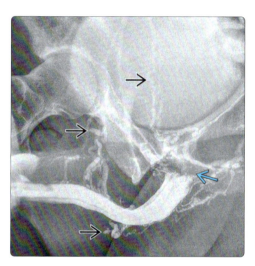

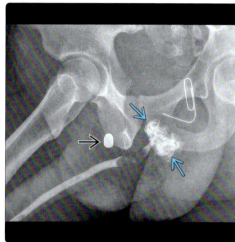

(Left) *Anterior oblique image during a RUG performed after crush injury shows abrupt truncation* ⇨ *of the urethra due to posterior urethral obstruction and venous filling* ⇨ *from site of injury. (Courtesy P. Ramchadani, MD, FACR.)* (Right) *Anterior oblique image during a RUG performed after gunshot wound shows contrast extravasation* ⇨ *due to membranous urethral injury. Note the bullet fragment* ⇨ *within the soft tissues. (Courtesy P. Ramchadani, MD, FACR.)*

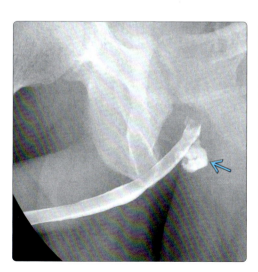

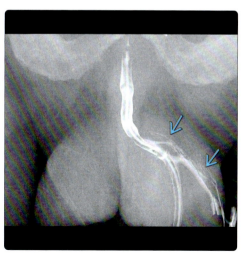

(Left) *Anterior oblique image during a RUG after a straddle injury shows contrast extravasation* ⇨ *due to a urethra injury at the bulbomembranous junction. (Courtesy P. Ramchadani, MD, FACR.)* (Right) *Anterior image obtained during a RUG due to a dog bite shows contrast extravasation* ⇨ *due to an injury of the pendulous segment of the urethra. (Courtesy P. Ramchadani, MD, FACR.)*

TERMINOLOGY

- Persistent inability to achieve or maintain penile erections of sufficient value to engage in satisfactory sexual activity

IMAGING

- Doppler ultrasound
  - Spectral Doppler interrogation of cavernosal arteries following injection of stimulant (e.g., prostaglandin derivative) should show ↑ peak systolic velocity and ↓ end diastolic velocity
  - Arterial insufficiency threshold range: PSV < 25-35 cm/s
  - Venous insufficiency threshold range: EDV > 5-7 cm/s
- Grayscale ultrasound
  - Peyronie disease: Hyperechoic plaques in corpora cavernosa
  - Penile fracture: Focal, linear defect in corpora cavernosa
- Measurement of penile: Branchial index
  - Measure ratio of peak systolic blood pressures
  - Abnormal is < 0.7

- Angiography
  - 2nd-line technique to evaluate for stenosis or occlusion in branches of internal pudendal artery
- Imaging recommendations
  - Best imaging tool
    - Penile Doppler ultrasonography
  - Protocol advice
    - Doppler sonography: Performed every 5 minutes after intracavernosal injection of stimulant agent (e.g., prostaglandin E1 derivative) over 20-30 minutes
    - Cavernosal arterial waveforms are sampled until peak systolic and end diastolic velocities are reached

CLINICAL ISSUES

- Patients typically given trial of phosphodiesterase inhibitors prior to any imaging
- Treatment
  - Medical: Phosphodiesterase inhibitors
  - Surgical: Revascularization vs. penile prosthesis

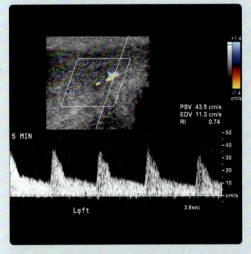 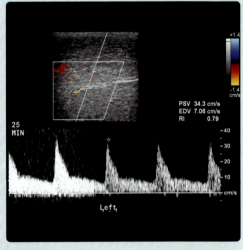

(Left) Transverse Doppler US at the left penile base obtained 5 minutes past intracavernosal injection shows a normal peak systolic velocity of 44 cm/s and an end diastolic velocity of 11 cm/s within the left cavernosal artery. (Courtesy M. Lockhart, MD.) (Right) Sagittal Doppler US in the same patient was obtained 20 minutes later at the left aspect of the penile base and shows that the end diastolic velocity has only decreased to 7 cm/s, consistent with venous insufficiency. (Courtesy M. Lockhart, MD.)

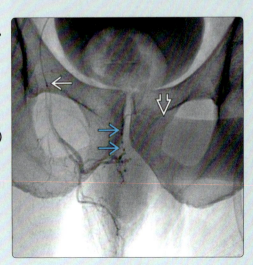 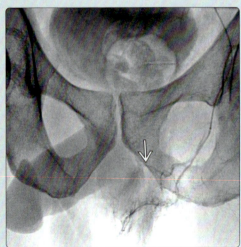

(Left) Anteroposterior view during angiography shows the catheter tip ⮕ in the right internal pudendal artery. The penile artery is irregular and shows multiple areas of narrowing ⮕. The dorsal penile artery ⮕ is diminutive, while the cavernosal artery could not be identified. (Right) AP view during left internal pudendal arteriogram in the same patient reveals that the penile artery ⮕ is diminutive and no flow was observed in the dorsal penile artery or cavernosal artery in this patient with advanced atherosclerosis.

SECTION 8

Testes

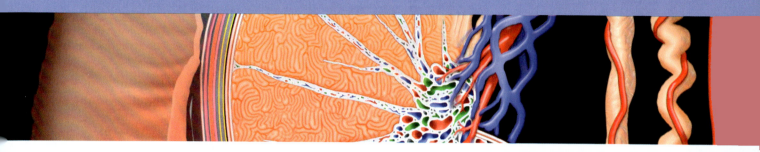

Nonneoplastic Conditions

Neoplasms

Introduction

High-frequency transducer sonography using gray-scale along with pulsed and color Doppler is the imaging modality of choice for evaluating patients presenting with scrotal pathology. Scrotal ultrasound (US) is often requested in an emergency setting in a case of acute scrotal pain. The leading differential diagnoses in such a scenario includes testicular torsion, acute epididymo-orchitis, and traumatic injury (in the setting of preceding trauma). In a nonacute setting, scrotal ultrasound is often requested for evaluation of chronic testicular pain or a palpable scrotal mass. The leading differential diagnoses in the nonacute setting when a mass is palpated includes a testicular neoplasm (benign or malignant) and extra testicular masses, including epididymal lesions and inguinal hernias.

Clinical correlation with history and symptoms is an extremely important aspect of scrotal sonography.

Ultrasound Technique for Scrotal Evaluation

Scrotal US is performed with the patient in the supine position and the scrotum supported by a towel placed between the thighs. Optimal results are obtained with a 10-14MHz high-frequency, linear-array transducer. Scanning is performed with the transducer in direct contact with the skin with copious amounts of gel; if necessary, a stand-off pad can be used for evaluation of superficial lesions.

The testes are examined in at least two planes (i.e., the longitudinal and transverse axes). The size and echogenicity of each testis and epididymis are compared with those on the opposite side. Scrotal skin thickness is evaluated for symmetricity as well as focal or diffuse edema. Color Doppler and pulsed Doppler parameters are optimized to display low-flow velocities and to demonstrate blood flow in the testes and surrounding scrotal structures. Color Doppler ultrasound should include comparison of right and left testicular spectral Doppler tracings. Power Doppler US may also be used to demonstrate intratesticular blood flow in patients with an acute scrotum, particularly if torsion is considered.

When evaluating patients presenting with an acute scrotum, the asymptomatic side should be scanned first in order to optimize gray-scale and color Doppler gain settings. This allows for comparison with the affected side (though a caveat is that testicular torsion can be a bilateral process in 2% of patients). Transverse images with portions of each testis on the same image should be acquired in gray-scale and color Doppler modes. Additional techniques, such as use of the Valsalva maneuver or upright positioning, can be used as needed for venous evaluation. Power Doppler sonography uses the integrated power of the Doppler signal to depict the presence of blood flow. Power Doppler sonography may be slightly more sensitive than standard color Doppler for detecting low-flow states and may provide essential information in the diagnosis of potential complete testicular torsion.

Clinical Perspective

Acute Scrotal Pain

In an emergency setting, acute scrotal pain should prompt an assessment of epididymo-orchitis, testicular torsion, and traumatic injury. Ultrasound features are correlated with history and physical examination findings. Although acute epididymo-orchitis and acute testicular torsion present similarly with acute onset of unilateral testicular pain,

epididymo-orchitis may be accompanied with fever &/or a Prehn sign (relief of pain with elevation of scrotum above the level of pubic symphysis). Moreover, the sonographic appearances for both diagnoses are very distinct: Edema with increased vascularity in epididymo-orchitis and edema with absent or reduced flow in torsion. A potential pitfall for testicular torsion is the torsion-detorsion syndrome, wherein the testis may detorse spontaneously: Detorsion results in reactive hyperemia, which can appear sonographically similar to epididymo-orchitis. An appropriate history preceding the clinical presentation may lead one to the correct diagnosis. Torsion-detorsion syndrome will typically present with intermittent symptoms of pain and discomfort. Epididymo-orchitis will present with constant or worsening pain. Associated findings of inflammation in the ipsilateral scrotum, such as scrotal skin thickening and pyocele, also favor epididymo-orchitis.

The diagnosis of a traumatic scrotal injury is usually not difficult with a prior history of trauma (blunt or penetrating). The purpose of performing an ultrasound after trauma is to determine whether surgical exploration is required. Most cases with testicular rupture (tunica albuginea disruption) will need to be surgically repaired. In addition, large hematoceles or large hematomas resulting in testicular ischemia may require surgical evacuation &/or debridement. The presences of color Doppler flow in the testis helps determine viability. It is extremely important to follow all such cases to resolution, as some hematomas may become infected and form an abscess.

Chronic/Nonacute Scrotal Pathology

In a nonacute setting, patients often present with an enlarged scrotum, palpable mass, or mild scrotal pain. An enlarged scrotum may be related to a hydrocele, spermatocele, scrotal wall edema, or inguinal hernia. In the setting of a palpable mass, ultrasound is extremely sensitive in detecting the presence of an intratesticular neoplasm, which is a malignancy until proven otherwise. Mild scrotal pain is often related to a varicocele, which can easily be diagnosed with color Doppler and Valsalva maneuvers.

Summary

The ability of ultrasound to diagnose the pathogenesis of the acute scrotum is unsurpassed by any other imaging modality. Ultrasound is the first-line imaging study performed in patients with acute scrotum. Knowledge of the normal and pathologic sonographic appearance of the scrotum and an understanding of the proper technique are essential for accurate diagnosis of an acute scrotum. High-frequency transducer sonography combined with color and power Doppler sonography provides information essential to reach a specific diagnosis in patients with testicular torsion, epididymo-orchitis, and scrotal trauma.

Selected References

1. Appelbaum L et al: Scrotal ultrasound in adults. Semin Ultrasound CT MR. 34(3):257-73, 2013
2. American Institute of Ultrasound in Medicine et al: AIUM practice guideline for the performance of scrotal ultrasound examinations. J Ultrasound Med. 30(1):151-5, 2011
3. Bhatt S et al: Role of US in testicular and scrotal trauma. Radiographics. 28(6):1617-29, 2008
4. Dogra V et al: Acute painful scrotum. Radiol Clin North Am. 42 (2): 349-63, 2004
5. Dogra VS et al: Sonography of the scrotum. Radiology. 227(1):18-36, 2003
6. Dogra V et al: Ultrasonography of the scrotum. J Ultrasound Med. 21(8):848, 2002

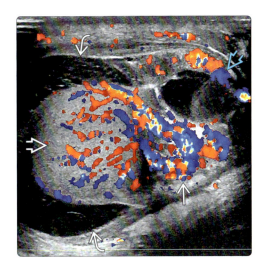

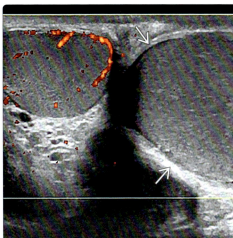

(Left) *Color Doppler ultrasound of an elderly male with acute scrotal pain and a history of urinary tract infections shows a hyperemic, epididymis* ➡ *and testis* ➡ *(an appearance compatible with epididymo-orchitis). Note the adjacent pyocele* ➡ *and debris filled epididymal cyst* ➡. **(Right)** *Power Doppler ultrasound of a 35-year-old man with acute left testicular torsion shows no flow within the left testis* ➡. *Technique should be optimized to detect slow flow when torsion is suspected; comparison to the asymptomatic testis is critical.*

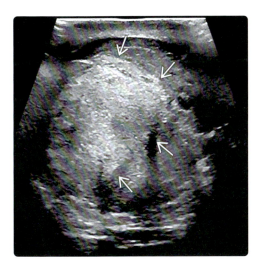

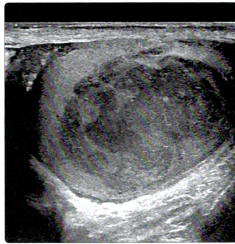

(Left) *Ultrasound performed on a young male, post blunt scrotal injury, shows a wide testicular fracture* ➡. *No flow was shown at color Doppler and the testis was not viable at exploration. The goal of ultrasound in these settings is to assess testicular flow and tunica integrity.* **(Right)** *Ultrasound shows a solid hypoechoic testicular mass (a finding indicating malignancy until proven otherwise). Most testicular tumors are either seminomas or mixed germ cell tumors, although lymphoma was confirmed in this HIV positive male.*

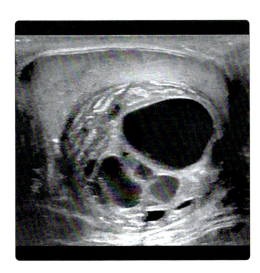

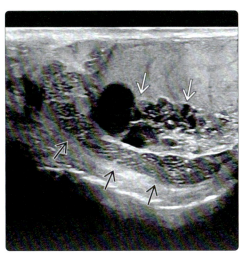

(Left) *Scrotal ultrasound of a 40-year-old man with a palpable mass shows a mixed cystic and solid testicular mass (a confirmed mixed germ cell tumor). Ultrasound is the imaging modality of choice for evaluation of scrotal contents.* **(Right)** *Ultrasound performed for evaluation of scrotal discomfort shows an elongated cystic mass* ➡ *composed of tubular components. Location within the mediastinum testis and the ultrasound appearance indicate dilated rete testes (a leave alone lesion). Note the post vasectomy epididymis* ➡.

TERMINOLOGY

- Incomplete descent of testis into scrotum

IMAGING

- Located anywhere from abdomen to inguinal canal
  - 10% bilateral: Inguinal canal most common (80%)
  - Imaging unable to distinguish retractile from fixed, cryptorchid inguinal testis
  - Role of imaging discounted in recent (2014) AUA guidelines: Physical exam typically suffices
  - Imaging utilized in equivocal cases, obesity, disorders of sexual differentiation
- Ultrasound: Study of choice for inguinal testis
  - Ovoid, homogeneous, well-circumscribed mass: Smaller than normally descended testis
  - Echogenic line of mediastinum testis helps differentiate from other soft tissues masses
- MR: Study of choice for potential intraabdominal testes not identified at laparoscopy
  - 94% accuracy for detection and characterization of undescended testes
  - T1WI: Low signal intensity ovoid mass; T2WI: high signal intensity ovoid mass
  - Decreased T2 signal secondary to fibrotic changes

TOP DIFFERENTIAL DIAGNOSES

- Retractile testis
- Inguinal masses (lymphadenopathy, hernia)
- Absent testis (anorchia): Congenital (rare) or prior resection

CLINICAL ISSUES

- ↑ risk of malignant neoplasm in both cryptorchid testis and contralateral testis
  - Increased risk likely from abnormal embryogenesis affecting both testes
  - 3.5-14.5% of testicular cancer patients have history of cryptorchidism
- ↑ incidence of infertility

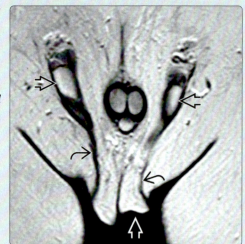
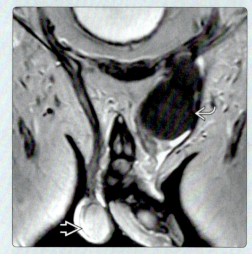

(Left) Coronal T2WI MR shows an empty scrotal sac ⊃ and bilateral undescended testes ⊃. The gubernaculum ➔, a ligament which extends from the lower pole of the testis to the scrotal sac, is well demonstrated. (Right) Coronal T2WI MR shows a low-signal tumor ➔ within an undescended testis. Compare this signal to the normally descended testis on the right ⊃. It is important to know that the increased risk of carcinoma does not just apply to the undescended side but also to the normally descended testis.

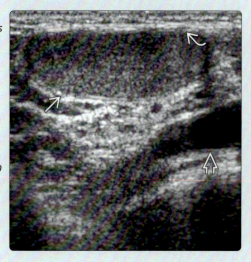
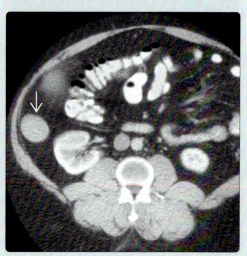

(Left) Oblique ultrasound along the inguinal canal shows an ovoid, hypoechoic testis ➔ deep to the subcutaneous tissue and fascia ➔. Note the femoral vessels ➔. The inguinal canal is the most common location for an undescended testis and may present as a palpable groin mass. (Right) Axial CECT shows ovoid soft tissue mass ➔ within the retroperitoneum just lateral to the kidney. This could easily be confused with other soft tissue masses or adenopathy, so history is essential. Lower images showed no spermatic cord.

KEY FACTS

IMAGING

- Absent or decreased abnormal testicular blood flow on color Doppler US
- Findings vary with duration and degree of rotation of cord
- Role of spectral Doppler is limited; may be helpful to detect partial torsion; in partial torsion of 360° or less, spectral Doppler may show diminished diastolic arterial flow
- Spiral twist of spermatic cord cranial to testis and epididymis causes torsion knot or whirlpool pattern of concentric layers: "whirlpool" sign
- Increased flow may be seen in affected testis if torsion-detorsion: Correlation with clinical history of preceding intermittent ipsilateral pain is helpful clue

PATHOLOGY

- Varying degrees of ischemic necrosis and fibrosis depending on duration of symptoms
- Undescended testes have increased risk of torsion

- Intravaginal ("bell clapper") torsion: Common type, most frequently occurs at puberty
- Extravaginal torsion: Neonates: Torsed testis is never viable, exploration performed for contralateral orchiopexy

CLINICAL ISSUES

- Acute scrotal/inguinal pain; swollen, erythematous hemiscrotum without recognized trauma; nausea/vomiting are classic
- Reducing time lag between onset of symptoms and time of surgical or manual detorsion is of utmost importance in preserving viable testis
- Nonviable testicle usually removed; higher risk of subsequent torsion on contralateral side; contralateral orchiopexy standard of care
- Venous obstruction occurs 1st, followed by obstruction of arterial flow, which leads to testicular ischemia

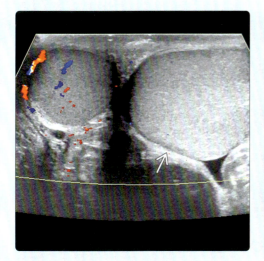

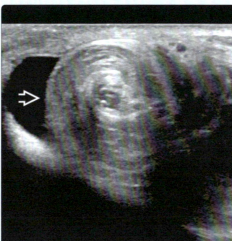

(Left) Color Doppler US performed on a young male patient with acute scrotal pain shows no flow within a relatively enlarged left testis ➡. Doppler parameters should be optimized to detect slow flow, and comparison to the contralateral (asymptomatic) testis is critical. (Right) US performed above the left testis in the same patient shows the "whirl" sign ➡ due to twisting of the spermatic cord. Direct visualization of the twisted cord may increase exam accuracy, particularly in cases of partial torsion.

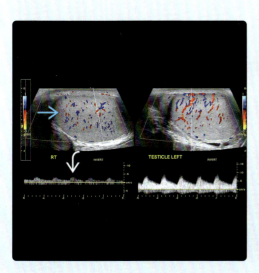

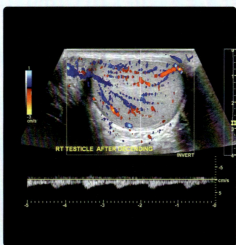

(Left) Sagittal color Doppler US of both testes in a young male patient with right testicular pain shows asymmetric blood flow with reduced flow to the right testis ➡, as seen on color flow and pulse wave Doppler ➡. This was surgically confirmed to be partial (180°) right testicular torsion. (Right) Transverse color Doppler US of the right testis of the same patient after detorsion shows characteristic Doppler hyperemia.

Segmental Infarction

IMAGING

- Rare lesion, but characteristic appearance suggests diagnosis in acute setting
  - Ultrasound: Elongated, geographic "mass" within superior aspect of testis
    - May be isoechoic in acute setting; hypoechoic lesion with peripheral echogenic rim is more typical
    - Avascular or hypovascular at color Doppler, peripheral hyperemic rim may be identified
  - MR: Utilize for confirmation or if ultrasound equivocal
    - Well-defined, geographic, peripheral "mass" with peripheral enhancement

TOP DIFFERENTIAL DIAGNOSES

- Testicular neoplasm
  - Round mass, rarely presents in acute setting
- Testicular hematoma
  - Hypovascular, hypoechoic mass: Typically post trauma
- Testicular abscess

- History (prior epididymo-orchitis, fever, leukocytosis, pyuria) aids diagnosis
- Testicular lymphoma and leukemia
  - Uni- or multifocal hypoechoic mass, post cessation of maintenance chemotherapy

CLINICAL ISSUES

- Rare cause for acute scrotum
  - Reported predisposing history: Vasculitis, sickle cell disease, hypercoagulable states, herniorrhaphy, varicocelectomy
  - Often idiopathic

DIAGNOSTIC CHECKLIST

- Ultrasound (and clinical) follow-up needed to confirm imaging impression (and exclude testicular tumor)
  - MR may increase diagnostic confidence

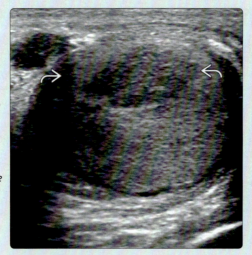
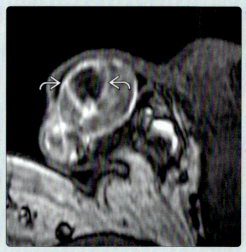

(Left) Transverse US performed on a 45-year-old man with acute scrotal pain shows an elongated, peripheral hypoechoic mass ➤. Although the appearance strongly suggests segmental infarction, as is often the case, no predisposing history was elicited. Ultrasound follow-up and a confirmatory MR were recommended. (Right) Axial gadolinium-enhanced T1 C+ fat-saturation MR on the same patient shows a triangular, avascular mass ➤ with peripheral rim enhancement, characteristic features of segmental infarction.

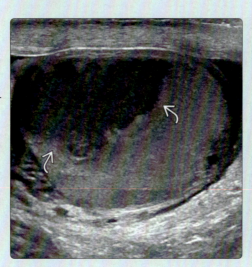
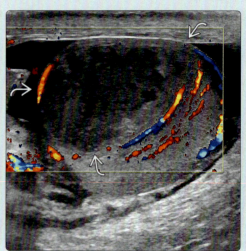

(Left) Sagittal US performed on a 47-year-old man with 2 weeks of scrotal pain shows a peripheral, wedge-shaped hypoechoic mass ➤. A prior US performed at the onset of pain was normal. (Right) Color Doppler US in the same patient shows the mass ➤ is avascular. Configuration of the lesion suggests segmental infarction, a diagnosis that prompted a work-up for vasculitis. Diagnosis of drug-induced (minocycline) vasculitis was ultimately confirmed, and symptoms resolved with steroids.

Torsion of Testicular Appendage

TERMINOLOGY

- Synonyms: Twisted appendage, torsed appendix testis, torsion of appendix epididymis, appendiceal torsion
- Definitions
  - Spontaneous twisting of pedunculated vestigial remnant along testicle or epididymis, causing ischemia & pain
  - Most common etiology of acute scrotal pain in children (more frequent than epididymoorchitis & testicular torsion)

IMAGING

- Ultrasound with Doppler best imaging modality
- Appendage size best indicator of torsion (> 5-6 mm acutely)
- Spherical shape suggests swelling (normally vermiform)
- Duration of symptoms determines echogenicity
  - < 24 hours: Hypoechoic with salt & pepper pattern
  - > 24 hours: Hypo-, iso-, or hyperechoic
  - Chronic: Calcified "scrotal pearl"
- Classically, ↓ or absent internal vascularity of torsed appendix with periappendiceal hyperemia
- Reactive hydrocele & scrotal wall edema common

TOP DIFFERENTIAL DIAGNOSES

- Testicular torsion
- Epididymoorchitis or orchitis

CLINICAL ISSUES

- Acute scrotal pain, swelling
  - Usually without nausea/vomiting present with testicular torsion
- ± small, tender, mobile lump at upper pole of testis
- ± blue dot sign of ischemic appendage seen through scrotal wall in minority of patients (< 30%)
- 80% of cases 7-14 years old; mean age: 9 years
  - vs. mean age of 14 years for testicular torsion, epididymoorchitis
- Absence of transverse lie present with testicular torsion

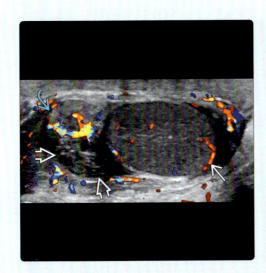
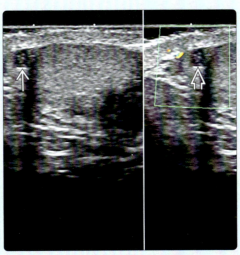

(Left) Longitudinal color Doppler US in a 10-year-old boy with left scrotal pain and swelling shows lack of blood flow in a heterogeneous round nodule ⇨ adjacent to the hyperemic, inflamed-appearing epididymal head ⇨. The testicular blood flow appears normal ⇨. (Right) Longitudinal US images of the epididymis in a 6-year-old boy show a hypoechoic nodule ⇨ superior to the testis, which is avascular on color Doppler ⇨. This was the point of maximal discomfort and likely a torsed appendage.

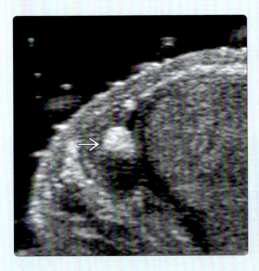
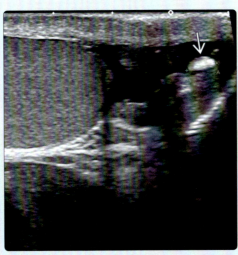

(Left) Oblique scrotal US shows an echogenic appendage ⇨ in a patient with a subacute history of pain. The increased echogenicity may reflect acute hemorrhage vs. more chronic fibrotic change or Ca^{2+} in a torsed appendage. (Right) Longitudinal US shows a hyperechoic ovoid focus ⇨ surrounded by a small hydrocele, consistent with a partially calcified, chronically torsed appendage. At this point in time, the patient was asymptomatic.

TERMINOLOGY

- Dilated rete testis
- Cystic transformation of rete testis

IMAGING

- Frequently bilateral
  - Usually asymmetric involvement
- Branching tubules converging at mediastinum testis
  - Dilated tubules create lace-like or fishnet appearance
- Adjacent parenchyma is normal
- Associated ipsilateral spermatoceles are common
- Tubules are avascular and fluid filled
  - No flow on color Doppler imaging
- MR performed for confirmation if cystic malignant neoplasm cannot be ruled out

TOP DIFFERENTIAL DIAGNOSES

- Testicular carcinoma

- Mixed germ cell tumors with teratomatous components will often have cystic areas
  - Does not form network of tubules
- Intratesticular varicocele
  - Characteristic color flow on Doppler
- Testicular infarct
  - Avascular, wedge-shaped area with sharp borders

CLINICAL ISSUES

- Generally nonpalpable and asymptomatic
- May be found when ultrasound performed for related issue, such as epididymal cyst

DIAGNOSTIC CHECKLIST

- Important to distinguish tubular ectasia from malignancy to prevent unnecessary orchiectomy

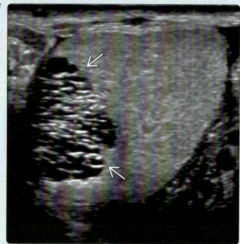
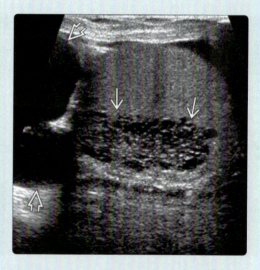

(Left) Transverse ultrasound of the left testis shows serpiginous, anechoic tubules ⇢ oriented along the mediastinum testis, a finding pathognomonic for dilated rete testis. The configuration and location should prompt a definitive imaging diagnosis of this benign entity. (Right) Sagittal ultrasound performed on an elderly man shows dilated rete testes ⇢ and large spermatoceles ⇢. Both entities are associated with efferent duct and epididymal duct obstruction.

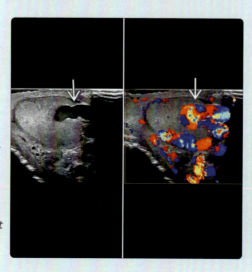
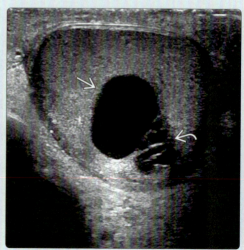

(Left) Sagittal ultrasound of an elderly man with severe right heart dysfunction shows a tubular anechoic structure within the mediastinum testis ⇢. Color Doppler confirms a huge varicocele with an intratesticular component, a potential mimic for dilated rete testis. (Right) Ultrasound of 31-year-old man with cystic fibrosis shows dilated rete testis ⇢ and a simple testicular cyst ⇢, potentially as a result of seminal vesicle agenesis and the abnormal epididymal fluid transport that is a characteristic feature of this patient population.

TERMINOLOGY

- Microcalcifications located within spermatic tubules

IMAGING

- Discrete, punctate, nonshadowing echogenic foci scattered within testicular parenchyma
- Majority are idiopathic; previous infection or trauma may also be responsible
- Adjacent hypoechoic foci, if seen, may represent neoplasia
- High-resolution US (≥ 7.5 MHz) is modality of choice

TOP DIFFERENTIAL DIAGNOSES

- Large cell calcifying Sertoli cell tumor
- Testicular granuloma
- Testicular vascular calcification
- "Burned-out" testicular cancer

PATHOLOGY

- Coexistent germ cell tumor in 18-75% of symptomatic male patients referred for US
- Associated with intratubular germ cell neoplasia: Germ cell version of breast carcinoma in situ

CLINICAL ISSUES

- Presence of microlithiasis alone in absence of other risk factors is not indication for further sonographic surveillance or biopsy
- US is recommended in follow-up of patients with ↑ risk of germ cell tumor: Personal/family history of germ cell tumor, maldescent or undescended testes, orchidopexy, testicular atrophy

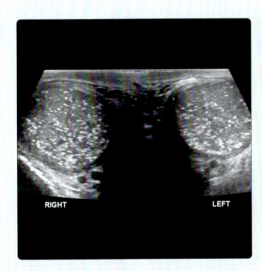

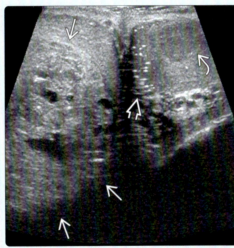

(Left) *Ultrasound of both testes demonstrates florid microlithiasis. Classic microlithiasis is strictly defined as ≥ 5 microliths per image. Without additional risk factors for germ cell tumor (GCT), follow-up by physical examination suffices.* (Right) *Ultrasound performed on a 43-year-old man with palpable masses and ↑ βHCG and aFP shows a huge right mixed GCT ➡, a left seminoma ➡, and surrounding microlithiasis ➡. Background intratubular germ cell neoplasia was also shown at pathology.*

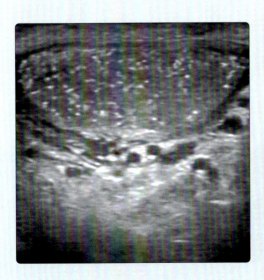

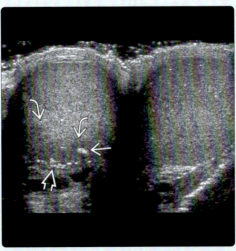

(Left) *Ultrasound of a young male patient with a history of a contralateral GCT shows an atrophic testis post orchiopexy with innumerable microliths. Ultrasound surveillance was performed because of the history of prior GCT and cryptorchidism and not microlithiasis per se.* (Right) *Scrotal ultrasound shows clustered macrocalcifications ➡, microcalcifications ➡, and vague background hypoechogenicity ➡. Massive retroperitoneal adenopathy (not shown) suggested a burned-out GCT (confirmed at orchiectomy).*

Testes

KEY FACTS

IMAGING

- Most common neoplasm in male patients aged 15-34 years
- Mostly unilateral; contralateral tumor develops eventually in 8%
- Seminoma is most common pure germ cell tumor of testis
- On US, seminomas are usually well defined, hypoechoic, and solid without calcification or tunica invasion
- Tumor < 1.5 cm is commonly hypovascular, and tumors > 1.6 cm are more often hypervascular
- Embryonal cell carcinomas are aggressive tumors, may invade tunica albuginea, and distort testicular contour
- US is used to identify and characterize scrotal mass; CT or MR for metastatic staging; PET to evaluate postchemotherapy seminoma
- Lymph nodes < 1 cm are suspicious if located in primary loading zones: Left-sided tumor→ paraaortic, left renal hilar nodes/right-sided tumor → paracaval, interaortocaval nodes

PATHOLOGY

- Associated with cryptorchidism, previous contralateral cancer; possible association with mumps orchitis and family history of tumor

CLINICAL ISSUES

- β-hCG is elevated in pure or mixed embryonal carcinoma or choriocarcinoma; also in 15-20% of those with advanced seminoma
- Elevated AFP levels above 10,000 µg/L are found almost exclusively in patients with nonseminomatous germ cell tumors (not seen with pure seminomas) and hepatocellular carcinoma
- Lactate dehydrogenase has independent prognostic significance: Increased levels reflect tumor burden, growth rate, and cellular proliferation

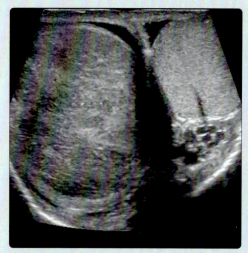
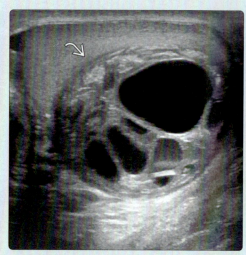

(Left) US of a 27-year-old man shows a hypoechoic mass that replaces & enlarges the right testis. The tunica was intact despite the size of the mass. Orchiectomy confirmed a pure seminoma. (Right) US shows a cystic & solid testicular mass ➡ (orchiectomy-confirmed MGCT composed of 90% teratoma & 10% embryonal tumor). Most testicular cancers are seminomas or MGCTs. Cystic change suggests nonseminomatous tumors. Tumor markers may ↑ specificity, but ultimate diagnosis occurs with orchiectomy.

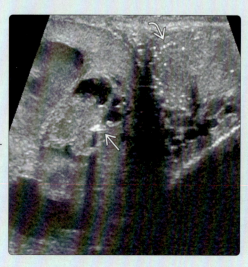
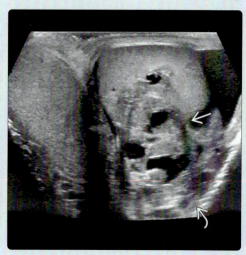

(Left) US of a 43-year-old man shows a large mixed cystic & solid right testicular mass containing calcifications ➡. Note the left microlithiasis ➡. Bilateral orchiectomy was performed for what was ultimately shown to be a tunica invasive right MGCT & small left seminoma (not shown). (Right) US of a 19 year old with back pain & a retroperitoneal mass shows a mixed cystic & solid left testicular lesion. It extends through the tunica ➡ & abuts up to the scrotal wall ➡. An MGCT was confirmed at orchiectomy.

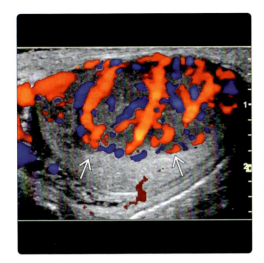

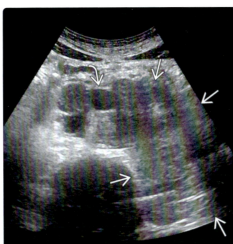

(Left) Scrotal color Doppler US of a young male patient with lung, liver, & brain metastases and ↑ LDH & β-HCG shows a vascular left testicular mass ➡. The Doppler appearance is nonspecific, but the elevated tumor markers indicate a MGCT. (Right) Transabdominal US of the same patient shows bulky paraaortic adenopathy ➡. The aorta ➡ is displaced anteriorly by tumor. Although identification of a testicular mass typically prompts a staging CT, gross adenopathy is easily assessed at initial sonography.

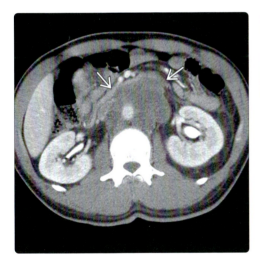

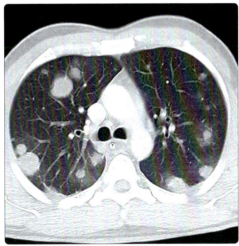

(Left) CECT of the same patient confirms bulky retroperitoneal adenopathy ➡. Awareness of patterns of nodal spread is critical, & even small nodes in characteristic locations should be viewed with concern. (Right) Chest CT of the same patient shows widespread lung metastases. Chest radiography and abdominal-pelvic CT are typically recommended for staging/surveillance of testicular carcinoma, but bulky adenopathy identified at initial sonography prompted up front chest CT examination.

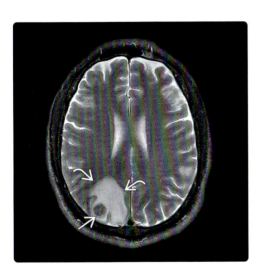

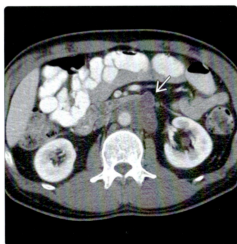

(Left) T2WI brain MR performed on the same patient because of neurological symptoms also shows an occipital lobe metastasis ➡ and surrounding edema ➡. (Right) Postchemotherapy CT of the same patient shows diminished enhancement of a smaller conglomerate nodal mass ➡. Residual mature teratoma was resected at retroperitoneal lymph node dissection.

(Left) *US performed on a 21-year-old man with a palpable testicular mass shows almost complete replacement of the right testis by a hypoechoic mass. Deformity of the tunica ➡ suggests tunica invasion. US performed in the same setting demonstrated retroperitoneal adenopathy (not shown).* **(Right)** *Staging CT of the same patient shows aortocaval adenopathy ➡, a characteristic nodal basin for right sided testicular tumors. A mixed germ cell tumor with tunica invasion was confirmed at orchiectomy.*

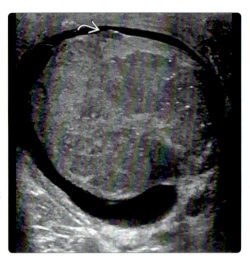
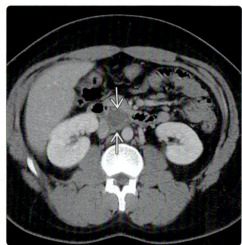

(Left) *Surveillance scrotal US of a male patient with known microlithiasis and a history of crytorchidism post orchiopexy shows a uniform isoechoic seminoma ➡ and background microlithiasis. A study performed 3 years prior was negative.* **(Right)** *Longitudinal grayscale US of the testis in a patient with a cystic teratoma shows a complex heterogeneous mass with cystic areas ➡ of varying sizes and small echogenic foci ➡.*

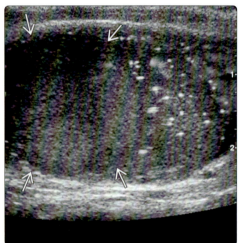
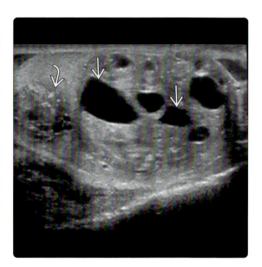

(Left) *US of a young black male patient shows bilateral testicular masses ➡. The differential diagnosis included multifocal germ cell tumor & lymphoma, but sarcoidosis was strongly suggested given characteristic mediastinal adenopathy on a prior CT. Sarcoid was (unfortunately) confirmed at orchiectomy.* **(Right)** *US of an infertile male patient shows bilateral hypoechoic masses ➡. The same differential as the prior patient may be considered, but a history of congenital adrenal hyperplasia indicates adrenal rests.*

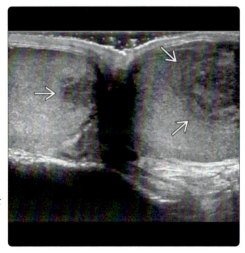
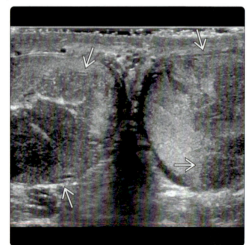

Testicular Lymphoma and Leukemia

TERMINOLOGY

- Infiltrative neoplasm of testis in which tumor cells surround and compress seminiferous tubules and normal testicular vessels

IMAGING

- Bilateral, solid, hypoechoic, hypervascular nodules/masses
- Diffuse hypoechoic testis with hypervascularity
- Striated pattern
- Testicular shape not altered
- Normal testicular vessels with straight course crossing through lesions
- Comparison of both testes to look for asymmetry in sizes and echogenicity

PATHOLOGY

- Most commonly secondary lymphomatous involvement of testis; rarely primary

- Lymphoma behaves similarly to leukemia with abnormal cells diffusely infiltrating interstitium with compression of seminiferous tubules without causing their destruction
- Testis is "sanctuary organ": Blood-gonad barrier limits accumulation of chemotherapeutic agents

CLINICAL ISSUES

- Stages IE and IIE: Orchidectomy
- Stages IIIE and IVE: Systemic chemotherapy using cyclophosphamide, doxorubicin, vincristine, and prednisolone
- Radiation in symptomatic and bulky deposits
- Lymphoma accounts for ~ 5% of all testicular tumors
- Most common bilateral testicular tumor
- Demographics: Testicular lymphoma typically in male patients > 50 years (germ cell tumor typically in male patients age 20-40)

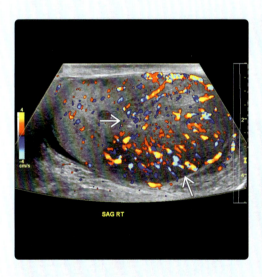

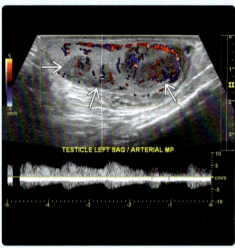

(Left) Sagittal color Doppler ultrasound of the right testis in a 56-year-old man with non-Hodgkin lymphoma shows a hypervascular focal mass ➡ in the inferior pole with focal enlargement of testis. Note that the shape of the testis is maintained. Pathology confirmed lymphoma. (Right) Sagittal color Doppler ultrasound of the left testis in a 65-year-old man shows multiple hypervascular hypoechoic masses ➡ in the testis. Pathology confirmed lymphoma.

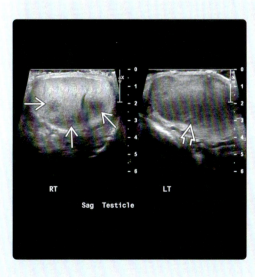

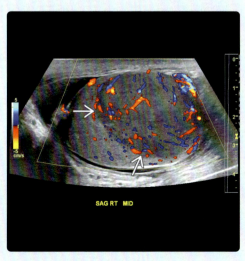

(Left) Sagittal grayscale ultrasound of the testes in a 60-year-old man with non-Hodgkin lymphoma shows bilateral hypoechoic masses, multifocal in the right ➡ and diffusely infiltrating in the left ➡. (Right) Sagittal color Doppler ultrasound of the right testis in a 51-year-old man with known history of acute myeloid leukemia shows a hypervascular focal hypoechoic mass ➡ in the inferior pole. Pathology confirmed acute myeloid leukemia.

T | Definition of Primary Tumor (T)

Category	Criteria
Clinical T (cT)	
cTX	Primary tumor cannot be assessed
cT0	No evidence of primary tumor
cTis	Germ cell neoplasia in situ
cT4	Tumor invades scrotum ± vascular/lymphatic invasion
Pathological T (pT)	
pTX	Primary tumor cannot be assessed
pT0	No evidence of primary tumor
pTis	Germ cell neoplasia in situ
pT1	Tumor limited to testis (including rete testis invasion) without lymphovascular invasion
pT1a*	Tumor < 3 cm in size
pT1b*	Tumor 3 cm or larger in size
pT2	Tumor limited to testis (including rete testis invasion) with lymphovascular invasion **or** tumor invading hilar soft tissue or epididymis or external surface of tunica albuginea ± lymphovascular invasion
pT3	Tumor invades spermatic cord ± lymphovascular invasion
pT4	Tumor invades scrotum ± lymphovascular invasion

Note: Except for Tis confirmed by biopsy and T4, the extent of the primary tumor is classified by radical orchiectomy. TX may be used for other categories for clinical staging.
*Subclassification of pT1 applies only to pure seminoma.

Adapted with permission from AJCC Cancer Staging Manual 8th ed., 2017.

N | Definition of Regional Lymph Node (N)

Category	Criteria
Clinical N (cN)	
cNX	Regional lymph nodes cannot be assessed
cN0	No regional lymph node metastasis
cN1	Metastases with lymph node mass 2 cm or smaller in greatest dimension **or** multiple lymph nodes, none > 2 cm in greatest dimension
cN2	Metastasis with lymph node mass > 2 cm but not > 5 cm in greatest dimension **or** multiple lymph nodes, any 1 mass > 2 cm but not > 5 cm in greatest dimension
cN3	Metastasis with lymph node mass > 5 cm in greatest dimension
Pathological N (pN)	
pNX	Regional lymph nodes cannot be assessed
pN0	No regional lymph node metastasis
pN1	Metastasis with lymph node mass 2 cm or smaller in greatest dimension and ≤ to 5 nodes positive, none > 2 cm in greatest dimension
pN2	Metastasis with lymph node mass > 2 cm but not > 5 cm in greatest dimension; or > 5 nodes positive, none > 5 cm; or evidence of extranodal extension of tumor
pN3	Metastasis with lymph node mass > 5 cm in greatest dimension

Adapted with permission from AJCC Cancer Staging Manual 8th ed., 2017.

M Definition of Distant Metastasis (M)

M Category	M Criteria
M0	No distant metastases
M1	Distant metastases
M1a	Non-retroperitoneal nodal or pulmonary metastases
M1b	Nonpulmonary visceral metastases

Adapted with permission from AJCC Cancer Staging Manual 8th ed., 2017.

S Definition of Serum Markers (S)

S category	S Criteria
SX	Marker studies not available or not performed
S0	Marker study levels within normal limits
S1	LDH < 1.5x N* **and** hCG (mIU/mL) < 5,000 **and** AFP (ng/mL) < 1,000
S2	LDH 1.5-10x N* **or** hCG (mIU/mL) 5,000-50,000 **or** AFP (ng/mL) 1,000-10,000
S3	LDH > 10x N* **or** hCG (mIU/mL) > 50,000 **or** AFP (ng/mL) > 10,000

*N indicates the upper limit of normal for the LDH assay.

Adapted with permission from AJCC Cancer Staging Manual 8th ed., 2017.

AJCC Prognostic Stage Groups

When T Is...	And N Is...	And M Is...	And S Is...	Then Stage Group Is...
pTis	N0	M0	S0	0
pT1-T4	N0	M0	SX	I
pT1	N0	M0	S0	IA
pT2	N0	M0	S0	IB
pT3	N0	M0	S0	IB
pT4	N0	M0	S0	IB
Any pT/TX	N0	M0	S1-3	IS
Any pT/TX	N1-3	M0	SX	II
Any pT/TX	N1	M0	S0	IIA
Any pT/TX	N1	M0	S1	IIA
Any pT/TX	N2	M0	S0	IIB
Any pT/Tx	N2	M0	S1	IIB
Any pT/Tx	N3	M0	S0	IIC
Any pT/TX	N3	M0	S1	IIC
Any pT/TX	Any N	M1	SX	III
Any pT/TX	Any N	M1a	S0	IIIA
Any pT/TX	Any N	M1a	S1	IIIA
Any pT/TX	N1-3	M0	S2	IIIB
Any pT/TX	Any N	M1a	S2	IIIB
Any pT/TX	N1-3	M0	S3	IIIC
Any pT/TX	Any N	M1a	S3	IIIC
Any pT/TX	Any N	M1b	Any S	IIIC

Adapted with permission from AJCC Cancer Staging Manual 8th ed., 2017.

pTis (Intratubular Germ Cell Neoplasia)

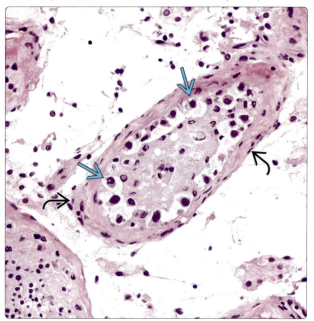

High-power magnification of an H&E stain shows a seminiferous tubule ⮕ with neoplastic intratubular germ cells ⮕. The neoplastic cells are large, pleomorphic with abundant vacuolated cytoplasm, and arranged in a single layer along the basement membrane.

pT1

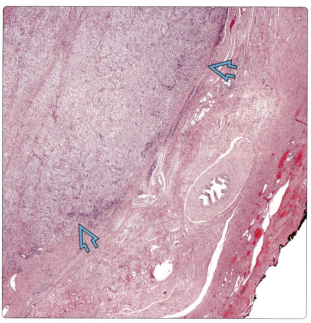

Low-power magnification of an H&E stain shows sheets of seminoma ⮕ that is replacing the testicular tissue but is limited to the testis without vascular or lymphatic invasion.

pT1

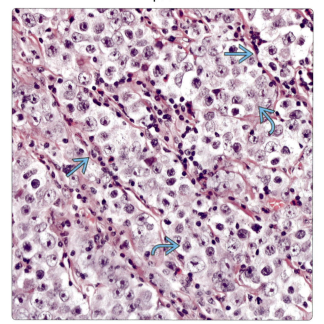

High-power magnification of an H&E stain of seminoma shows diffuse sheets of tumor cells ⮕ with intervening branching fibrous septa ⮕. The neoplastic cells are polyhedral and have pale to clear cytoplasm with round to oval nuclei and 1-2 prominent nuclei.

pT1

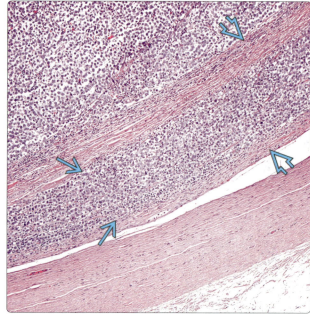

Intermediate-power magnification of an H&E stain shows seminoma tumor cells ⮕ that focally infiltrate into the tunica albuginea ⮕ without involvement of the tunica vaginalis.

pT2

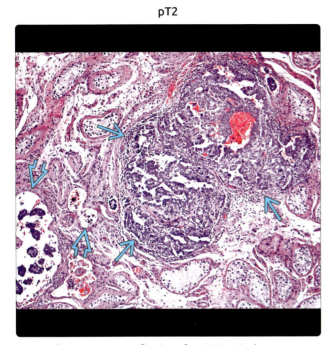

Intermediate-power magnification of an H&E stain shows an embryonal carcinoma component of a germ cell tumor ➡ infiltrating the seminiferous tubules with intravascular invasion in lymphatic/blood vessel spaces ➡.

pT2

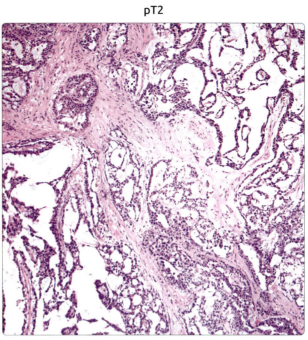

In an H&E-stained specimen from the same patient, other areas of the mixed germ cell tumor show yolk sac component.

pT3

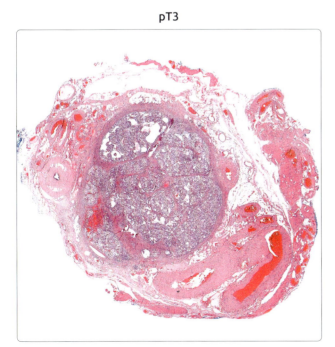

H&E stain of a cross section from a spermatic cord shows spermatic cord involvement by a testicular tumor.

pT3

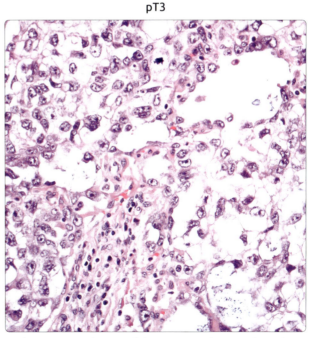

High-power magnification of the H&E-stained section shows the yolk sac tumor, which expands the spermatic cord with a microcystic (most common) pattern giving a reticular or lace-like appearance.

T1

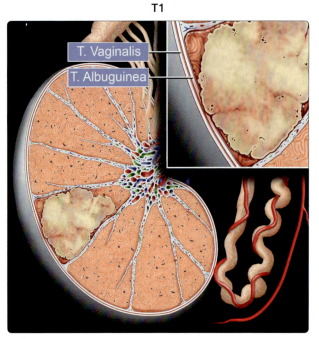

Graphic illustrates tumor limited to the testis and epididymis without vascular/lymphatic invasion. The tumor may invade into the tunical albuginea but not the tunica vaginalis (as seen in the inset). Both are classified as T1 disease.

T2

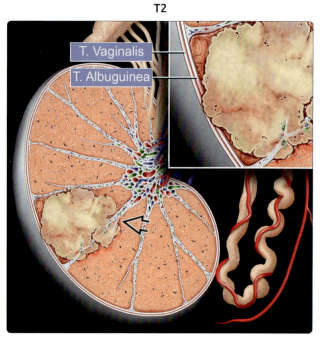

Graphic illustrates tumor limited to the testis and epididymis with vascular/lymphatic invasion ⇒. Tumor extending through tunica albuginea and involving tunica vaginalis (as seen in the inset) is also classified as T2 disease.

T3

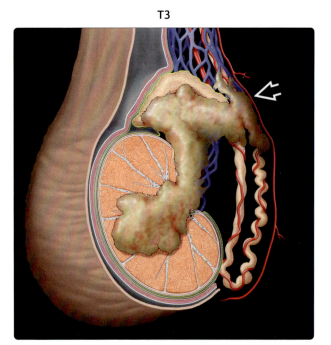

Graphic illustrates tumor invading the spermatic cord ⇒ (± vascular/lymphatic invasion), compatible with T3 disease.

T4

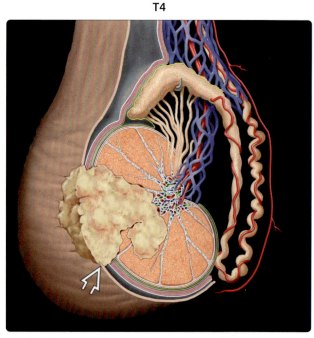

Graphic illustrates tumor invading the scrotum ⇒ (± vascular/lymphatic invasion), which is considered T4 disease.

N Staging

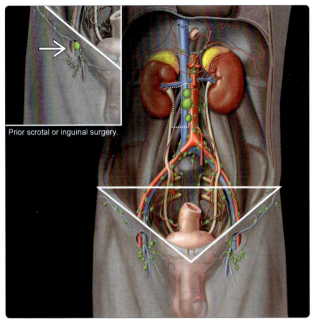

Prior scrotal or inguinal surgery.

Right testicular nodal spread initially involves nodes around the inferior vena cava (IVC), including retroperitoneal, aortocaval, and paracaval nodes (dotted white line). If there has been disruption of lymphatics from prior scrotal or inguinal surgery or tumor invasion of scrotum, then spread is to inguinal nodes ➡.

N Staging

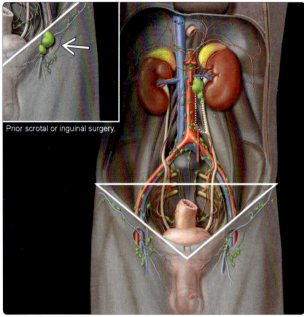

Prior scrotal or inguinal surgery.

Left testicular spread involves the retroperitoneal area bounded by renal vein, aorta, ureter, and IVC (dotted line). If lymphatics are disrupted by prior scrotal or inguinal surgery or tumor invasion of scrotum, then spread is to inguinal nodes ➡. Size of nodes determines N stage: < 2 cm = N1, 2-5 cm = N2, > 5 cm = N3.

Metastases, Organ Frequency

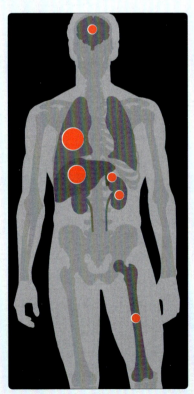

Lung	89%
Liver	73%
Brain	31%
Bone	30%
Kidney	30%
Adrenal gland	29%

Data from Bredael JJ et al: Autopsy findings in 154 patients with germ cell tumors of the testis. Cancer. 50(3):548-51, 1982.

TERMINOLOGY

- Gonadal stromal tumors arise from nongerm cell elements

IMAGING

- May be indistinguishable from germ cell tumors on grayscale US
  - Leydig cell tumors: Small, solid, hypoechoic intratesticular mass (consider if ↑ testosterone, ↓ follicle-stimulating hormone, ↓ luteinizing hormone)
  - Sertoli cell tumors: Small, hypoechoic mass with occasional hemorrhage, which may lead to heterogeneity and cystic components
  - Gonadoblastoma: Stromal tumor in conjunction with germ cell tumor, usually mixed sonographic features; associated with disorders of sexual differentiation
- High-resolution US (≥ 7.5 MHz) is best imaging tool for detection of gonadal stromal neoplasms

CLINICAL ISSUES

- 30% of patients with gonadal stromal tumors have endocrinopathy secondary to testosterone or estrogen production by tumor
  - Children: Precocious puberty and gynecomastia
  - Adults: Impotence, ↓ libido
- Majority of these tumors are benign
- Orchidectomy is preferred treatment; partial orchiectomy may be feasible if confident that lesion is not germ cell tumor

DIAGNOSTIC CHECKLIST

- Consider stromal tumor in any patient with endocrinopathy and testicular mass

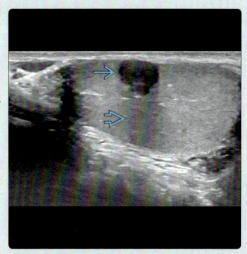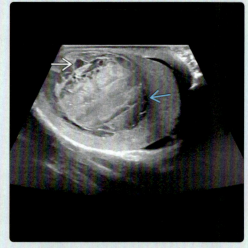

(Left) Sagittal grayscale ultrasound of the right testis in a 16-year-old boy demonstrates a well-defined hypoechoic mass ➡ with mild posterior acoustic shadowing ➡. Pathology after orchiectomy confirmed it to be a benign sex cord-stromal tumor (unclassified type). (Right) Sagittal grayscale ultrasound in a 16-year-old boy demonstrates a well-defined, predominantly solid mass ➡ with interspersed cystic areas ➡. Pathology confirmed it to be a granulosa cell tumor (adult type).

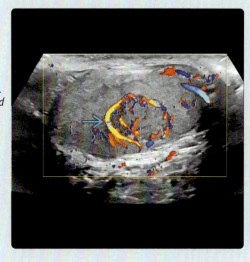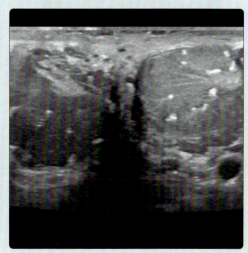

(Left) Sagittal color Doppler ultrasound of the right testis in this 33-year-old man demonstrates a hypoechoic solid mass with internal vascularity ➡. Pathology confirmed a Leydig cell tumor. (Right) Surveillance ultrasound performed on a 20-year-old man with a history of Carney complex shows innumerable echogenic foci throughout both testes. The appearance was stable over many years. Though exceedingly rare, the patient's clinical history and stability at surveillance imaging indicate large-cell calcifying Sertoli cell tumors.

Epidermoid Cyst

TERMINOLOGY

- Rare, benign, keratin-containing lesion of controversial origin

IMAGING

- High-resolution US (≥ 7.5 MHz) is imaging modality of choice
- **Grayscale Ultrasound**
  - Characteristic onion skin or target/bull's-eye appearance of avascular testicular "mass"
  - Unilocular cyst containing keratin; fibrous wall
  - Sharply circumscribed, encapsulated round "mass"
- **Color Doppler Ultrasound**
  - Avascular, no blood flow demonstrable
- Most commonly intratesticular but rarely may be extratesticular

TOP DIFFERENTIAL DIAGNOSES

- Tunica albuginea cyst
  - Located within tunica: Solitary, unilocular, and anechoic
- Germ cell tumor
  - Heterogeneous mass with vascularity seen on Doppler
- Testicular granuloma
  - Most probably due to tuberculosis, usually multiple

CLINICAL ISSUES

- May occur at any age; 2nd-4th decades most common
- 1-2% of all testicular tumors
- No malignant potential
- Enucleate 1st if lesions < 3 cm with characteristic US appearance and no color flow; testis can be spared if
  - Frozen sections of lesion are consistent with epidermoid cyst
  - No evidence of malignancy within or surrounding lesion
  - Negative tumor markers (AFP, β-HCG)

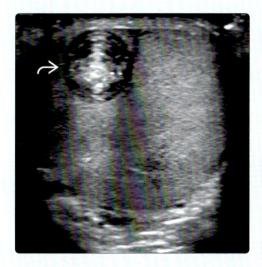
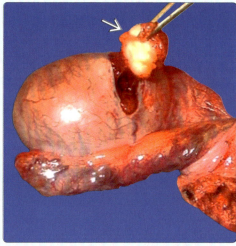

(Left) Scrotal ultrasound of a young male patient shows a testicular mass ⟳ composed of concentric rings of alternating echogenicity and an echogenic core. The onion skin appearance is due to lamellated keratin layers and strongly suggests an epidermoid cyst. (Right) Tumor markers were negative, and the mass ⟳ was enucleated. Frozen sectioning confirmed an epidermoid cyst. Recognition of classic sonographic features should prompt an attempt at testis-sparing surgery.

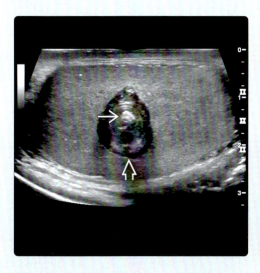
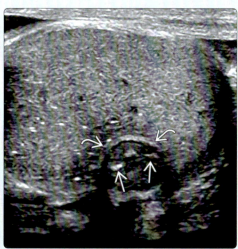

(Left) Ultrasound of the testis demonstrates a well-demarcated intratesticular epidermoid cyst ⟳. Central echogenicity ⟳ is due to keratin. (Right) Scrotal ultrasound performed on a different patient to assess for a residual abscess post-scrotal wall incision and drainage shows a solid mass with an echogenic rim ⟳ and several internal echogenic reflectors ⟳, an appearance suggestive of an epidermoid cyst. Intraoperative frozen sectioning was inconclusive. Orchiectomy confirmed a foreign body granuloma.

SECTION 9
Epididymis

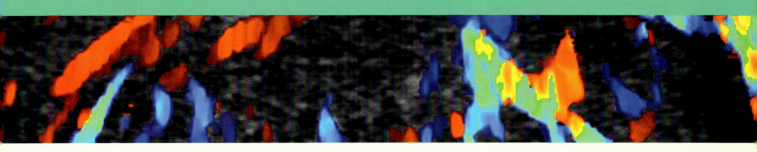

TERMINOLOGY

- Inflammation of epididymis &/or testis

IMAGING

- Test of choice: Color Doppler US; high-frequency transducers (≥ 10 MHz)
- Diffuse or focal hyperemia in body and tail of epididymis ± increased vascularity of testis (compare with contralateral testis if subtle)
- Starts within tail of epididymis → body → head → testis
- Orchitis is usually secondary, occurring in 20-40% of epididymitis due to contiguous spread of infection
  - Can cause vascular compromise → ischemia → testicular infarction → sonographic features indistinguishable from testicular torsion
  - Reversal of arterial diastolic flow of testis is ominous finding associated with testicular infarction

TOP DIFFERENTIAL DIAGNOSES

- Testicular torsion
- Testicular lymphoma
- Testicular trauma

CLINICAL ISSUES

- Most common cause of acute scrotal pain in adolescent boys and adults (15-35 years)
- Males 14-35 years of age: Most commonly caused by *Neisseria gonorrhoeae* and *Chlamydia trachomatis*
- Scrotal swelling, erythema; fever; dysuria
  - Associated lower urinary tract infection and its symptoms, urethral discharge
  - In elderly males, infection due to urinary tract pathogens; pathway: Ejaculatory duct reflux (vasectomy offered in recurrent cases)
- Prognosis excellent if treated early with antibiotics; follow-up scans to exclude abscess if no improvement

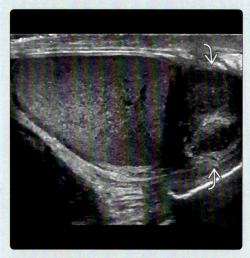 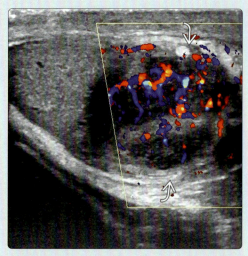

(Left) *US performed on a 39-year-old man with subacute scrotal pain shows a relatively enlarged, hypoechoic left epididymal tail* ➡️*. (Right) Color Doppler US performed on the same patient shows that the epididymal tail mass is hyperemic* ➡️*. The patient ultimately reported a recent history of treated sexually transmitted disease. Clinical symptoms and vascularity improved after a course of antibiotics. The clinical history and Doppler appearance are classic for early, uncomplicated epididymitis.*

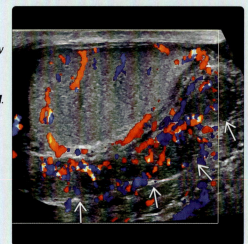 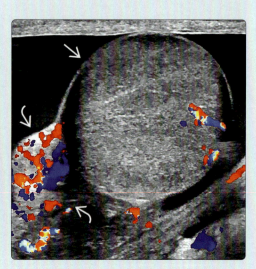

(Left) *Color Doppler US performed on an elderly man with persistent severe scrotal pain despite antibiotic therapy for epididymitis following a prostate biopsy shows a persistently enlarged, hyperemic right epididymis* ➡️*. (Right) Color Doppler US of the same patient shows a hyperemic left epididymis* ➡️ *and minimal flow within a heterogeneous testis* ➡️*. Aggressive or poorly treated epididymitis may result in testicular venous infarction (confirmed in this case post orchiectomy).*

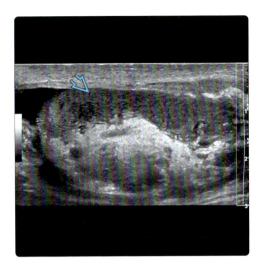
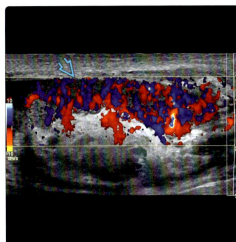

(Left) *Sagittal grayscale US of the right scrotum demonstrates a thickened heterogeneous and hypoechoic epididymis ➡️.* (Right) *Color Doppler US of the epididymis in the same patient reveals marked hyperemia ➡️ of the epididymis, consistent with acute epididymitis. Side-to-side grayscale and Doppler comparison is useful for more equivocal cases.*

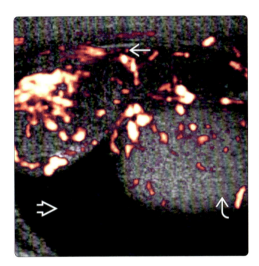
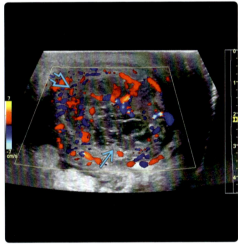

(Left) *Oblique power Doppler US shows a markedly enlarged, hypoechoic epididymis with increased vascularity ➡️, suggesting acute epididymitis. Note the normal testis ➡️ and hydrocele ➡️.* (Right) *Color Doppler US of the left epididymis reveals a markedly hyperemic tail ➡️ with a central heterogenous hypoechoic lesion ➡️. The findings are consistent with epididymitis complicated by an epididymal abscess.*

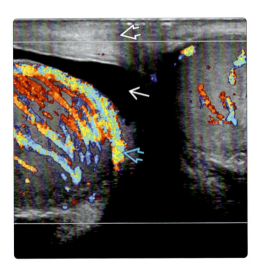
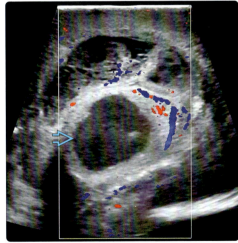

(Left) *Transverse color Doppler US of bilateral testicles shows the right testicle is markedly hypervascular ➡️ in appearance compared with the left, consistent with right-sided orchitis. In addition, there are associated findings of scrotal wall thickening ➡️ and a small hydrocele ➡️.* (Right) *Color Doppler US of the left testis in a patient who presented with acute epididymo-orchitis reveals a hypoechoic, thick-walled lesion within the testicle ➡️, consistent with a testicular abscess.*

TERMINOLOGY

- Benign solid paratesticular tumor of mesenchymal origin

IMAGING

- Solid intrascrotal mass, usually extratesticular
- Location
  - Epididymis: Most common location overall
  - May arise in tunica albuginea
  - Rarely intratesticular or other locations, such as spermatic cord and prostate
- Imaging appearance
  - Rounded or ovoid
  - Well circumscribed
  - Varying echogenicity
  - Gentle transducer pressure may show mass can move independent of testis
  - Refractive edge shadows on grayscale US
  - Hypovascular or avascular on color Doppler US
  - Size: 5 mm to 5 cm

- MR may confirm extratesticular mass; ↓ T2 signal intensity compared to testis

TOP DIFFERENTIAL DIAGNOSES

- Leiomyoma
- Lipoma
- Cystadenoma

CLINICAL ISSUES

- Most common solid mass in epididymis
  - 36% of all paratesticular tumors
- Slowly enlarges over years
- Most surgically excised to confirm diagnosis
- Some urologists and patients elect surveillance
- Age: 20 years and older
  - Mean age: 36
  - Rarely seen in boys

DIAGNOSTIC CHECKLIST

- Consider leiomyoma

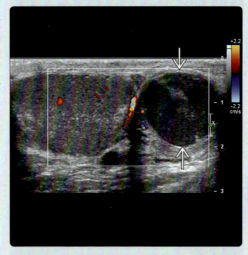
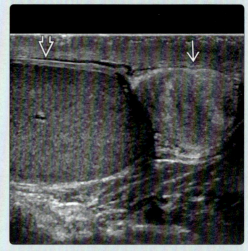

(Left) Longitudinal US in a 41-year-old man with a history of a palpable scrotal mass shows a hypoechoic adenomatoid tumor ➡, with no internal flow, within the epididymal tail. (Right) Sagittal scrotal US of a 63-year-old man with a palpable, nontender, but slowly growing paratesticular mass shows a solid, slightly echogenic epididymal tail lesion ➡ adjacent to normal testis ➡ (was surgically confirmed an adenomatoid tumor).

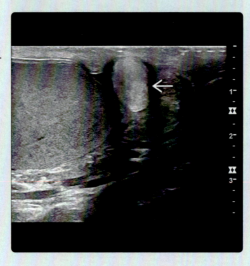
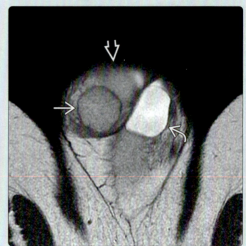

(Left) Longitudinal US in a 37-year-old man shows an incidental hyperechoic ovoid mass ➡ in the epididymal tail. The tumor was resected and was compatible with an adenomatoid tumor. (Right) T2 MR performed on a 38-year-old man with a slowly growing scrotal mass shows a paratesticular, epididymal lesion ➡ (a surgically confirmed adenomatoid tumor). Note adjacent testis ➡ and a T2-bright, fluid-containing a contralateral epididymal head cyst ➡.

Spermatocele/Epididymal Cyst

TERMINOLOGY

- Spermatocele: Retention cyst of rete testis or epididymis containing spermatozoa
- Epididymal head cyst: Collection of simple fluid

IMAGING

- US findings
  - Simple or complex cystic mass, classically within epididymal head: May contain diffuse, low-level echoes due to spermatozoa
  - "Falling snow" sign: 2° color Doppler mechanically moving particular matter within cyst

TOP DIFFERENTIAL DIAGNOSES

- Hematocele: History of trauma, complex fluid within tunica vaginalis
- Pyocele: Associated epididymo-orchitis, hyperemia, and enlargement of epididymis &/or testis

- Hydrocele: Simple fluid within tunica vaginalis; conforms to testis
- Tunica albuginea cyst: Tiny (2- to 5-mm) cyst between tunica layers

PATHOLOGY

- Etiology: Unknown, may reflect scarring 2° to either epididymitis, trauma, or vasectomy
- Associated abnormalities: Dilated rete testis

CLINICAL ISSUES

- Most common signs/symptoms: Painless scrotal mass
- Treatment: Most can be observed if asymptomatic/resection if discomfort

DIAGNOSTIC CHECKLIST

- Cystic extratesticular lesions almost always benign; if no vascularized soft tissue elements, not neoplasm

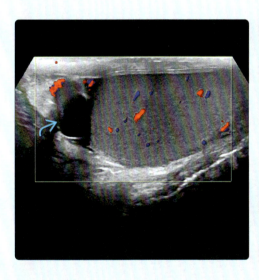

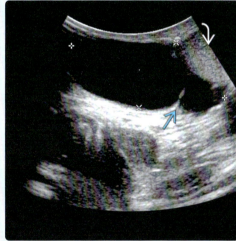

(Left) Typical appearance of an incidentally discovered and clinically unimportant epididymal cyst is shown. Note the well-circumscribed, anechoic, avascular lesion ⇨ in the epididymal head. (Right) Large epididymal cyst (calipers) is shown with a single thin septation ⇨ in the right hemiscrotum, displacing the testis ⇨ inferiorly. Note that an abdominal probe rather than a high-frequency linear probe was needed to capture this large lesion. A hydrocele (a diagnostic mimic) envelopes, rather than displaces, the testis.

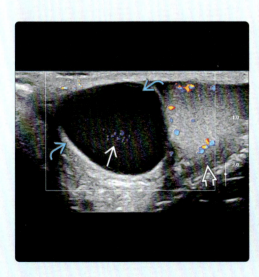

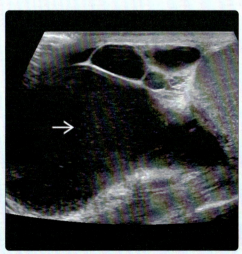

(Left) Large spermatocele ⇨ superior to right testis ⇨ contains punctate low-level echoes with corresponding Doppler artifact ⇨. These punctate foci were mobile in real time. (Right) Longitudinal grayscale ultrasound demonstrates a complex, multiseptate cystic mass with numerous locules containing debris ⇨, characteristic findings for a spermatocele.

Sperm Granuloma

IMAGING

- Ultrasound: Solid, well-circumscribed, hypoechoic epididymal lesion
- Nonspecific appearance, though clinical history, vasectomy, or other causes of epididymal tubular obstruction (trauma, infection) may prompt diagnosis

TOP DIFFERENTIAL DIAGNOSES

- Adenomatoid tumor
  - Solitary, varying echogenicity lesion: Most common solid epididymal tumor
- Chronic epididymitis
  - Enlarged, heterogeneous epididymis: Elicit history of prior bacterial epididymitis
  - Other causes (drug induced, traumatic) possible
- Leiomyoma
  - 2nd most common solid epididymal tumor

PATHOLOGY

- Foreign body giant cell reaction to extravasated sperm after epididymal obstruction, most commonly post vasectomy

CLINICAL ISSUES

- Benign inflammatory process: Typically asymptomatic palpable mass
- Pathophysiology of sperm granulomas (tubular obstruction) may lead to postvasectomy pain syndrome in 10% of male patients, 5-7 years post procedure

DIAGNOSTIC CHECKLIST

- Consider if small, solid, hypoechoic epididymal mass, post vasectomy
- Physical examination &/or ultrasound follow-up may suffice

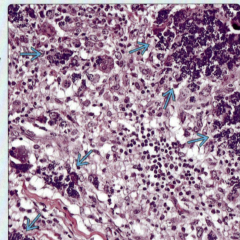
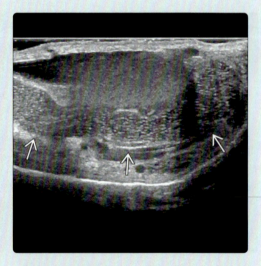

(Left) H&E stain of an epididymal mass shows aggregates of extravasated sperm ⮕ surrounded by inflammatory cells, typical of a sperm granuloma. (From DP: Genitourinary.) (Right) Ultrasound of the left testis in a man with pain post vasectomy shows an enlarged epididymis ⮕ and tubular ectasia. Obstruction after vasectomy (or due to trauma, infection) results in sperm extravasation and localized foreign body reactions (sperm granuloma).

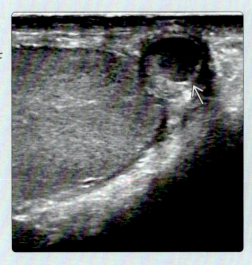
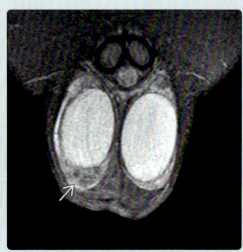

(Left) Ultrasound performed to evaluate a palpable mass 4 years post vasectomy shows a well-circumscribed hypoechoic right epididymal tail mass ⮕. Epididymectomy performed because of lesion growth showed fibrosis, granulation, and a sperm granuloma. (Right) Preoperative coronal T2 MR of the same patient shows a corresponding T2-hypointense epididymal tail lesion ⮕. Scrotal MR is typically reserved for evaluation of large masses, though ↑ epididymal T1 intensity may suggest a poor vasectomy reversal outcome.

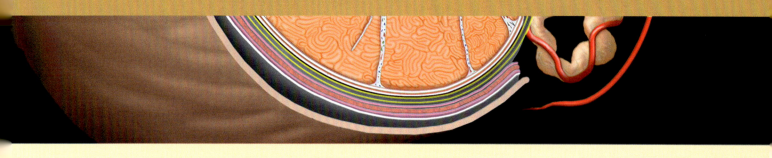

SECTION 10

Scrotum

Hydrocele

TERMINOLOGY

- Congenital or acquired serous fluid contained within layers of tunica vaginalis

IMAGING

- Best diagnostic clue: Scrotal fluid collection surrounding testis except for "bare area" where tunica vaginalis does not cover testis and is attached to epididymis
- Ultrasound: Crescentic anechoic fluid collection surrounding testis, avascular at color Doppler
- "Physiologic hydrocele": Scant anechoic fluid surrounding testis is normal finding
- Consider MR if growth of extremely large, complex, hydrocele

TOP DIFFERENTIAL DIAGNOSES

- Pyocele/hematocele
- Spermatocele

PATHOLOGY

- Congenital or communicating hydrocele secondary to failure of processus vaginalis to close
  - "Hydrocele/hernia" reducibility indicates patent processus vaginalis and requires repair
- Secondary condition in adults due to epididymitis or surgery for varicocele, though often idiopathic

CLINICAL ISSUES

- Typically painless, transilluminating scrotal fluid collection
- Hydrocelectomy if discomfort: Excellent prognosis with surgical repair
  - Surgical resection of hydrocele sac with oversewing of edges; tunica everted so scrotal skin can absorb fluid

DIAGNOSTIC CHECKLIST

- Image interpretation pearl: Simple hydrocele envelopes rather than displaces testis

(Left) Scrotal ultrasound of a 28-year-old male patient with scrotal discomfort shows a simple hydrocele. Note how with the exception of the "bare" area ➡, the fluid envelopes the testis. Secondary hydroceles in this age group may be due to prior epididymitis, though hydroceles are often idiopathic. (Right) Ultrasound performed on a 45-year-old male patient with a palpable left scrotal mass shows a large epididymal cyst ➡ and a small adjacent hydrocele ➡. The cyst displaces the testis rather than enveloping it.

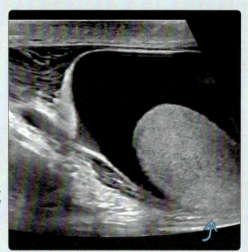
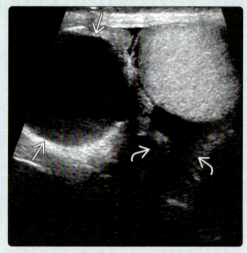

(Left) Power Doppler ultrasound of a 27-year-old male patient who presented with a fever and scrotal pain shows a simple hydrocele ➡ adjacent to the testis ➡, which is hyperemic due to orchitis. Note the numerous engorged vessels radiating from the mediastinum testis. (Right) T2 MR of a male patient with scrotal swelling shows huge, septated (communicating) hydroceles that conform to the scrotal sac but displace the testes ➡. A prior CT showed complex ascites and carcinomatosis due to peritoneal mesothelioma.

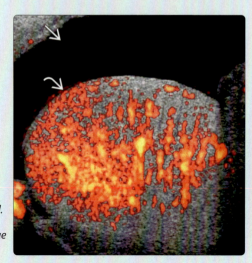
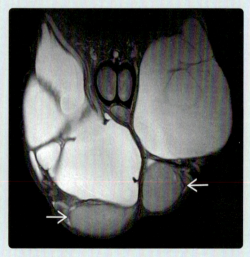

Varicocele

TERMINOLOGY

- Dilatation of veins of pampiniform plexus > 2-3 mm in diameter secondary to retrograde flow in gonadal (testicular) vein

IMAGING

- Best diagnostic clue
  - Dilated serpiginous veins behind superior pole of testis on color Doppler US
  - Prominent color flow within vessels with Valsalva secondary to retrograde flow
- Protocol advice: Resting and Valsalva color Doppler images of epididymis
- Distention secondary to retrograde flow with Valsalva

TOP DIFFERENTIAL DIAGNOSES

- Tubular ectasia/rete testis
- Hematocele/pyocele
- Epididymitis
- Hernia

CLINICAL ISSUES

- Most common signs/symptoms
  - Vague scrotal discomfort or pressure, primarily when standing ("flicking" pain)
- Majority (80%) are left sided, bilateral in 15% of patients
- Most frequent reversible cause of male infertility
- Fertility outcomes after varicocele treatment (embolization, ligation) are mixed: treatment may be less effective than previously thought

DIAGNOSTIC CHECKLIST

- Consider renal vein occlusion/compression by retroperitoneal tumor in elderly man
- Check retroperitoneum, particularly if isolated right-sided varicocele
- Valsalva essential for diagnosis of small varicoceles

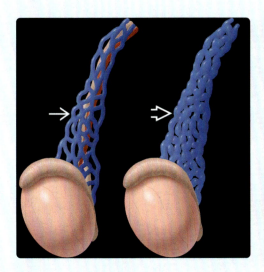

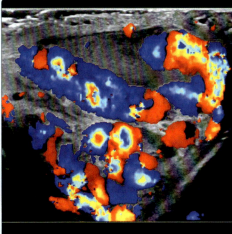

(Left) Graphic of the veins of the pampiniform plexus depicts the normal appearance ➡ on the left, while the depiction on the right demonstrates the abnormally dilated veins characteristic of a varicocele ⇨. (Right) Color Doppler ultrasound performed on an elderly male patient with scrotal discomfort shows a huge left varicocele. The late onset prompted imaging of the retroperitoneum, which demonstrated marked dilatation of the cava and renal veins due to severe right heart dysfunction.

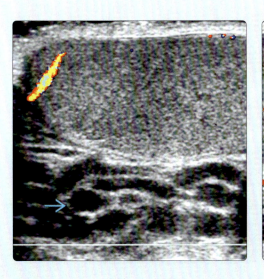

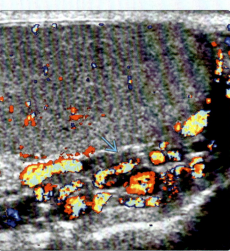

(Left) Longitudinal color Doppler ultrasound without a Valsalva maneuver demonstrates little flow in the dilated pampiniform veins ➡. (Right) Longitudinal color Doppler ultrasound obtained while the patient performed a Valsalva maneuver illustrates a marked increase in flow within the varicocele ⇨, the characteristic finding in the setting of a varicocele. Visualization of flow on color Doppler ultrasound during a Valsalva maneuver is particularly beneficial in diagnosing small varicoceles.

Pyocele

TERMINOLOGY

- Complex peritesticular fluid, complication of epididymo-orchitis

IMAGING

- Best imaging tool: Ultrasound with color Doppler
- Complex fluid collection within tunica vaginalis on ultrasound
  - Linear septations due to fibrinous strands
  - Low-level echoes from pus, white cell debris
- Color Doppler findings
  - Hyperemia of epididymis and testis 2° to epididymo-orchitis
  - Avascular complex paratesticular fluid collection

TOP DIFFERENTIAL DIAGNOSES

- Hematocele
- Spermatocele
- Hydrocele
- Epididymal cyst
- Fournier gangrene

CLINICAL ISSUES

- Most common signs/symptoms: Acute scrotal pain
- Other signs/symptoms: Fever, dysuria, scrotal skin thickening
- Most respond to antibiotic therapy
  - Empiric antibiotic choice based upon patient age
    - Prepubescent, middle-aged men: Coliform bacteria
    - Patients 14-35 years of age: Gonococcus/chlamydia
- Drainage rarely needed
- Rarely evolves into loculated scrotal abscess

DIAGNOSTIC CHECKLIST

- Consider repeat ultrasound if no clinical improvement with empiric antibiotic therapy
- Assess for complications (testicular abscess, infarction) or atypical infection (mycobacterium)

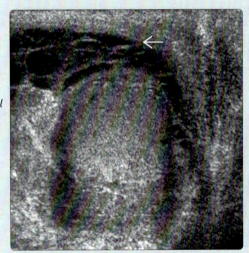
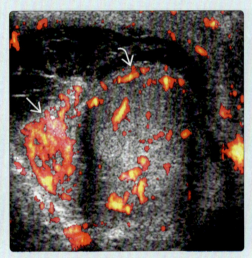

(Left) Sagittal grayscale ultrasound of the scrotum in a 19-year-old man presenting with fever and acute scrotal pain demonstrates linear strands of pus ➡ within the tunica vaginalis, consistent with a pyocele. (Right) Sagittal power Doppler ultrasound in the same patient reveals epididymal ➡ and testicular ➡ hyperemia (hallmarks of epididymo-orchitis).

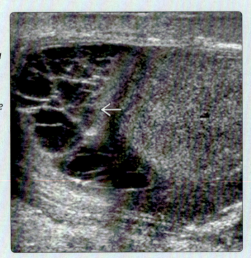
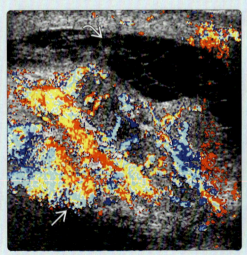

(Left) Sagittal grayscale ultrasound in a 37-year-old man presenting with acute scrotal pain, fever, and dysuria demonstrates a large pyocele with numerous septations ➡. (Right) Sagittal color Doppler ultrasound of epididymis in the same patient illustrates hyperemia from epididymitis ➡ as well as the adjacent pyocele ➡.

Paratesticular Rhabdomyosarcoma

TERMINOLOGY

- Paratesticular rhabdomyosarcoma (PT-RMS) refers only to intrascrotal rhabdomyosarcoma (RMS), not other GU sites

IMAGING

- Large, lobulated paratesticular mass with variable echogenicity; often heterogeneous & hypervascular compared to testis
  - Usually arises in epididymis; may arise from or invade tunica, testis, or spermatic cord
  - Can be ill defined or well defined; may encase testicle
- Look for retroperitoneal adenopathy

TOP DIFFERENTIAL DIAGNOSES

- Epididymitis
- Inguinal hernia
- Hematoma
- Lipoma

PATHOLOGY

- Malignant solid tumor of mesenchymal origin; arises from skeletal muscle precursors
- Most PT-RMS are embryonal subtypes
- Most cases sporadic
- ↑ risk with *TP53* mutations, *DICER1* mutations, RASopathies

CLINICAL ISSUES

- Gradual, painless scrotal swelling, ± palpable mass
- 2 age peaks: < 5 years & 2nd decade
- Most common extratesticular solid mass in boys
  - ~ 50% of solid extratesticular masses are malignant in boys
- PT-RMS accounts for ~ 5% of childhood RMS but has much better prognosis than other forms of genitourinary RMS
  - > 90% survival rate for localized (nonmetastatic) PT-RMS
  - Age < 1 or > 10 years, tumor size ≥ 5 cm, & lymph node involvement portend worse prognosis

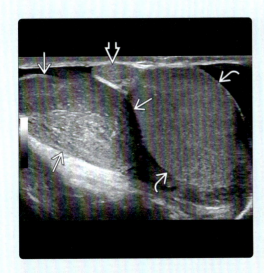

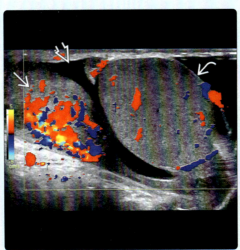

(Left) Longitudinal oblique US through the left hemiscrotum shows a slightly heterogeneous & hyperechoic paratesticular soft tissue mass ➡. Note the normal testis ➡ & epididymis ➡. (Right) Color Doppler US from the same study reveals markedly increased blood flow within the mass ➡ compared to the testis ➡; also note the small hydrocele ➡. This mass was a localized paratesticular rhabdomyosarcoma (PT-RMS).

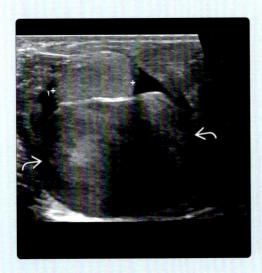

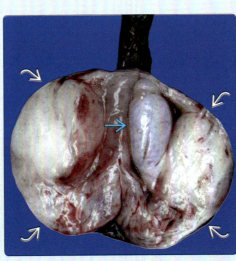

(Left) Scrotal US in a 5 year old with 1 week of right scrotal swelling shows a large, slightly heterogeneous paratesticular mass ➡, ultimately proven to be a PT-RMS. Real-time imaging showed the mass to almost completely surround the testis (shown with calipers). (Right) Gross pathologic bivalved specimen from the same patient status post orchiectomy shows a large, bland, tan-white PT-RMS almost completely surrounding ➡, but not invading, the testis ➡.

TERMINOLOGY

- **Incarcerated (irreducible) hernia**: Entrapment of hernia content within hernia sac
- **Strangulated hernia**: Compromised blood flow to hernia content resulting in ischemia/necrosis

IMAGING

- **Direct inguinal hernia**
  - Acquired hernia caused by weakness of fascia transversalis
  - Hernia sac emerges **superomedial** to origin of inferior epigastric vessels & protrudes through Hesselbach triangle
  - **Lateral crescent sign**: Compression, flattening, & lateral displacement of inguinal canal content
- **Indirect inguinal hernia**
  - Most common type of groin hernia; more common in males

- Hernia sac protrudes lateral to Hesselbach triangle, **superolateral** to course of inferior epigastric vessels
- Inguinal canal is expanded, & its content might not be well visualized
- **Femoral hernia**
  - Due to narrow neck, it has high rate of complications (obstruction, strangulation)
  - Femoral hernia neck is **inferior** to inguinal ligament & inferior epigastric vessels
  - Hernia sac runs craniocaudal course & is closely associated with femoral vein & causing flattening of vein
- **Obturator hernia**
  - Rare; usually seen in older females/associated with radical or robotic prostatectomies in males
  - Hernia sac extends through obturator canal & commonly protrudes between obturator externus (posteriorly) & pectineus muscle (anteriorly)
  - High risk of obstruction; ~ 90% of patients present with bowel obstruction

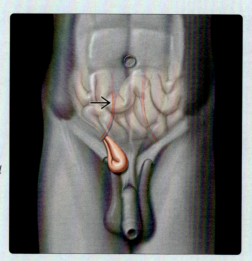 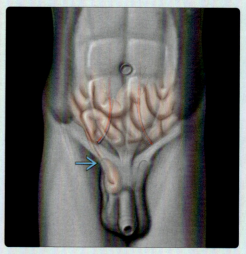

(Left) Graphic shows a direct inguinal hernia protruding through the roof of the inguinal canal. Note the location of the hernia sac above the inguinal ligament and medial to the inferior epigastric vessels ⟶. Direct inguinal hernia results in flattening of inguinal canal. (Right) Graphic of an indirect inguinal hernia shows a hernia sac extending into the inguinal canal and exiting through the superficial inguinal ring ⟶ into the scrotum.

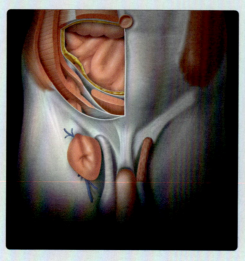 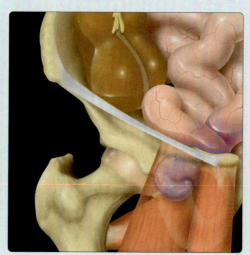

(Left) Graphic of a femoral hernia shows close association between the hernia sac and femoral vessels, commonly resulting in compression and concavity of the vein. The femoral hernia sac originates below the inguinal ligament and below the origin of the inferior epigastric artery. (Right) Graphic shows location of obturator hernia deep to the pectineus muscle.

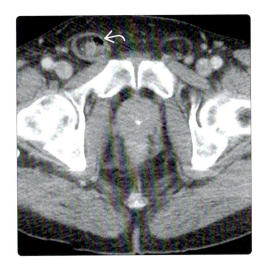
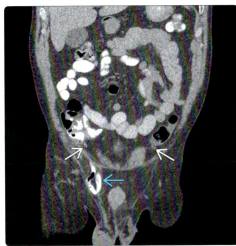

(Left) Axial CECT in this elderly man shows bilateral indirect inguinal hernias with the right hernia sac containing the bowel ➔. (Right) Coronal NECT in the same patient shows that the hernia sac contains the appendix ➔. This type of hernia is termed an Amyand hernia. The hernia sac originated lateral to the inferior epigastric vessels ➔.

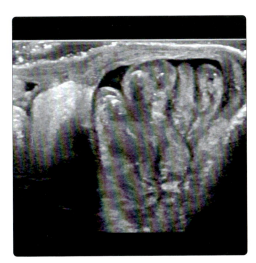
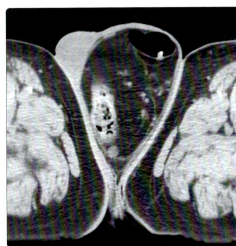

(Left) Grayscale US in a patient with history of scrotal mass shows multiple bowel loops and free fluid within the left hemiscrotum. Real-time scan also showed peristalsis. (Right) Axial NECT in the same patient confirms a large scrotal hernia containing bowel loops and mesenteric fat.

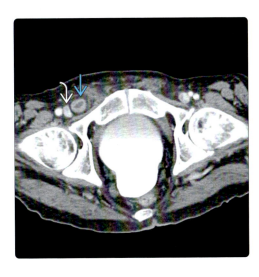
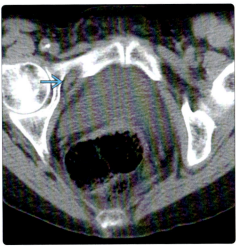

(Left) Axial CECT shows a loop of thickened, hyperemic bowel ➔ herniating into the femoral canal, medial to the femoral vein. Notice that the femoral vein ➔ is compressed. The herniated bowel lies posterolateral to the pubic tubercle. (From DI3: GI.) (Right) Axial NECT in this elderly female patient shows bowel herniation ➔ through the obturator canal. The hernia sac lies lateral to the obturator internus muscle.

TERMINOLOGY

- Life-threatening, polymicrobial, necrotizing soft tissue infection of perineal, perianal, or genital regions

IMAGING

- NECT: Most useful modality for depicting extent of soft tissue infection and gas in emergent setting
  - Fascial thickening, subcutaneous fat stranding, subcutaneous gas correlate with extent of affected tissue at debridement
  - Infection spreads along superficial (Scarpa, Colle, dartos) pelvic fascial planes to scrotum, anterior abdominal wall, buttocks
  - Untreated, overwhelming infection may extend into deep pelvic extraperitoneal space
- Ultrasound may be employed as initial test for males with acute scrotal pain and early (subclinical) manifestations of Fournier gangrene
  - Scrotal wall edema

- Scrotal wall gas: Echogenic foci with posterior "dirty" shadowing

TOP DIFFERENTIAL DIAGNOSES

- Scrotal edema
  - Reflection of 3rd spacing: Local, systemic manifestations of inflammation absent
- Scrotal cellulitis
  - Less aggressive, localized soft tissue infection
  - Subcutaneous gas absent (though absence does not entirely exclude Fournier gangrene)
- Perianal fistula/abscess

CLINICAL ISSUES

- Predisposing factors: Impaired host immunity and local tissue hypoxia (diabetes)
- High mortality rate even with aggressive, rapid treatment: Sepsis, multisystem organ failure
- CT guides extent of often repeated debridements

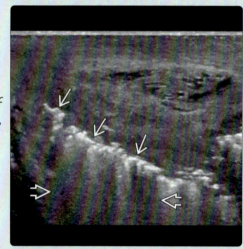

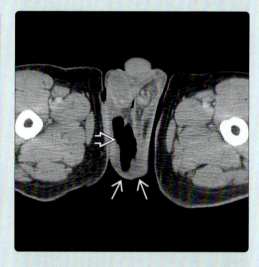

(Left) Transverse ultrasound performed on a 54-year-old diabetic man with a 2-day history of scrotal pain and erythema shows posterior scrotal wall echogenicity ➡ and "dirty" posterior shadowing ➡, a characteristic appearance of soft tissue gas. (Right) Axial CECT of the same patient shows scrotal wall edema ➡ and extensive gas ➡. Fournier gangrene is a surgical emergency. This patient was successfully treated with broad spectrum antibiotics, partial scrotectomy, and ultimately flap reconstruction.

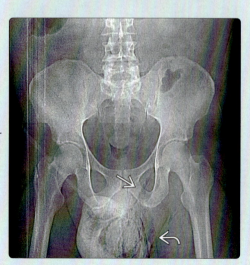

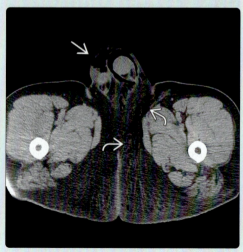

(Left) Digital scout image of a 43-year-old man with scrotal pain, erythema, and leukocytosis shows scrotal ➡ and inguinal ➡ subcutaneous emphysema. (Right) Axial NECT performed on the same patient shows scrotal wall ➡ and left medial buttock ➡ subcutaneous gas. Serial NECT studies guided the extent of multiple debridements. Predisposing causes of Fournier gangrene include impaired immunity and local tissue hypoxia. The inciting event for overwhelming infection may be minor local trauma.

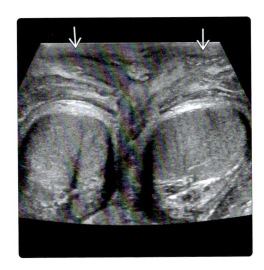

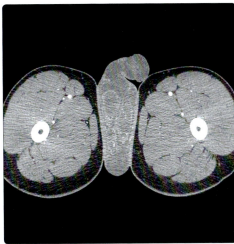

(Left) *Scrotal ultrasound performed on a 21-year-old man transferred with scrotal pain, purulent drainage, mild leukocytosis, and concern for Fournier gangrene shows diffuse scrotal wall edema* ➡. (Right) *NECT performed on the same patient confirms marked scrotal wall edema, but no soft tissue gas. Although the absence of gas does not entirely exclude a necrotizing infection, a lack of a predisposing history, and a rapid clinical response to antibiotics and superficial incision and drainage indicate scrotal cellulitis.*

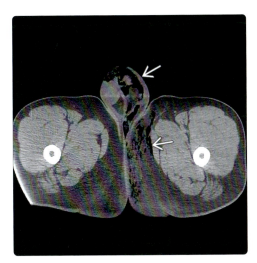

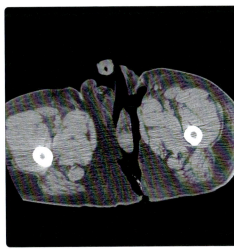

(Left) *NECT of a 41-year-old diabetic man presenting with scrotal pain, sepsis, and acute kidney injury shows scrotal wall and ischioanal fossa-buttock gas* ➡ *findings compatible with Fournier gangrene.* (Right) *NECT of the same patient 5 days after an initial debridement. The patient had a protracted clinical course that included 16 debridements and skin flaps. CT is utilized to guide debridement, particularly if infection extends to pelvic extra peritoneal compartments.*

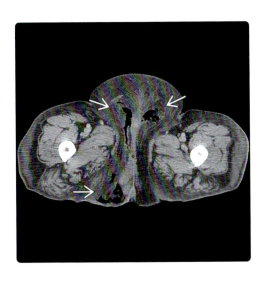

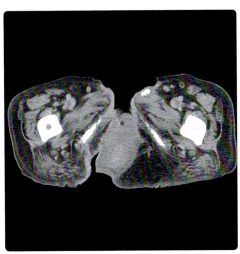

(Left) *Emergent NECT performed on a 55-year-old diabetic woman with sepsis and respiratory failure shows diffuse perineal edema, mons pubis, and ischianal gas* ➡. *A Fournier gangrene severity index incorporating clinical and lab parameters is used to assess mortality risk.* (Right) *NECT of the same patient performed 6 weeks after admission shows the result of extensive mons and ischoanal debridements. Mortality rates of > 30% have been reported despite aggressive resuscitation, IV antibiotics, and soft tissue debridement.*

Scrotal Trauma

IMAGING

- Heterogeneous testicular parenchyma or contour abnormality of testis in setting of scrotal trauma
  - Disruption of tunica albuginea is very specific for testicular rupture
- Extratesticular hematocele: Most common finding in scrotum after blunt injury
- US appearance of hematoma depends on time elapsed since trauma
- Intra- or extratesticular gas in scrotum, missile track, &/or foreign bodies (bullet/pellet) is indicative of penetrating injury
- Spermatic cord hematoma appears as heterogeneous avascular mass superior to testis
- Color Doppler is useful to determine viable portions of testis

PATHOLOGY

- Sports injuries (> 50%), vehicular and ballistic trauma, and iatrogenic

CLINICAL ISSUES

- Unless repaired within 72 hours, salvage rate is only 45%
- Follow-up of conservatively treated testicular hematomas is essential due to increased risk of infection, which may obviate orchiectomy
- Orchiectomy (total or partial) is performed for nonviable testis
- Surgical exploration and drainage must be performed for large intratesticular hematomas (large traumatic hematocele should prompt exploration regardless of ultrasound findings)

DIAGNOSTIC CHECKLIST

- Irregularity of testicular contour, heterogeneous parenchyma and echogenic collection in tunica vaginalis

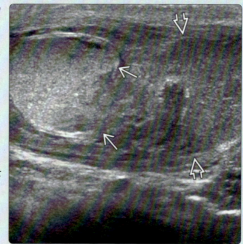
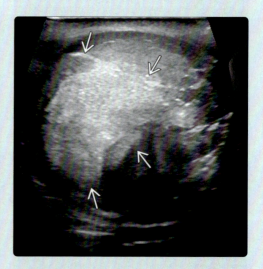

(Left) Scrotal US performed on a 23-year-old man post-MVA shows a widely disrupted lower pole tunica ➡ and adjacent hypoechogenicity ➡ (a combination of extruded seminiferous tubules and acute clot). Flow within the upper pole (not shown) suggested residual viable testis and emergent partial orchiectomy was performed. (Right) Transverse US shows a mid testicular fracture ➡ post blunt trauma. The testis was entirely necrotic despite emergent exploration, and an orchiectomy was performed.

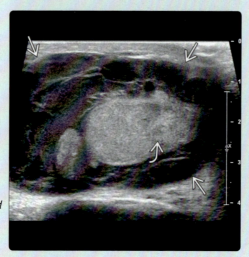
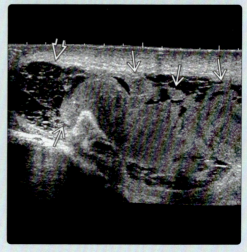

(Left) US post trauma shows a complex extratesticular fluid collection ➡ with an appearance consistent with a hematocele. Mild testicular heterogeneity ➡ also suggests contusion/hematoma. (Right) US performed 1 week post MVA shows a deformed heterogenous testis, extruded parenchyma ➡, and a hematocele ➡. The combination of testicular heterogeneity and tunica disruption is both sensitive and specific for rupture. The testis was not viable at exploration.

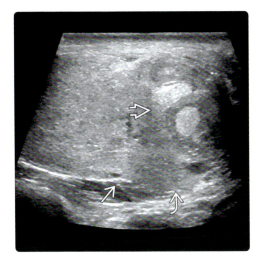

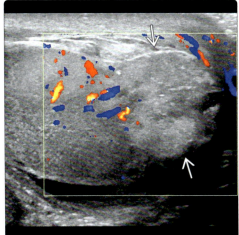

(Left) *US of the testis after a lacrosse ball injury demonstrates a disrupted tunica albuginea ➡, testicular heterogeneity ⇉, and a contour abnormality ⬈, a constellation of findings sensitive and specific for testicular rupture.* **(Right)** *Corresponding color Doppler US in the same patient shows avascular, nonviable, extruded testicular parenchyma ➡. Salvage of perfused viable testis may be possible immediately post injury.*

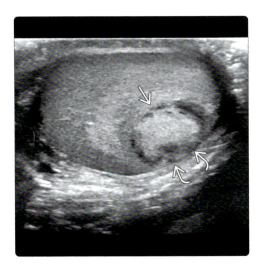

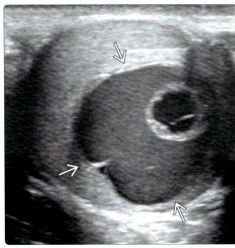

(Left) *US performed post blunt trauma shows a well-defined intraparenchymal lesion ➡ and intact adjacent tunica ⬈. Resolution of the "lesion" at follow-up US confirmed the impression of a contained testicular hematoma.* **(Right)** *US performed on a patient with a history of scrotal trauma and 3-week history of scrotal pain shows a complex cystic testicular mass ➡. Lack of change at short-term surveillance imaging prompted orchiectomy for what was confirmed to be a mixed germ cell tumor.*

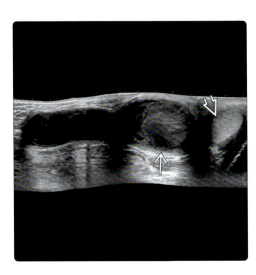

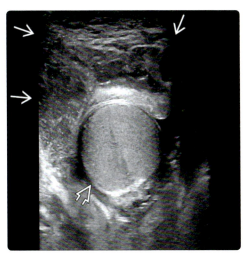

(Left) *Sagittal panoramic US of the right scrotum after inguinal herniorrhaphy shows a large, complex fluid collection ➡ extending from the superior pole of the testis ⇉ into the groin. Surgery confirmed a spermatic cord hematoma.* **(Right)** *US performed on a patient with multiple pelvic fractures and extensive extraperitoneal hemorrhage shows an intact testis ⇉ and a large scrotal wall hematoma ➡.*

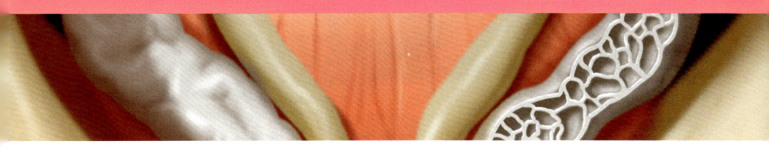

SECTION 11
Seminal Vesicles

IMAGING

- **Infectious/inflammatory conditions**
  - **Acute seminal vesiculitis**
    - Usually caused by bacterial infection and seen in association with prostatitis &/or epididymitis
    - Imaging: Enlarged seminal vesicles (SVs); diffuse wall thickening with diffuse enhancement; complex fluid content; surrounding inflammatory changes
  - **Chronic seminal vesiculitis**
    - Rare entity caused by chronic or repetitive bacterial infection of SV, usually in association with chronic prostatitis
    - Imaging: Enlargement of SVs or atrophy and loss of convolutions; thickening (± enhancement) of SV septations and walls
  - **Amyloidosis**
    - Localized SV amyloidosis, common finding in elderly; usually incidental finding with no clinical significance

- Imaging: **Nodular** (more common) or diffuse (less common) wall thickening with markedly ↓ T2 signal of convolutions; ± SV hemorrhage
- May mimic tumoral invasion by prostate cancer
- **Degenerative processes**
  - **Acquired SV cyst**
    - Obstruction at level of excretory duct or ejaculatory duct can result in acquired cystic dilatation of SV
  - **SV calcification**
- **Neoplastic lesions**
  - **Primary neoplasms**: Exceedingly rare
    - Benign: Cystadenoma, papillary adenoma, leiomyoma, teratoma
    - Malignant: Adenocarcinoma, leiomyosarcoma, cystosarcoma phyllodes, angiosarcoma, seminoma, carcinoid
  - **Secondary neoplasms**
    - Secondary involvement by local invasion or metastasis

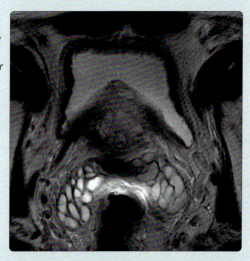
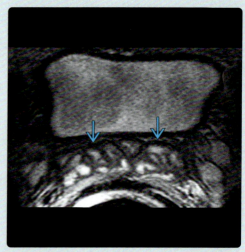

(Left) Axial T2WI MR, with use of endorectal coil, shows the normal appearance of seminal vesicles with thin-walled convolutions. Note the bladder wall thickening, which is presumably secondary to prostatomegaly. (Right) Axial T2WI MR, with use of endorectal coil, shows diffuse seminal vesicular wall thickening ➡. In the absence of clinical findings of acute seminal vesiculitis, these findings were thought to be due to chronic seminal vesiculitis or amyloidosis.

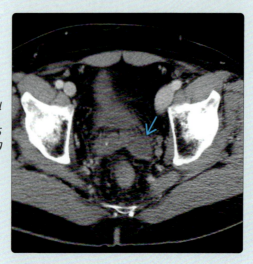
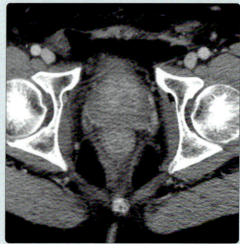

(Left) Axial CECT in a 52-year-old man with a history of perineal pain shows asymmetric enlargement and hypodensity of the left seminal vesicle ➡ with stranding in rectovesical and perirectal spaces. (Right) Axial CECT (same patient) shows prostatomegaly (volume of 65 cc) and periprostatic stranding that were new since a prior CT. The patient had new elevated PSA, CRP, and WBC. He was diagnosed with acute prostatovesiculitis. PSA returned to normal after treatment with systemic antibiotics.

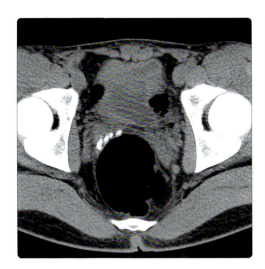

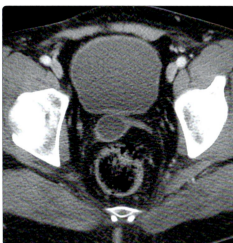

(Left) *NECT through seminal vesicles shows discrete calcified calculi in distribution of right vas deferens. Similar to prostate calculi, the majority of vas deferens and seminal vesicle calculi have urinary composition and are thought to be due to reflux of urine and stasis.* (Right) *Axial CECT in 40-year-old male patient with a history of repeated epididymitis shows a right seminal vesicle cyst. Given the history and absence of renal anomalies, this cyst was felt to be sequela of prior infections. Note the marked atrophy of left seminal vesicle.*

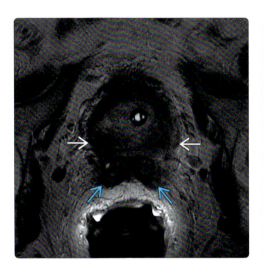

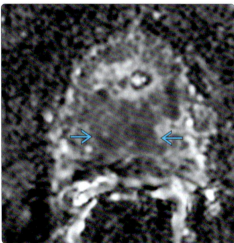

(Left) *Axial T2WI MR in a 77-year-old patient with a history of biopsy-proven Gleason 8 prostate cancer shows abnormal signal in the prostate base peripheral zone ➡ as well as distortion and signal alteration of seminal vesicles ➡.* (Right) *ADC map in the same patient shows corresponding restricted diffusion in areas of tumoral invasion ➡. The patient had extracapsular extension and involvement of neurovascular bundles (not shown).*

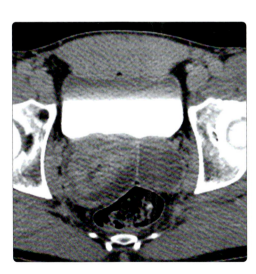

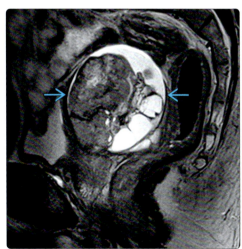

(Left) *Axial NECT in a 52-year-old patient with a history of hematospermia shows a large mixed solid and cystic mass in the rectovesical space.* (Right) *Sagittal T2WI MR in the same patient better shows the mixed solid/cystic nature of tumor ➡. There was no invasion to adjacent organs. The mass was resected and pathology result was consistent with low-grade sarcoma. (Courtesy P. Woodward, MD.)*

KEY FACTS

TERMINOLOGY

- Seminal vesicle (SV)

IMAGING

- Embryology
  - Development of SV, vas deferens, and urinary system closely associated to each other
  - **Mesonephric (wolffian) duct** gives rise to SV and vas deferens
- SV agenesis/hypogenesis
  - Absent, or markedly small, SV
  - Agenesis more common than hypogenesis
  - Usually unilateral
  - Due to interruption of normal SV development (occurs before 7th week of gestation)
  - High association with renal and vas deferens anomalies
  - Bilateral SV agenesis strongly associated with *CFTR* gene mutation (64-73%)
    - Considered genital form of cystic fibrosis

- Congenital SV cyst
  - Can be isolated or associated with other genitourinary anomalies
  - Bilateral SV cysts have high association with autosomal dominant polycystic kidney disease (44-60%)
  - SV cysts usually < 5 cm
  - MR: ↑ T2, variable T1 signal
    - SV cyst may show high T1 signal due to proteinaceous or hemorrhagic cyst content

TOP DIFFERENTIAL DIAGNOSES

- Acquired SV cysts
  - Any obstructive process in SV, ejaculatory duct, or excretory duct can result in acquired SV cyst
- **Müllerian duct cyst (prostatic utricle)**
  - Usually in midline prostate
- **Cyst-like intrapelvic structures (mimics)**
  - Ureterocele, dilated ectopic ureter, bladder diverticulum, urethral diverticulum

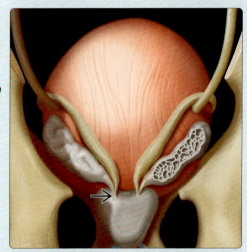
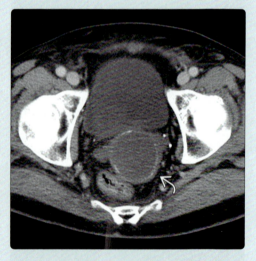

(Left) Coronal posterior graphic of the bladder shows the relationship between the seminal vesicles, vas deferens, and prostate gland. The vas deferens and the excretory duct of the seminal vesicle join each other to form the ejaculatory duct ➡, which, through the verumontanum, drains into prostatic urethra. (Right) Axial CECT in a patient with a history of left renal agenesis shows a large, rim-calcified, left seminal vesicle cyst ➡.

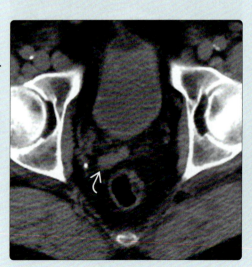
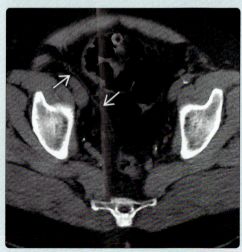

(Left) Axial NECT in patient with a history of left renal agenesis shows an absent ipsilateral, left seminal vesicle. Note the normal right SV ➡. (Right) Axial NECT obtained more superiorly in the same patient shows the left vas deferens agenesis as well. The right vas deferens is annotated ➡. Because of the common pathway of development, there is a high association between anomalies of these organs.

SECTION 12
Prostate

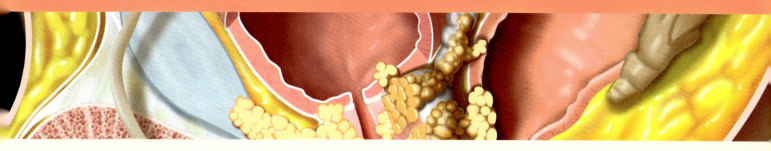

Prostatitis and Abscess

TERMINOLOGY

- National Institutes of Health classified into 4 types
  - Type 1: Acute bacterial prostatitis
  - Type 2: Chronic bacterial prostatitis
  - Type 3: Chronic prostatitis/chronic pelvic pain syndrome
  - Type 4: Asymptomatic inflammatory prostatitis

IMAGING

- Prostatitis is clinical diagnosis
- Imaging generally reserved to evaluate for abscess formation
  - Rim-enhancing, unilocular or multilocular, low-attenuation mass in prostate
- Focal or diffuse low signal intensity of peripheral zone on T2WI MR

TOP DIFFERENTIAL DIAGNOSES

- Congenital prostatic cyst
- Cystic degeneration of benign prostatic hypertrophy

- Prostate carcinoma

PATHOLOGY

- Acute bacterial prostatitis
  - Ascending colonization of urinary tract or post biopsy
- Predisposing risk factors
  - Bladder outlet obstruction due to benign prostatic hyperplasia
  - Prior instrumentation
  - Chronic indwelling bladder catheters
  - Immunocompromised states, such as diabetes

CLINICAL ISSUES

- Treatment
  - Antibiotics
  - Transurethral or transrectal drainage may be necessary

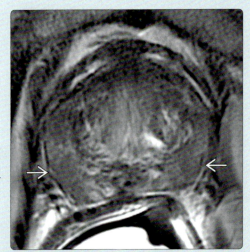
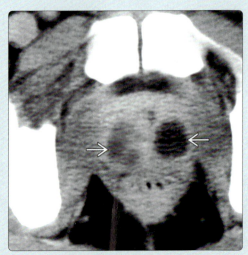

(Left) Axial T2WI MR shows diffuse low signal intensity of the peripheral zone ➡ in this patient with prostatitis. When the inflammatory process affects the peripheral gland focally, it may be difficult to distinguish from cancer, and a biopsy may be required. (Right) Axial CECT shows multiple rim-enhancing low-density regions ➡ within the prostate, consistent with abscesses. Although antibiotic therapy may suffice for uncomplicated prostatitis, surgical drainage is typically employed for imaging apparent abscesses.

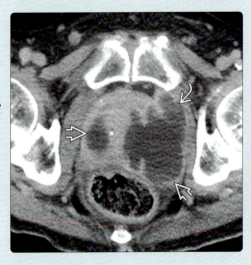
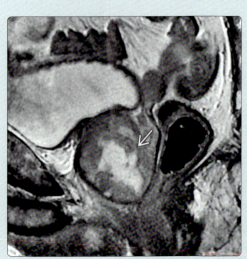

(Left) Axial CECT shows multiple abscesses ➡ within an enlarged prostate. The abscess on the left ➡ has extended beyond the capsule into the periprostatic tissues. (Right) Sagittal T2WI MR in a patient with a history of acute prostatitis shows an irregular fluid collection ➡ in the midportion of the prostate, compatible with abscess.

Prostatic Cyst

TERMINOLOGY
- Spectrum of cystic lesions in prostate
  - May be either congenital or acquired

IMAGING
- Best imaging technique
  - Transrectal ultrasound
  - MR
- Subtypes
  - Degenerative cyst
    - Most common prostatic cyst
    - Cystic degeneration of benign prostatic hyperplasia
    - Small cysts in background of hyperplastic nodules
  - Müllerian duct cyst
    - Typically large, extending above prostate
    - Oval or teardrop-shaped
  - Prostatic utricle cyst
    - Arises from midline and rarely extends beyond prostate

- Commonly communicates with urethra
  - Ejaculatory duct cyst
    - Located along course of ejaculatory duct
  - Retention cyst
    - Obstruction of prostatic gland ducts
    - Away from midline

TOP DIFFERENTIAL DIAGNOSES
- Prostatic abscess
  - Cystic lesion with thick walls and septa

CLINICAL ISSUES
- Prostatic cysts reported in 7.6% of asymptomatic men
- May be symptomatic
  - Pelvic pain, hematuria, rectal pain, dysuria, ejaculatory pain, hematospermia
- Often no treatment; may drain and inject with sclerosing agent if symptomatic

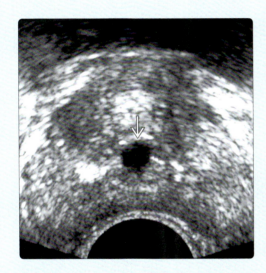
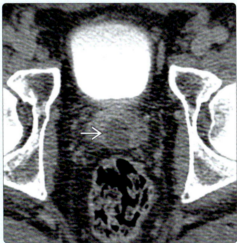

(Left) Axial transrectal ultrasound shows a midline cyst ➡. Communication with the urethra favors a utricle cyst. (Right) Axial CECT shows a well-defined, low-density lesion in the midline of the prostate ➡. The location suggests a utricle cyst.

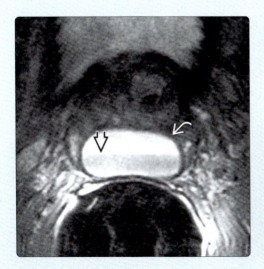
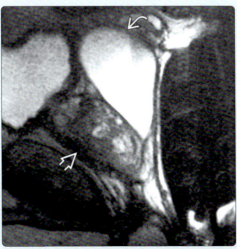

(Left) Axial T2WI MR shows a hemorrhagic midline cyst ➡ within the peripheral zone of the prostate gland. Note the fluid-fluid level ➡ created by the layering blood products. (Right) Sagittal T2WI MR shows the same teardrop-shaped cyst ➡ extending cephalad to the prostate gland ➡. Müllerian duct cysts are typically midline and large, extending above the base of the prostate, and only rarely communicate with the urethra. This patient presented with acute pain from the intracystic hemorrhage.

Prostate

IMAGING

- **Multiparametric MR (mpMR)**
  - Combination of anatomical and functional imaging
  - Anatomical imaging
    - T2WI
      - Lesion detection and characterization; gland volume and extraprostatic extension
    - T1WI
      - Rule out prostatic hemorrhage (tumor mimicker)
  - Functional imaging
    - Diffusion-weighted imaging (DWI)
    - Apparent diffusion coefficient map (ADC)
      - Interpretation of combined high b-value (≥ 1,400 s/mm²) DWI and ADC map
      - Lesion detection and characterization
    - Dynamic contrast-enhanced (DCE) study
      - Multiple T1WI obtained during and after IV injection of contrast

- Key sequence for assessment of tumor recurrence
  - MR spectroscopy (MRS)
    - Key metabolic compounds in prostate gland: Citrate [2.60 parts per million (ppm)]; creatine (3.04 ppm); choline (3.20 ppm)
  - Technical notes
    - Scanner: ≥ 1.5T
    - Coils: Surface multichannel phased array ± endorectal
    - At least 6 weeks after prostate biopsy
- **Normal prostate gland**
  - Peripheral zone
    - 70% of gland volume
    - High and homogeneous signal intensity (SI) on T2WI
  - Transition zone
    - 5% of gland volume
    - In benign prostatic hyperplasia (BPH), volume increases and SI on T2WI is heterogeneous ("organized chaos")
  - Central zone: 25% of gland volume (↓ in BPH)

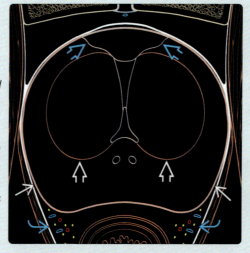

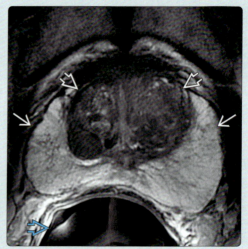

(Left) Medical illustration shows an axial view through the midprostate. The visualized key anatomical structures include peripheral zone ➡, transition zone ➡, neurovascular bundles ➡, and anterior fibromuscular stroma ➡. (Right) Axial T2WI MR of the prostate through the midgland is shown. The peripheral zone ➡ shows high signal intensity (SI) given the water content in the normal gland. The transition zone ➡ shows heterogeneous SI in this subject with mild BPH. This image was obtained using an endorectal coil ➡.

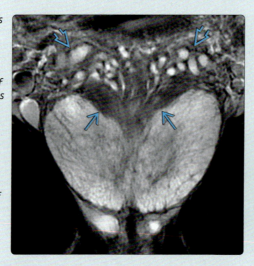

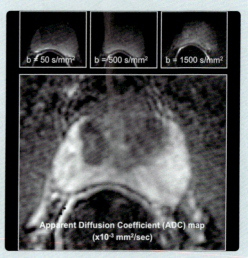

(Left) Coronal T2WI MR shows the prostate in the same patient. Central zone appears as a triangular or V-shaped hypointense structure ➡ in the posterosuperior portion of the gland. The seminal vesicles ➡ appears as hyperintense tubular structures. (Right) Composite figure shows axial DWI MR (at different b-value) and ADC map. The SI on DWI reflects the motility of water molecules. It is key for cancer detection. The ↑ cellularity of tumor restricts water diffusion, resulting in ↑ SI on high b-value DWI and ↓ SI on ADC map.

TERMINOLOGY

Abbreviations

- Multiparametric MR (mpMR)
- Signal intensity (SI)
- Peripheral zone (PZ)
- Transition zone (TZ)
- Central zone (CZ)
- Diffusion-weighted imaging (DWI)
- Apparent diffusion coefficient (ADC)
- Magnetic resonance spectroscopy (MRS)

Definitions

- MR study composed of anatomical and functional imaging

IMAGING

MR Findings

- T1WI
  - Main role: Exclusion of postbiopsy hemorrhage is potential mimicker for malignancy
  - Evaluation of pelvic lymphadenopathy
- T2WI
  - Anatomical imaging
  - Multiplanar acquisition
  - Key role in tumor detection and staging
    - Normal prostate
      - PZ: 70% of gland volume, high and homogeneous SI
      - TZ: 5% of gland volume, in benign prostatic hyperplasia (BPH), volume increases and SI on T2WI is heterogeneous ("organized chaos")
      - CZ: 25% of gland volume ($\downarrow$ in BPH)
    - Cancer: Mass with low SI
- DWI
  - Functional imaging
    - SI based on motion restriction of water molecules
  - Key role in lesion characterization and detection
    - Interpretation of combined high b-value ($\geq$ 1,400 s/mm²) DWI and ADC map
    - Cancer: High SI on high b-value DWI and low SI on ADC map
      - ADC values correlate with tumor grading (lower ADC value in higher Gleason score)
- T1WI C+
  - Dynamic contrast-enhanced (DCE) study
    - Multiple T1WI obtained during and after IV injection of contrast
  - Role in lesion characterization/detection
  - Key role in assessment of tumor recurrence after prostatectomy
  - Imaging interpretation
    - Qualitative analysis: Most commonly used, based on assessment of enhancement of lesion compared to surrounding gland
      - Cancer typically shows higher and earlier enhancement than surrounding gland
    - Semiquantitative analysis: Curves of enhancement
      - Type 1: Progressive enhancement
      - Type 2: Upslope followed by plateau
      - Type 3: Upslope followed by decline, most specific for cancer
    - Quantitative analysis: Pharmacokinetic modeling
      - K-trans (volume transfer constant) and K-ep (reverse reflux rate constant) are increased in cancer
- MRS
  - Role in assessment of tumor aggressiveness and response to treatment
    - Limited role in tumor detection (compared to T2WI+DWI and DCE)
  - Key metabolic compounds in prostate gland
    - Citrate [2.60 parts per million (ppm)]
    - Creatine (3.04 ppm)
    - Choline (3.20 ppm)
  - Cancer
    - $\uparrow$ choline and $\downarrow$ citrate; $\uparrow$ choline-plus-creatine to citrate ratio (CC:C)
- **Common cancer mimickers**
  - Prostatitis
    - Inflammation in PZ reduces SI on T2WI
    - Helpful tip: Inflammation usually shows a non-mass-like and ill-defined appearance
  - BPH nodules
    - Stromal nodules may restrict diffusion
      - Helpful tip: Benign nodules are usually well-defined on T2WI
  - Hemorrhage (post biopsy)
    - Hemorrhage may appear as low SI on T2WI
    - Helpful tip: High SI on T1WI
  - CZ
    - On axial T2WI at base of gland, it may appear with round/oval shape and low SI
    - Helpful tip: Coronal images demonstrate triangular (teardrop- or butterfly-shaped) appearance

Imaging Recommendations

- Protocol advice
  - Scanner: $\geq$ 1.5T
  - Coil: Surface multichannel phased array $\pm$ endorectal
  - Timing: At least 6 weeks after biopsy
  - Sequences
    - Multiplanar high resolution T2WI
    - DWI with multiple b-values, high b-value $\geq$ 1400 s/mm²
    - DCE with temporal resolution < 10 sec

DIAGNOSTIC CHECKLIST

Reporting Tips

- Prostate Imaging Reporting and Data System (PI-RADS)
  - Current version: PI-RADS v2
  - Main aim: Standardization of acquisition and interpretation of mpMR of prostate
  - Findings are classified in 5 categories of risk for clinically significant cancer (from PI-RADS 1: Very low risk, to PI-RADS 5: Very high risk) based on appearance on T2WI, DWI, and DCE

(Left) *Axial T2WI MR (top) and ADC map (bottom) show symmetric ovoid structures ➡ of low signal intensity projecting over the peripheral zone of the base.* (Right) *Coronal T2WI in the same patient confirms those structures to be the central zone ➡. The central zone typically appears as a symmetric V-shaped structure on coronal images. On axial images, the central zone may mimic cancer because of low signal intensity on T2WI and ADC map.*

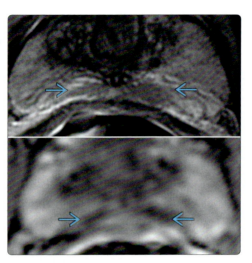
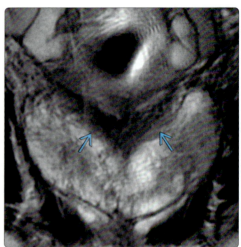

(Left) *Axial T2WI MR shows the prostate in a 66-year-old man presenting with increased PSA (6.8 ng/mL). The peripheral zone shows ill-defined, decreased signal intensity ➡.* (Right) *Axial postcontrast T1WI MR at the same level reveals diffuse hyperenhancement of the peripheral zone ➡. Prostate biopsy demonstrated acute on chronic prostatitis. Inflammation is a common cancer mimicker because it is associated with decreased signal intensity on T2WI.*

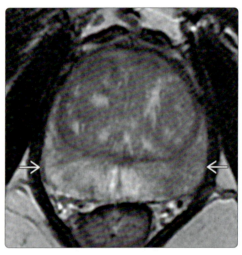
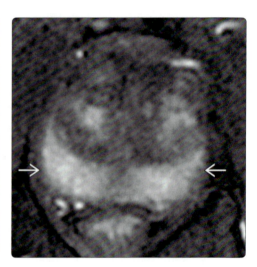

(Left) *Axial T2WI MR shows the prostate in a 67-year-old man with history of prostate cancer (Gleason score 3+4 = 7) on a recent systematic biopsy. The cancer is a low signal intensity mass located in the posterolateral aspect of the peripheral zone ➡.* (Right) *Axial T1WI MR obtained at the same level shows an area of high signal intensity corresponding to postbiopsy hemorrhage ➡. Note that the area with cancer does not show high signal intensity ➡. This appearance, defined as a halo sign, is highly specific for cancer.*

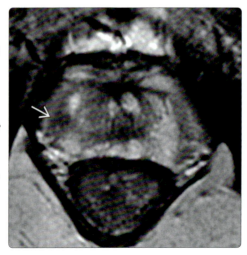
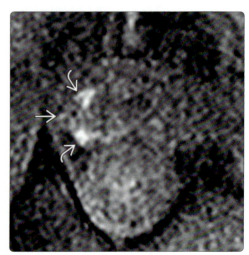

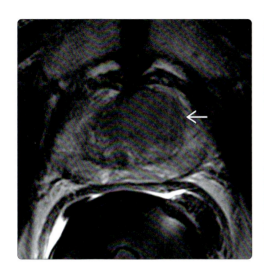
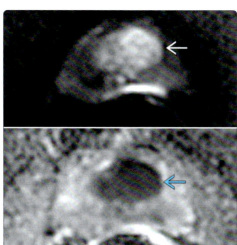

(Left) Axial T2WI MR of the prostate in a 64-year-old man presenting with elevated PSA (24 ng/mL) shows a large mass of low signal intensity ➡ in the anterior transition zone. Target biopsy revealed adenocarcinoma, Gleason score 5+4 = 9. (Right) The cancer shows high signal intensity on the high b-value DWI ➡ (top) and low signal intensity on the ADC map ⇨ (bottom portion). DWI/ADC represents the key functional technique in an mpMR study of the prostate.

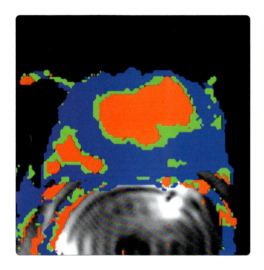
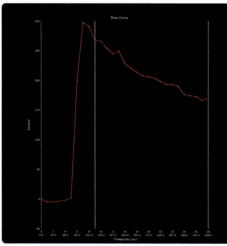

(Left) Color-coded map is based on curves of enhancement. The cancer is displayed with the color red corresponding to a type 3 curve (upslope followed by decline). Cancer typically shows a higher and earlier enhancement than the normal gland. (Right) Type 3 curve of enhancement (wash-in followed by washout) is the most specific for cancer.

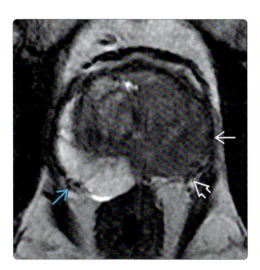
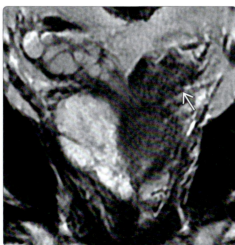

(Left) Axial T2WI MR of the prostate in a 70-year-old man presenting with elevated PSA (16.8 ng/mL) shows a large mass ➡ of low signal intensity in the peripheral zone of the left midgland. At prostatectomy, the mass was adenocarcinoma, Gleason score 5+4 = 9 with extraprostatic extension. Note the tumor involvement of the left neurovascular bundle (NVB) ➡. The right NVB is normal ⇨. (Right) Coronal T2WI MR of the prostate in the same patient reveals tumor extension into the left seminal vesicle ➡.

Benign Prostatic Hypertrophy

TERMINOLOGY

- Benign prostatic hyperplasia (BPH)
  - Glandular and stromal hyperplasia leading to enlargement of transition and periurethral zones and increased prostatic volume

IMAGING

- Best imaging tools: transrectal US and multiparametric (mp) MR
- US: Enlarged gland: Nodules are hypoechoic (80%) or isoechoic/echogenic (20%)
- mpMR: Enlarged transition zone with multiple nodules of different signal intensity on T2WI
  - Glandular BPH nodule: ↑ signal intensity
  - Stromal BPH nodule: ↓ signal intensity
- CT: Enlarged prostate with extrinsic impression on base of bladder
- IVP: Extrinsic impression on bladder base, "J-hooking" of distal ureters

TOP DIFFERENTIAL DIAGNOSES

- Prostate cancer
- Prostate abscess
- Bladder carcinoma

CLINICAL ISSUES

- Prostate volume increases with age and peaks in 6th/7th decade
- Lower urinary tract symptoms: Obstructive (e.g., incomplete voiding), irritative (e.g., urgency)
- Medical therapy: α blockers; 5-α reductase inhibitors; anticholinergics; PDE5 inhibitors
- Surgery: e.g., transurethral resection, open prostatectomy

DIAGNOSTIC CHECKLIST

- Among available imaging tests, mpMR is most helpful to differentiate BPH nodule from prostatic cancer
  - Morphologic features on T2WI
  - Signal intensity on DWI/ADC map

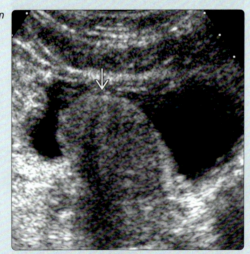
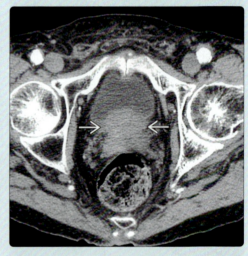

(Left) Transabdominal US in an 82-year-old man presenting with symptoms of bladder outlet obstruction reveals marked enlargement of the prostate ➡ due to benign prostatic hyperplasia. (Right) Axial CECT in a 78-year-old man presenting with urinary frequency demonstrates an enlarged prostate gland ➡ protruding into the bladder lumen.

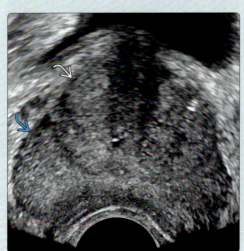
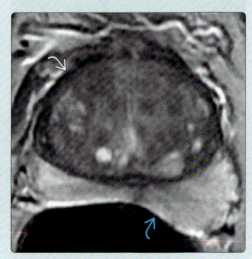

(Left) Transrectal US of benign prostatic hyperplasia (BPH) is shown. The transition zone ➡ is enlarged and heterogeneous. The peripheral zone ➡ appears homogeneous. (Right) Axial T2 MR of the prostate in the same patient shows an enlarged transition zone ➡ with heterogeneous signal intensity, findings compatible with BPH. Note a normal peripheral zone ➡ with homogeneous signal intensity.

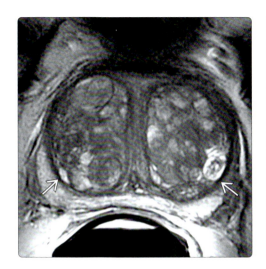

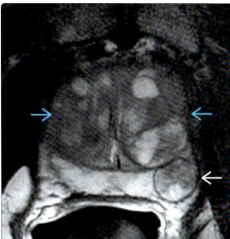

(Left) Axial T2 MR shows an enlarged transition zone ➡ with multiple nodules of different signal intensity, consistent with BPH. Nodules with high signal intensity are glandular rich. Nodules with low signal intensity are stromal rich. (Right) Axial T2 MR of the prostate shows BPH ➡ and an exophytic nodule ➡ projecting on the left peripheral zone. Exophytic BPH nodules can be distinguished from cancer based on the well-defined margins and the signal intensity similar to other BPH nodules.

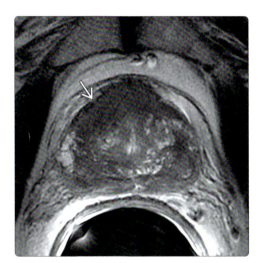

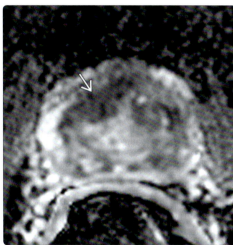

(Left) Axial T2 MR through the midgland shows a lenticular, hypointense mass ➡ with ill-defined borders (erased charcoal drawing sign) in the anterior right transition zone, corresponding to biopsy-proven prostate adenocarcinoma. The transition zone is the origin of 20-25% of prostate cancers, which may be difficult to differentiate from benign prostatic hypertrophy nodules. (Right) Axial apparent diffusion coefficient map shows the tumor in the transition zone as a hypointense mass ➡.

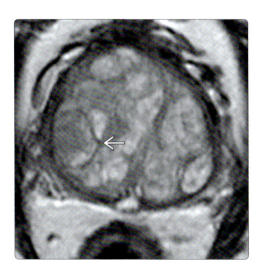

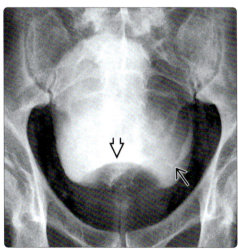

(Left) Axial T2 MR through an enlarged prostate with BPH is shown. Benign stromal nodules have low signal intensity on T2 MR, thus potentially mimicking cancer. Benign nodules usually have well-defined borders ➡, while tumors in the transition zone tend to present with ill-defined margins. (Right) IVP shows an extrinsic impression ➡ on the base of the bladder with "J-hooking" of the left ureter ➡ in this patient with BPH.

Prostate Carcinoma

IMAGING

- 70% of prostate carcinomas occur in peripheral zone
- Transrectal ultrasonography (TRUS)
  - Hypoechoic lesion in peripheral zone
- Multiparametric MR imaging
  - Classification of lesions according to Prostate Imaging Reporting and Data System (PI-RADS)
    - 5 categories of risk for clinically significant cancer from PI-RADS 1 = very low, to PI-RADS 5 = very high
  - T2WI
    - Peripheral zone: Hypointense mass ± extracapsular extension
    - Transition zone: Hypointense lenticular, noncircumscribed mass
  - DWI
    - Focal, markedly hypointense on ADC and markedly hyperintense on high (> 1,400) b-value DWI
  - DCE
    - Focal enhancement earlier or contemporaneous with adjacent gland
  - MRS
    - ↓ citrate level; ↑ choline level
    - ↑ choline + creatine:citrate ratio

TOP DIFFERENTIAL DIAGNOSES

- Benign prostatic hyperplasia (BPH)
- Bladder carcinoma
- Prostatitis

PATHOLOGY

- > 95% of tumors are adenocarcinoma

CLINICAL ISSUES

- Most common noncutaneous cancer in American men
- Most important factor affecting choice of treatment is establishing likelihood of clinically localized disease

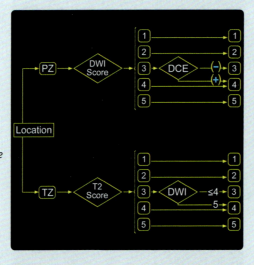
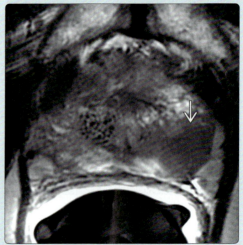

(Left) *Graphic shows the Prostate Imaging Reporting and Data System (PI-RADS, version 2) algorithm to assign each lesion to 1 of 5 categories of risk for clinically significant cancer. DWI is the dominant sequence in the peripheral zone. T2WI is the dominant sequence in the transition zone.* (Right) *Axial T2WI MR through the prostate apex shows a 2.0-cm hypointense lesion ➡ in the left peripheral zone (T2 score = 5).*

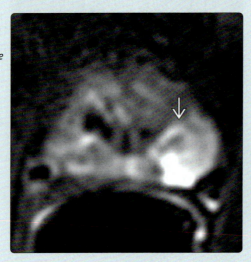
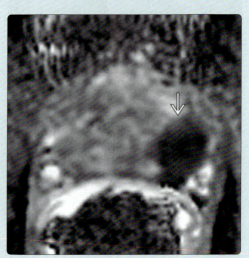

(Left) *Axial DWI (b = 1,500 s/mm²) MR demonstrates the mass in the left peripheral zone as markedly hyperintense ➡. (Right) Axial ADC map shows the mass in the left peripheral zone as markedly hypointense ➡ (DWI score = 5). The lesion is assigned a category of PI-RADS 5, corresponding to a very high risk of clinically significant cancer. At biopsy, the mass was proven to be adenocarcinoma (Gleason score 3+4 = 7).*

TERMINOLOGY

Abbreviations

- Prostate cancer (PC)
- Peripheral zone (PZ)
- Transition zone (TZ)
- Central zone (CZ)
- Diffusion-weighted imaging (DWI)
- Apparent diffusion coefficient (ADC)
- Dynamic contrast enhanced study (DCE)

Definitions

- Malignancy of prostate gland
  - > 95% of tumors are adenocarcinoma

IMAGING

General Features

- Location
  - 70% in PZ, 20-25% in TZ, 5-10% in CZ

Ultrasonographic Findings

- **Transrectal ultrasonography (TRUS)**
  - Hypoechoic lesion in PZ
  - Primary use
    - Assessment of prostate size
    - Guide for biopsy
    - Brachytherapy seed placement

CT Findings

- Limited role in detecting and staging PC
  - Evaluation of advanced disease; lymphadenopathy; bone metastases

MR Findings

- Multiparametric MR (mpMR) imaging
  - Anatomic imaging
    - T2WI; T1WI
  - Functional imaging
    - DWI
    - DCE study
    - Magnetic resonance spectroscopy (MRS)
- **Prostate Imaging Reporting and Data System (PI-RADS)**
  - Version 2 (released in 2015)
  - System aimed at standardizing performance and interpretation of mpMR of prostate
  - Classification of prostate findings in 5 categories of risk for clinically significant cancer
    - PI-RADS 1: Very low risk
    - PI-RADS 2: Low risk
    - PI-RADS 3: Intermediate risk
    - PI-RADS 4: High risk
    - PI-RADS 5: Very high risk
  - Clinically significant cancer
    - Gleason score ≥ 7
    - &/or volume ≥ 0.5 cc
    - &/or extraprostatic extension
  - Classification is based on imaging appearance on T2WI, DWI/ADC, DCE, and application of algorithm
- T2WI
  - PC appearance
    - Low signal intensity mass
    - PZ
      - □ Score 4 (PI-RADS v2): Circumscribed, homogeneous moderate hypointense focus/mass confined to prostate and < 1.5 cm
      - □ Score 5 (PI-RADS v2): Same as 4 but ≥ 1.5 cm &/or presence of extraprostatic extension
    - TZ
      - □ Score 4 (PI-RADS v2): Moderately hypointense, lenticular or noncircumscribed, and < 1.5 cm
      - □ Score 5 (PI-RADS v2): Same as 4 but ≥ 1.5 cm &/or presence of extraprostatic extension
  - Advantages
    - Lesion detection and characterization; assessment of extraprostatic extension
  - Limitations
    - False-positives: e.g., hemorrhage, inflammation
- DWI
  - PC appearance: Focal area of high SI on DWI (b-value > 1,400 s/mm²) and low SI on ADC map
    - Score 4 (PI-RADS v2): Focal, markedly hypointense on ADC and markedly hyperintense on high b-value DWI and < 1.5 cm
    - Score 5 (PI-RADS v2): Same as 4 but ≥ 1.5 cm &/or presence of extraprostatic extension
  - Advantages
    - Increased sensitivity for tumor detection in PZ and TZ
  - Limitations
    - Limited specificity in TZ
      - □ Stromal-rich benign prostatic hyperplasia (BPH) nodule can show restricted diffusion
- MRS
  - PC appearance
    - ↓ citrate level; ↑ choline level
    - ↑ choline + creatine:citrate ratio
  - Limitations
    - Increased total acquisition time; high expertise required
- DCE
  - PC appearance
    - Qualitative (visual) analysis: Early hyperenhancement; rapid washout
    - Semiquantitative analysis: Type III curve (increase followed by decline) most suspicious for cancer
    - Quantitative analysis: ↑ K-trans (volume transfer constant)
  - Advantages
    - Key sequence for detection of tumor recurrence
  - Limitations
    - False-positive: Inflammation in PZ and BPH in TZ
  - Role in PI-RADS v2
    - Limited; presence of focal enhancement earlier or contemporaneous to gland receives positive score that can upgrade indeterminate lesion in PZ to category PI-RADS 4

Nuclear Medicine Findings

- Bone scan
  - ↑ uptake in bone metastases
  - Indications

- Gleason score ≥ 8; prostate-specific antigen (PSA) ≥ 20 ng/mL; T ≥ 3
- Advanced prostate cancer and bone pain
- Posttreatment follow-up

Imaging Recommendations

- Best imaging tool
  - mpMR
    - Tumor detection and staging
    - Guidance for biopsy
    - Active surveillance
    - Posttreatment follow-up

DIFFERENTIAL DIAGNOSIS

Benign Prostatic Hyperplasia

- Stromal: Well-defined nodules with discrete margins

Bladder Carcinoma

- Large tumor involving base of bladder may mimic PC

Prostatitis

- Distribution: Lobar; diffuse

PATHOLOGY

Gross Pathologic & Surgical Features

- > 95% of PCs are adenocarcinoma
- Gleason score
  - Score 1-5 (5 being worst) for 2 most common areas of tumor
  - Prognostic grade groups
    - Group I: Gleason score < 7
    - Group II: Gleason score 3+4 = 7
    - Group III: Gleason score 4+3 = 7
    - Group IV: Gleason score 8
    - Group V: Gleason score 9-10
- Tumor spread
  - Hematogenous
    - Prostatic venous plexus drains into internal iliac veins and communicates with vertebral venous plexus
    - Sacrum and lumbar spine most common site of bone metastases (osteoblastic)
  - Lymphatic
    - Primary drainage to internal iliac nodes, then to retroperitoneal nodes
  - Local
    - Seminal vesicles, bladder, rectum

CLINICAL ISSUES

Presentation

- Most common signs/symptoms
  - Symptoms
    - Clinically localized disease is typically asymptomatic
    - Urinary symptoms: Hesitancy, urgency, ↑ frequency
    - Bone pain from metastases
  - Abnormal digital rectal exam (DRE)
- Laboratory data
  - Increased PSA level
    - PSA density (PSAD) > 0.15 ng/mL/cc
    - PSA velocity > 0.75 ng/mL/year

- Percent-free PSA < 25%
  - PSA derivatives & novel biomarkers may assist in diagnosis
- Screening
  - United States Preventative Task Force recommends individualized patient approach (C recommendation)
  - Cutoff of 4.0 ng/mL before referral to urologist

Demographics

- Age
  - ↑ risk with age; rare < 50 years
  - Median age at diagnosis: 68 years old
- Ethnicity
  - African Americans > Caucasians
- Epidemiology
  - Most common noncutaneous malignancy

Treatment

- Options, risks, complications
  - Active surveillance
    - Risk stratification according to Gleason grade, PSA, PSAD, number of cores, & percentage of involved core
    - Very low-risk prostate cancer (cT1c, G3+3=6, PSA < 10, PSAD < 0.15, 1-2 cores and < 50% core involvement) associated with very low mortality
  - Watchful waiting
    - Await development of advanced symptoms and treat palliatively
    - May be utilized in patients for whom radical therapy is inappropriate
  - Surgery
    - Radical prostatectomy (open, laparoscopic, robotic) with bilateral pelvic lymphadenopathy
    - Ideal for patients with clinically localized disease and long life expectancy
    - Risks: Erectile dysfunction, stress urinary incontinence, anastomotic stricture, lymphocele, rectal injury, bladder injury
  - Radiation therapy
    - Poor surgical candidates, locally advanced disease, salvage therapy
    - External beam radiotherapy, intensity-modulated radiotherapy, sterotactic body radiation therapy, brachytherapy (for localized disease)
    - Risks: Erectile dysfunction, radiation cystitis, proctitis
  - Localized therapies: e.g., cryotherapy; high-intensity focused ultrasound
  - Hormonal therapy: Node positive disease, induction for radiotherapy, metastatic disease
  - Metastatic disease: Hormonal therapy, docetaxel, cabazetaxel, abiraterone/prednisone, enzalutamide, sipuleucel-T, radium-223, ketoconazole, mitoxantrone
    - Castration-resistant metastatic prostate cancer defined as radiographic evidence of metastatic disease despite testosterone < 50 ng/mL

SELECTED REFERENCES

1. Weinreb JC, Barentsz JO, Choyke PL, Cornud F, Haider MA, Macura KJ, Margolis D, Schnall MD, Shtern F, Tempany CM, Thoeny HC, Verma S. Weinreb JC. PI-RADS Prostate Imaging-Reporting and Data System:2015,Version 2. Eur Urol 2016;69(1):16-40. PI-RADS Assessment Categories (page 17) Lexicon/Definitions (T2W; DWI; DCE) reported in tables on page 23, 25, 27 reproduced with permission from ACR.

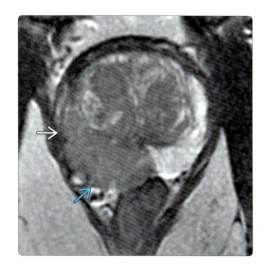

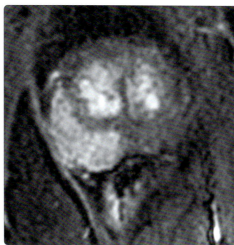

(Left) *Axial T2WI MR of the prostate through the midgland shows a 2.2-cm hypointense mass* ➡ *replacing the right peripheral zone with extraprostatic extension into the rectoprostatic angle and right neurovascular bundle* ➡ *(T2 score 5).* (Right) *Axial postcontrast T1WI MR at same level reveals enhancement of the lesion (positive score). The lesion appeared markedly hyperintense on DWI and hypointense on an ADC map (not shown), resulting in a DWI score of 5 and a PI-RADS category 5 (Gleason score 9 adenocarcinoma at biopsy).*

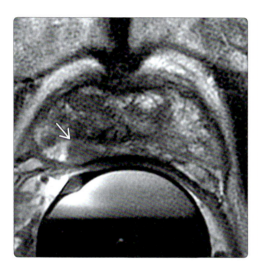

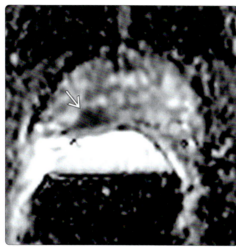

(Left) *Axial T2WI MR shows a 1-cm low signal intensity focus confined to the prostate (score 4)* ➡ *corresponding to biopsy-proven prostate cancer. Of prostate cancers, 70% occur in the peripheral zone.* (Right) *Axial ADC map shows the cancer in the right peripheral zone as a low signal intensity lesion (score 4)* ➡. *A focal lesion in the peripheral zone that is hyperintense on high b-value DWI and hypointense on ADC is highly suspicious for cancer. This lesion received a final PI-RADS score of 4 because of its size (< 1.5 cm).*

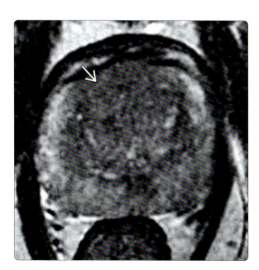

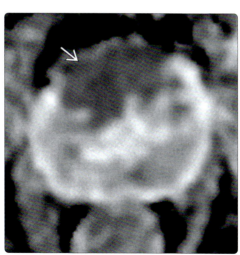

(Left) *Axial T2WI MR shows the prostate through the midgland in a patient presenting with elevated PSA and PSA density (0.5 ng/mL²) and prior negative biopsies. A noncircumscribed lenticular and hypointense mass* ➡ *is in the anterior gland (T2 score 5).* (Right) *Axial ADC map at same level shows the lesion as markedly hypointense* ➡ *(DWI score 5). At biopsy, the mass was proven to be an adenocarcinoma (Gleason 4+3). The characterization of lesions in the transition zone strongly relies on the morphologic appearance.*

(Left) *Axial T2WI MR of the prostate (midgland) shows multiple linear and wedge-shaped hypointensities* ➔ *corresponding to a T2 score = 2.* (Right) *Axial ADC map at the same level shows no focal abnormalities in the peripheral zone (score 1) resulting in a PI-RADS score 1. Linear or wedge-shaped abnormalities in the peripheral zone are usually inflammation or fibrosis.*

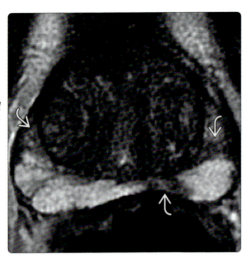
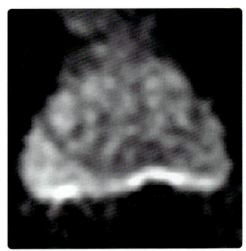

(Left) *Axial T2WI MR of the prostate through the midgland shows a large hypointense mass* ➔ *affecting both lobes with extension into the left neurovascular bundle* ➔. (Right) *Axial CECT of advanced disease shows an enhancing mass* ➔ *within the prostate with obliteration of the fat plane between the mass and the bladder. There is also inguinal adenopathy* ➔.

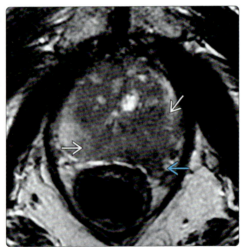
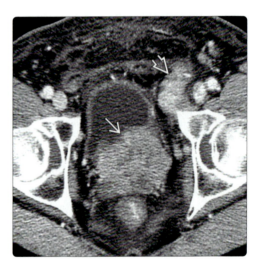

(Left) *Sagittal T2WI MR shows a large mass in the base of the prostate* ➔ *invading the left seminal vesicle* ➔. *The mass corresponds to a biopsy-proven adenocarcinoma (Gleason score: 4+5 = 9).* (Right) *Graphic of the prostate gland shows tumor invasion into the surrounding tissues, including the rectum* ➔ *and seminal vesicles* ➔.

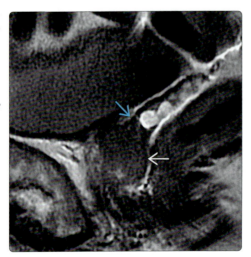
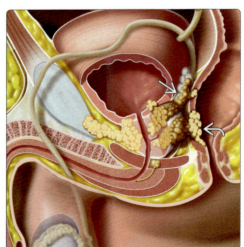

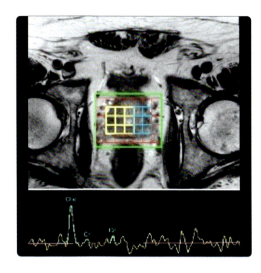

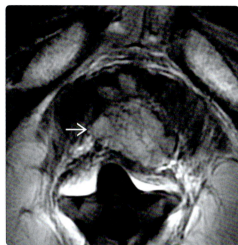

(Left) *Axial MRS of the prostate shows typical composition of prostate cancer with increased choline level and increased choline + creatine:citrate ratio. (Courtesy R. Girometti, MD.)* (Right) *Axial T2WI MR through the lower pelvis in a postprostatectomy patient with biochemical relapse reveals a large mass ⮕ at the base of the bladder. Biopsy confirmed recurrent adenocarcinoma.*

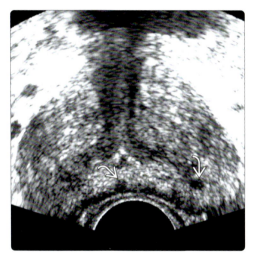

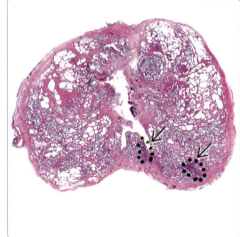

(Left) *Transverse transrectal ultrasonography shows a mildly enlarged prostate with small, hypoechoic lesions ⮕ in the peripheral zone. The PSA level was elevated (14.2 ng/mL). Biopsy of the lesions confirmed carcinoma.* (Right) *Resected prostate (whole-mount section) shows the tumor inked ⮕.*

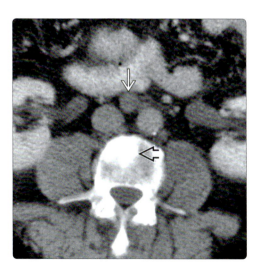

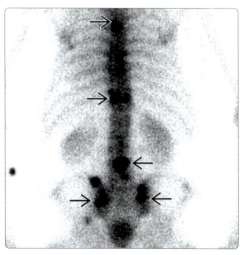

(Left) *Axial CECT in a patient with metastatic prostate cancer shows retroperitoneal lymphadenopathy ⮕ and a blastic vertebral metastasis ⮕.* (Right) *Bone scan in patient with prostate cancer shows multiple metastases ⮕, predominately in the lumbar spine and pelvis. Because there is drainage from the prostatic venous plexus to the vertebral venous plexus, the lower spine is a common site of involvement. Bone metastases are generally osteoblastic.*

T | Definition of Primary Tumor (T)

T Category	T Criteria
TX	Primary tumor cannot be assessed
T0	No evidence of primary tumor
T1	Clinically inapparent tumor that is not palpable
T1a	Tumor incidental histologic finding in ≤ 5% of tissue resected
T1b	Tumor incidental histologic finding in > 5% of tissue resected
T1c	Tumor identified by needle biopsy found in 1 or both sides, but not palpable
T2	Tumor is palpable and confined within prostate
T2a	Tumor involves 1/2 of 1 side or less
T2b	Tumor involves more than 1/2 of 1 side but not both sides
T2c	Tumor involves both sides
T3	Extraprostatic tumor that is not fixed or does not invade adjacent structures
T3a	Extraprostatic extension (unilateral or bilateral)
T3b	Tumor invades seminal vesicle(s)
T4	Tumor is fixed or invades adjacent structures other than seminal vesicles such as external sphincter, rectum, bladder, levator muscles, &/or pelvic wall

Adapted with permission from AJCC Cancer Staging Manual 8th ed., 2017.

N | Definition of Regional Lymph Node (N)

N Category	N Criteria
NX	Regional nodes were not assessed
N0	No positive regional nodes
N1	Metastases in regional nodes(s)

Adapted with permission from AJCC Cancer Staging Manual 8th ed., 2017.

Pathologic T (pT)

T Category	T Criteria
T2	Organ confined
T3	Extraprostatic extension
T3a	Extraprostatic extension (unilateral or bilateral) or microscopic invasion of bladder neck
T3b	Tumor invades seminal vesicle(s)
T4	Tumor is fixed or invades adjacent structures other than seminal vesicles such as external sphincter, rectum, bladder, levator muscles, &/or pelvic wall

Note: There is no pathological T1 classification.
Note: Positive surgical margin should be indicated by an R1 descriptor, indicating residual microscopic disease.

Adapted with permission from AJCC Cancer Staging Manual 8th ed., 2017.

M | Definition of Distant Metastasis (M)

M Category	M Criteria
M0	No distant metastasis
M1	Distant metastasis
M1a	Nonregional lymph node(s)
M1b	Bone(s)
M1c	Other site(s) with or without bone disease

Note: When more than one site of metastasis is present, the most advanced category is used. M1c is most advanced.

Adapted with permission from AJCC Cancer Staging Manual 8th ed., 2017.

G Definition of Histologic Grade Group (G)

Grade Group	Gleason Score	Gleason Pattern
1	≤ 6	≤ 3 + 3
2	7	3 + 4
3	7	4 + 3
4	8	4 + 4
5	9 or 10	4 + 5, 5 + 4, or 5 + 5

The Gleason system has been compressed into so-called Grade Groups.

Adapted with permission from AJCC Cancer Staging Manual 8th ed., 2017.

AJCC Prognostic Stage Groups

When T is...	And N is...	And M is...	And PSA is...	And Grade Group is...	Then the stage group is...
cT1a-c, cT2a	N0	M0	< 10	1	I
pT2	N0	M0	< 10	1	I
cT1a-c, cT2a	N0	M0	≥ 10 < 20	1	IIA
cT2b-c	N0	M0	< 20	1	IIA
T1-2	N0	M0	< 20	2	IIB
T1-2	N0	M0	< 20	3	IIC
T1-2	N0	M0	< 20	4	IIC
T1-2	N0	M0	≥ 20	1-4	IIIA
T3-4	N0	M0	Any	1-4	IIIB
Any T	N0	M0	Any	5	IIIC
Any T	N1	M0	Any	Any	IVA
Any T	N0	M1	Any	Any	IVB

Note: When either PSA or Grade Group is not available, grouping should be determined by T category &/or either PSA or Grade Group as available.

Adapted with permission from AJCC Cancer Staging Manual 8th ed., 2017.

T1 (Gleason Score 3 + 3 = 6)

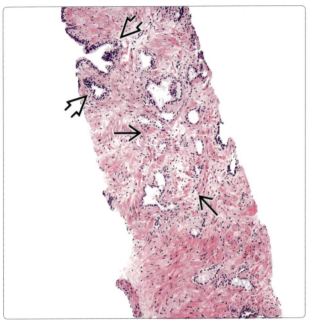

Low-power H&E stain from a core needle prostate biopsy sample shows a small focus of cancer ⇨. Normal prostatic glands are also present ⇨. The tumor represented < 5% of both the core biopsy and the final prostatectomy specimen. (Original magnification, 100x.)

T1 (Gleason Score 3 + 3 = 6)

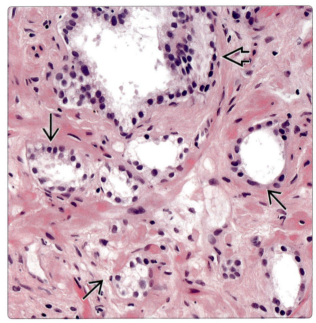

Higher magnification of the same sample shows the numerous invasive neoplastic glands ⇨ lacking basal epithelial cells. Normal prostatic glandular tissue ⇨ has normal benign luminal epithelial cells as well as basal epithelial layer. (Original magnification, 400x.)

T1 (Gleason Score 3 + 3 = 6)

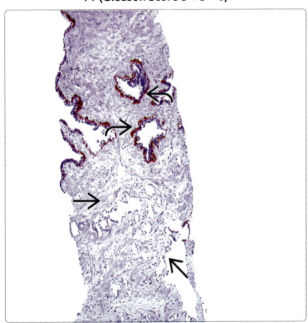

High molecular weight cytokeratin immunostain in the same case demonstrates absence of basal cell layer in the atypical glands ⇨, supporting the diagnosis of adenocarcinoma. The benign glands ⇨ show positive staining, which indicates intact basal cell layer. (Original magnification, 100x.)

T1 (Gleason Score 3 + 3 = 6)

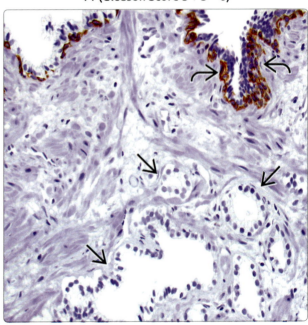

Higher magnification shows malignant glands ⇨ and total absence of staining with keratin antibody. The basal cell layer is intact (brown staining) in benign glands ⇨. (Original magnification, 600x.)

T2b (Gleason Score 3 + 4 = 7)

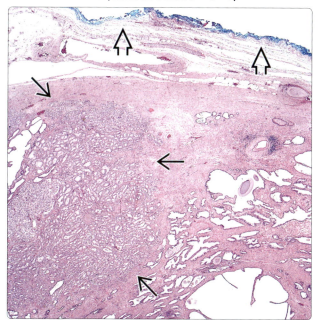

Low-power H&E-stained section from a prostatectomy specimen shows sheets of invasive prostatic adenocarcinoma ▣ on the left. The adenocarcinoma is confined to the prostate tissue and is away from the prostatic capsule or the blue-inked resection margin ▣. (Original magnification, 40x.)

T2b (Gleason Score 3 + 4 = 7)

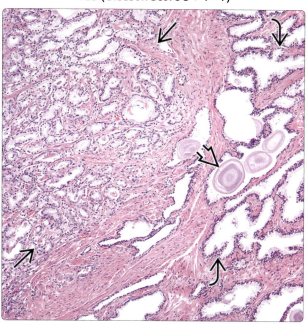

High-power view of the previous slide shows sheets of neoplastic glands in the left upper corner ▣ and benign prostatic glands ▣ with numerous pink round structures ▣, (corpora amylacea) representing laminated concretions of prostatic secretions within glandular lumina. (Original magnification, 400x.)

T3a (Gleason Score 4 + 3 = 7)

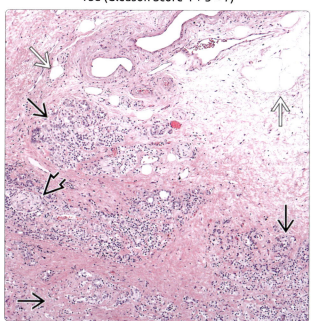

Low-power H&E stain from prostatectomy specimen shows the tumor ▣ extending into the periprostatic tissue in proximity to the periprostatic fat ▣. Note also the perineural invasion (tumor surrounding nerve tissue) ▣. (Original magnification, 40x.)

T3b (Gleason Score 3 + 4 = 7)

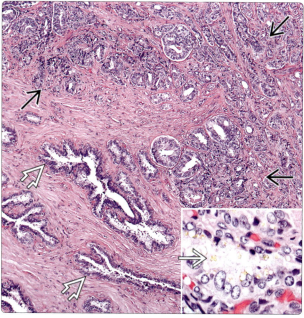

H&E stain of a tumor invading seminal vesicles shows the tumor ▣ and seminal vesicle tissue ▣. (Original magnification, 400x) The inset highlights the golden yellow pigment ▣ (lipofuscin) that is characteristically found abundantly in seminal vesicle tissue.

T2a

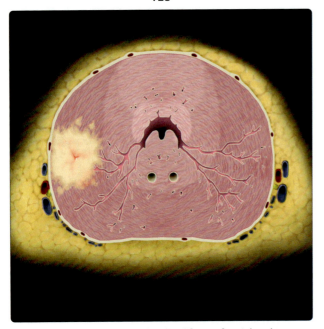

Axial graphic demonstrates a localized focus of peripheral zone tumor that involves less than 1/2 of 1 lobe of the prostate. This is consistent with T2a disease. T1 disease is neither clinically apparent nor visible on imaging.

T2b

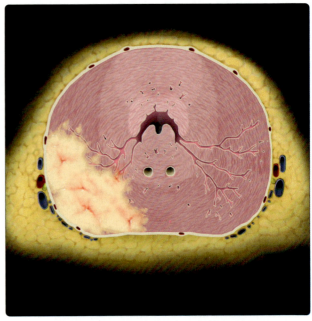

Axial graphic demonstrates a larger focus of peripheral zone tumor that involves more than 1/2 of 1 lobe of the prostate but does not cross the midline. The prostatic capsule is intact, and the neurovascular bundle is unaffected by tumor. This is consistent with T2b disease.

T2c

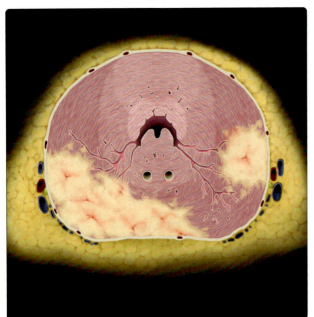

Axial graphic demonstrates a larger focus of peripheral zone tumor that involves more than 1/2 of 1 lobe of the prostate and crosses the midline. An additional focus of tumor is present on the contralateral side of the gland. Both of these findings fulfill the criteria for T2c disease.

T3a

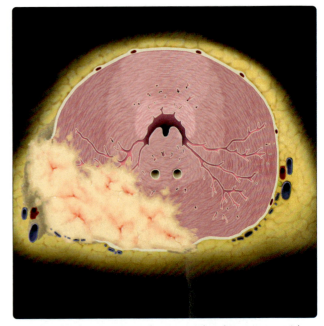

Axial graphic demonstrates a larger peripheral zone tumor with focal bulging of the prostatic contour posteriorly. Additionally, in the posterolateral margin, the capsule is invaded and tumor spills into the surrounding periprostatic fat and surrounds the neurovascular bundle. This is consistent with T3a disease.

N1

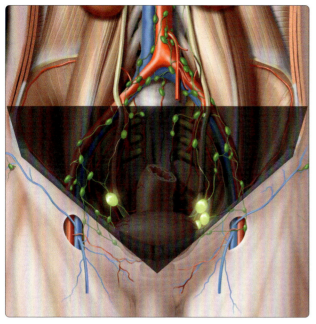

Coronal graphic shows regional lymph nodes shaded in black. Enlarged bilateral internal iliac nodes are present, indicating N1 disease. N1 disease is considered stage IV, regardless of the T stage.

M1a

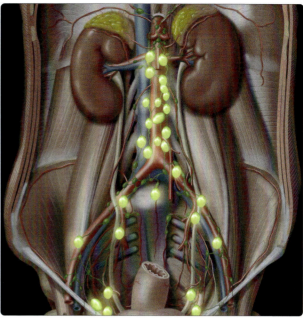

Coronal graphic shows enlarged regional lymph nodes in the pelvis and enlarged nonregional nodes in the common iliac and paraaortic lymph node stations. The presence of nonregional lymph node metastases upgrades disease to M1a.

Metastases, Organ Frequency

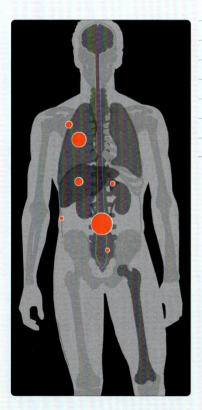

Bone	*90%*
Lung	*46%*
Liver	*25%*
Pleura	*21%*
Adrenal gland	*13%*
Peritoneum	*7%*
Meninges	*6%*

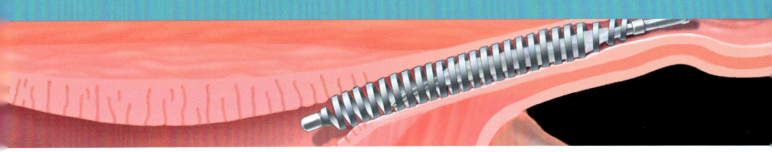

SECTION 13
Procedures

PREPROCEDURE

- Indications
  - Upper tract decompression
  - Nephrolithotomy
  - Urinary diversion
  - Whitaker test for evaluation of obstruction
- Preprocedure imaging
  - Assess degree of hydronephrosis
  - Evaluate position/anatomy of kidney

PROCEDURE

- US-guided initial access in hydronephrosis
- Direct fluoroscopic guidance can be used for
  - Retrograde contrast injection
  - Target calculus or indwelling stent
  - IV contrast ± Lasix (helpful in nondilated system)
  - Direct puncture using anatomic landmarks
- 1-puncture technique if targeted calyx visualized/accessed at outset of procedure; otherwise, 2-puncture technique

- Avascular plane of Brödel: 20-30° off sagittal plane
  - Decreases likelihood of vascular injury

POST PROCEDURE

- Technical success rate in hydronephrosis: 95-98%
  - 80-85% success in nondilated systems
- Transient hematuria common after placement
  - Often resolves within 24-48 hours

OUTCOMES

- Complications
  - Vascular injury and gross hematuria
  - Consider angiography/embolization if persists
  - Bowel transgression with suprapubic tube
- Follow-up imaging for urolithiasis can include
  - Abdominal and pelvic radiography
  - Ultrasound (US)
  - Nonenhanced CT (NECT)

Percutaneous Nephrostomy

Preferred Needle Position (Avascular Plane of Brödel)

(Left) *Clinical photograph shows the typical sagittal position of the US probe during percutaneous nephrostomy. The US probe is cloaked in a sterile cover for use in the sterile field.* (Right) *Graphic shows a needle ➡ entering the renal collecting system via a posterior calyx ➡ along the relatively avascular plane of Brödel. This plane is located between the anterior ➡ & posterior ➡ divisions of the renal artery & lies 20-30° from the sagittal plane. Access via this plane minimizes bleeding and potential vascular injury.*

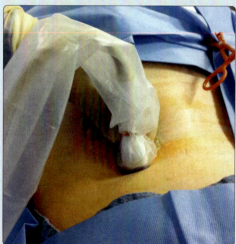

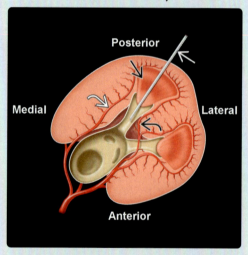

Nephrostomy Catheter

Nephroureteral Catheter

(Left) *Graphic shows that a nephrostomy catheter ➡ has been percutaneously introduced into the left renal collecting system ➡ via a superior pole calyx ➡. The pigtail coil ➡ of the catheter is positioned in the renal pelvis.* (Right) *Graphic shows that a nephroureteral catheter ➡ has been percutaneously placed into the left renal collecting system via a posterior calyx ➡; the distal pigtail coil ➡ of the catheter is in the bladder, and the proximal pigtail ➡ is in the renal pelvis.*

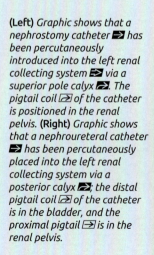

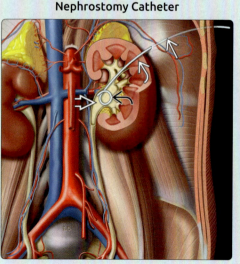

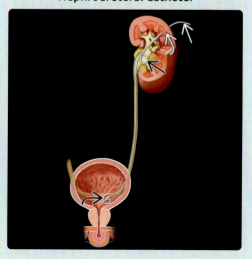

Percutaneous Nephrostomy (Initial CT Imaging)

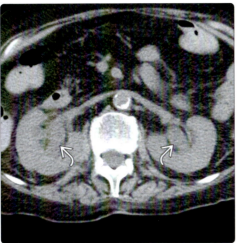

Percutaneous Nephrostomy (Preliminary Ultrasound Planning)

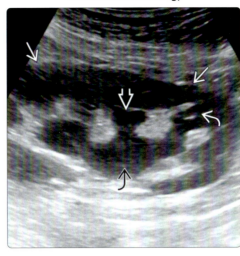

(Left) *Axial NECT obtained in a 68-year-old man who presented with fever & leukocytosis following radical cystectomy & ileal conduit formation shows moderate bilateral hydronephrosis ➘, which was due to recurrent tumor at the ureteral-conduit anastomosis. (Right) Sagittal US of the left kidney ➔ demonstrates moderate dilatation of the calyces ➘ & the renal pelvis ➘. A posterior calyx ➘ of the inferior pole has been selected for percutaneous nephrostomy access.*

Percutaneous Nephrostomy (Preparation of Access Site)

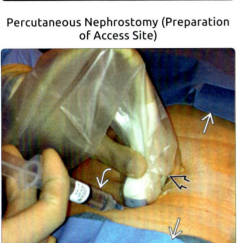

Percutaneous Nephrostomy (US-Guided Needle Placement)

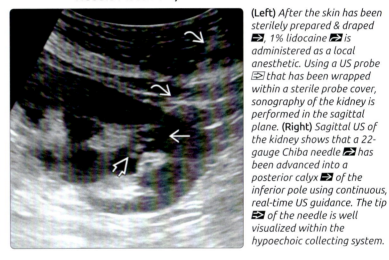

(Left) *After the skin has been sterilely prepared & draped ➔, 1% lidocaine ➘ is administered as a local anesthetic. Using a US probe ➘ that has been wrapped within a sterile probe cover, sonography of the kidney is performed in the sagittal plane. (Right) Sagittal US of the kidney shows that a 22-gauge Chiba needle ➘ has been advanced into a posterior calyx ➘ of the inferior pole using continuous, real-time US guidance. The tip ➘ of the needle is well visualized within the hypoechoic collecting system.*

Percutaneous Nephrostomy (US-Guided Needle Placement)

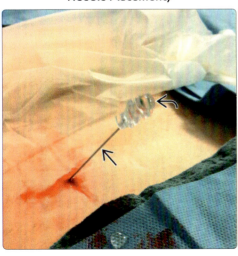

Percutaneous Nephrostomy (Antegrade Nephrostogram)

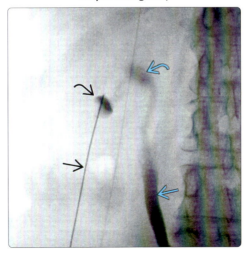

(Left) *After advancing the Chiba needle ➔ into the targeted calyx, the inner stylet is removed & efflux of urine ➘ is noted, thereby confirming access into the collecting system. (Right) Fluoroscopic AP image shows that contrast injected via the Chiba needle ➔ confirms access in the inferior pole calyx ➘ & propagates into the renal pelvis ➘ & proximal ureter ➔. A 1-puncture technique or 2-puncture technique (using a Ring needle) may be used to access a calyx under fluoroscopic guidance.*

Percutaneous Nephrostomy (Transition to Larger Guidewire)

Percutaneous Nephrostomy (Guidewire Placement in Renal Pelvis)

(Left) *Photograph shows that a 0.035-inch 3-J guidewire ➦ has been introduced into the sheath ➥ & is being advanced into the renal collecting system. The larger guidewire is needed to provide more stability for nephrostomy catheter placement.* (Right) *Fluoroscopic radiograph shows that the 0.035-inch 3-J guidewire ➥ has been advanced through the 6-Fr sheath ➥ using fluoroscopic guidance & has been allowed to form a loop within the renal pelvis. The tip of the guidewire ➥ is in a superior pole calyx.*

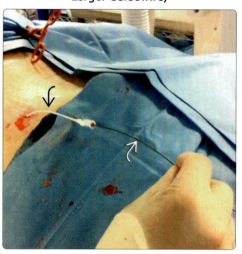

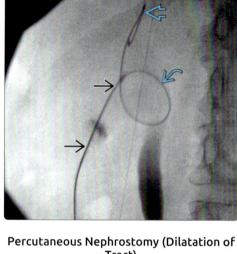

Percutaneous Nephrostomy (Dilatation of Tract)

Percutaneous Nephrostomy (Dilatation of Tract)

(Left) *The access sheath is exchanged for an 8-Fr dilator ➥ to expand the soft tissue tract. The fascial dilator is advanced over the 3-J guidewire into the renal collecting system. Care is taken not to kink the guidewire during tract dilation.* (Right) *Fluoroscopic AP image obtained during tract dilatation shows that the 8-Fr dilator ➥ has been advanced over the 3-J guidewire ➥, so that the dilator tip is within the lower pole calyx ➥. The guidewire position should remain stable during all exchanges.*

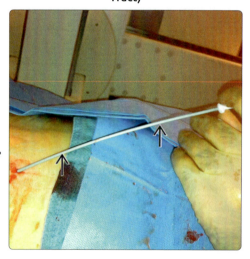

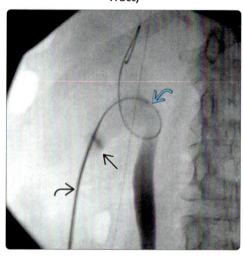

Percutaneous Nephrostomy (Nephrostomy Catheter Placement)

Percutaneous Nephrostomy (Nephrostomy Catheter Placement)

(Left) *The dilator is removed, & an 8-Fr locking nephrostomy catheter, which is mounted on an inner stiffener, is advanced. Once within the renal collecting system, the inner stiffener is unscrewed ➦ & held still while the catheter ➥ is advanced over the wire further into the collecting system.* (Right) *Fluoroscopic AP image shows that the 8-Fr nephrostomy catheter ➥ has been advanced into the collecting system ➥. Once a turn in the guidewire ➥ is reached, the inner stiffener is unscrewed.*

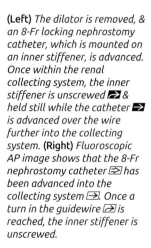

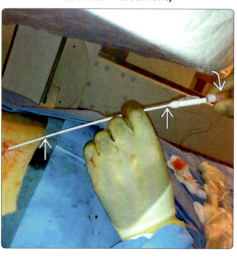

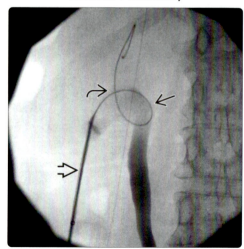

Percutaneous Nephrostomy (Nephrostomy Catheter Placement)

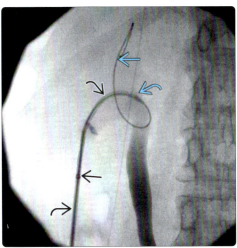

Percutaneous Nephrostomy (Nephrostomy Catheter Placement)

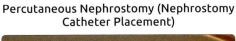
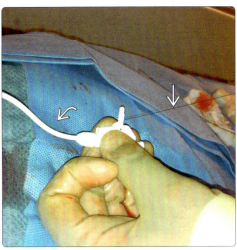

(Left) *After the inner stiffener is unscrewed, it is held in a stationary position, & the catheter ➡ is advanced over the guidewire ➡ further into the collecting system ➡. A radiopaque marker ➡ demarcates the last sidehole of the nephrostomy catheter, which should reside within the collecting system.* (Right) *After the nephrostomy catheter has been satisfactorily positioned under fluoroscopy, the guidewire is removed & the string ➡ is pulled to form the distal pigtail of the catheter ➡.*

Percutaneous Nephrostomy (Nephrostomy Catheter Placement)

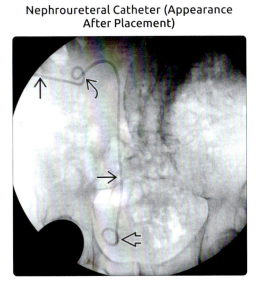

Percutaneous Nephrostomy (Aspiration of Urine)

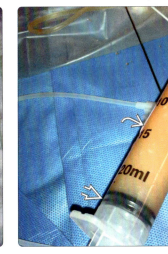

(Left) *Fluoroscopic image demonstrates the final position of the nephrostomy catheter. The pigtail portion ➡ of the catheter & the radiopaque marker ➡ lie within the renal pelvis ➡. Injection of contrast confirms positioning in the collecting system.* (Right) *Photograph shows that a syringe ➡ has been attached to the nephrostomy catheter, allowing aspiration & decompression of the collecting system. In this example, purulent urine ➡ was present, reflecting clinically suspected urosepsis.*

Nephroureteral Catheter (Appearance After Placement)

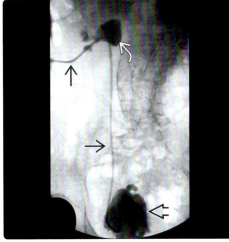

Nephroureteral Catheter (Contrast Injection Evaluation)

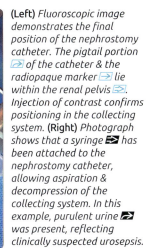

(Left) *Fluoroscopic AP image prior to catheter exchange shows the typical course of a nephroureteral catheter ➡. The proximal pigtail ➡ is in the upper quadrant (renal pelvis), & the distal pigtail ➡ is in the pelvis (urinary bladder). Nephroureteral catheters are useful in patients prone to catheter dislodgement or in cases of ureteral stenosis or injury.* (Right) *Contrast injection demonstrates catheter patency ➡. There is opacification of the renal pelvis ➡ & the urinary bladder ➡.*

Evaluation of Cause of Obstruction (Distal Ureteral Stricture)

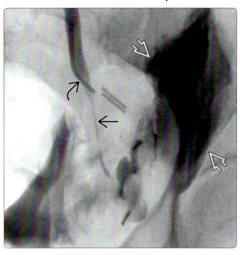

Traversing Cause of Obstruction (Distal Ureteral Stricture)

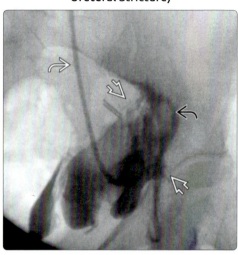

(Left) *Fluoroscopic AP image shows contrast injection via a 5-Fr Kumpe catheter ➡ that has been advanced into the distal ureter. The injected contrast reveals a distal ureteral stricture ➡ that results in ureteral obstruction in this patient who has undergone radical cystectomy & ileal conduit ➡ formation.* **(Right)** *The distal ureteral stricture was crossed with a 0.035-inch angled hydrophilic guidewire followed by an 8-Fr nephroureteral catheter ➡ with the distal pigtail ➡ placed into the conduit ➡.*

Suprapubic Cystostomy (Trocar Technique)

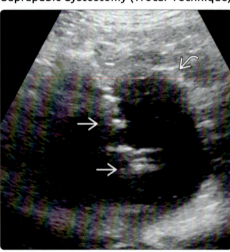

Suprapubic Cystostomy (Trocar Technique)

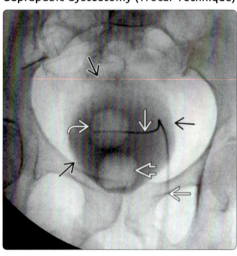

(Left) *Transverse US reveals a urinary bladder ➡ that has been distended by saline administered via a transurethral catheter. A trocar ➡ mounted with a 14-Fr Foley catheter is advanced into the bladder. A strong thrust is used to puncture, rather than "tent," the bladder wall.* **(Right)** *Fluoroscopic AP image shows contrast injected through the suprapubic cystostomy catheter ➡, confirming location of the catheters in the bladder ➡. The Foley balloons of the suprapubic ➡ & transurethral catheters ➡ are seen.*

Suprapubic Cystostomy (Seldinger Technique)

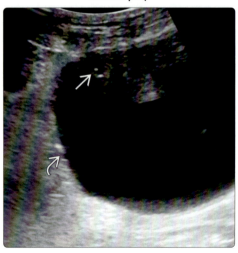

Suprapubic Cystostomy (Seldinger Technique)

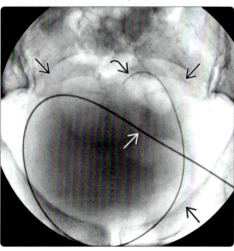

(Left) *Transverse US shows that a 19-g ultrathin Chiba needle ➡ has been advanced into a distended bladder ➡. A Longdwell needle could also have been used to access the bladder.* **(Right)** *Fluoroscopic image shows that after accessing the urinary bladder contrast is injected via the needle to confirm positioning ➡. A 0.035-inch Amplatz guidewire ➡ is then advanced via the Chiba needle ➡ & allowed to coil in the bladder. The needle is removed & the tract is dilated, followed by suprapubic catheter placement.*

Suprapubic Cystostomy (Seldinger Technique)

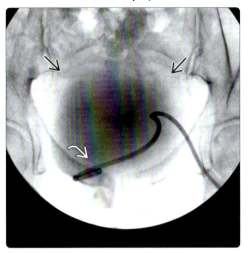

Antegrade Ureteral Stent (Appearance After Placement)

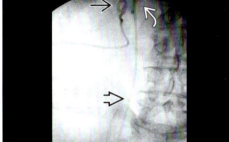
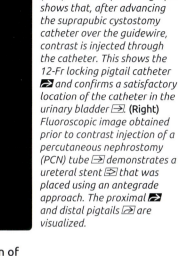

(Left) *Fluoroscopic radiograph shows that, after advancing the suprapubic cystostomy catheter over the guidewire, contrast is injected through the catheter. This shows the 12-Fr locking pigtail catheter ➤ and confirms a satisfactory location of the catheter in the urinary bladder ➡. (Right) Fluoroscopic image obtained prior to contrast injection of a percutaneous nephrostomy (PCN) tube ➡ demonstrates a ureteral stent ➡ that was placed using an antegrade approach. The proximal ➤ and distal pigtails ➡ are visualized.*

Antegrade Ureteral Stent (Injection of Safety PCN)

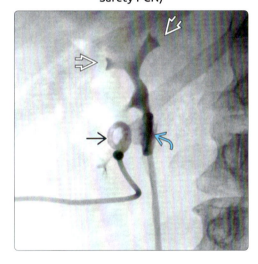

Antegrade Ureteral Stent (Injection of Safety PCN)

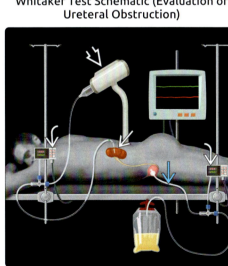

(Left) *Fluoroscopic radiograph shows injection of contrast via the nephrostomy catheter ➡ to assess the ureteral stent prior to PCN removal. The renal pelvis & calyces ➤ are opacified, & the proximal pigtail ➡ of the ureteral stent is seen. (Right) Fluoroscopic image of the pelvis following contrast injection of the safety nephrostomy catheter shows an opacified bladder ➡ containing the distal pigtail ➤ of the ureteral stent ➡. As this confirmed stent patency, the safety PCN was removed.*

Whitaker test (Evaluation of Ureteral Obstruction)

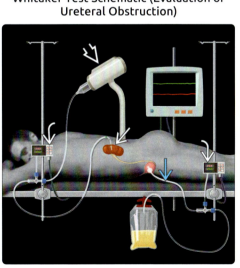

Whitaker Test Schematic (Evaluation of Ureteral Obstruction)

(Left) *Coronal CECT shows mild pelvicaliectasis of the right kidney. A subsequent Whitaker test showed that this finding was not due to obstruction. (Right) Whitaker test schematic shows that a needle ➤ in the renal pelvis is infused with saline via an injector ➡. Pressures are measured there & in the bladder via a Foley catheter ➡, using transducers ➤, to evaluate for ureteral stasis vs. obstruction.*

PREPROCEDURE

- **Indications for ablation**
  - Small (< 3 cm), exophytic, posterior renal mass ideal
  - Traditional indications: Elderly patient, comorbidities
  - Evolving management paradigm: Favorable safety profile, lower long-term costs, recurrence rates may be comparable to open/laparoscopic nephron-sparing surgery
  - Approach also changing with recognition of biology of incidental "small" (< 3 cm) renal mass
  - > 20% "small" (≤ 3 cm) renal masses are benign
  - Very low chance of metastases of renal cell carcinoma < 3 cm
  - Biology prompts less aggressive approach
    - Active surveillance
    - Percutaneous ablation, particularly if growth
- **Indications for embolization**
  - Angiomyolipoma (AML) > 4 cm; nonruptured aneurysms > 5 mm
- Review prior imaging
  - Thermal ablation injury risk if tumor near collecting system; consider pyeloperfusion
  - Determine vascularity of AML before treating

PROCEDURE

- **Ablation**: CT guidance used for most renal ablations
  - Goal: Ablation zone completely encompasses tumor plus 0.5- to 1.0-cm margin
- **Embolization**: Perform as selectively as possible
  - Devascularize AML; preserve normal renal tissue

POST PROCEDURE

- **Ablation**: ≥ 90% complete necrosis in mass ≤ 4 cm
  - CT/MR nonenhancement correlates with necrosis
- **AML embolization**: Success rate of 90-100%
  - Tumor does not disappear; decreases by 40-66%

RFA of RCC: Small Target Lesion Identified at CECT

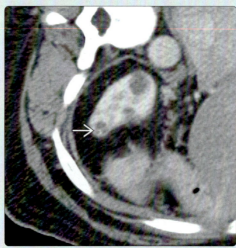

RFA of RCC: Targeting via NECT

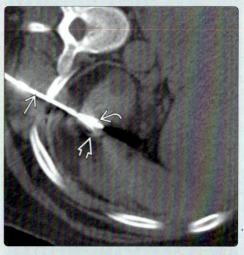

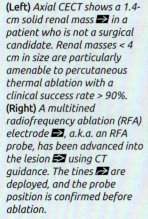

(Left) Axial CECT shows a 1.4-cm solid renal mass ➡ in a patient who is not a surgical candidate. Renal masses < 4 cm in size are particularly amenable to percutaneous thermal ablation with a clinical success rate > 90%. *(Right)* A multitined radiofrequency ablation (RFA) electrode ➡, a.k.a. an RFA probe, has been advanced into the lesion ⇨ using CT guidance. The tines ➡ are deployed, and the probe position is confirmed before ablation.

Cryoablation of RCC: Targeting via CECT

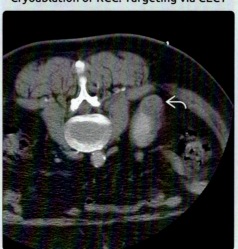

Cryoablation of RCC: "Ice Ball" Monitor

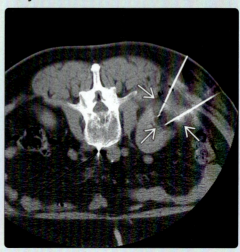

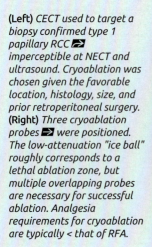

(Left) CECT used to target a biopsy confirmed type 1 papillary RCC ➡ imperceptible at NECT and ultrasound. Cryoablation was chosen given the favorable location, histology, size, and prior retroperitoneal surgery. *(Right)* Three cryoablation probes ➡ were positioned. The low-attenuation "ice ball" roughly corresponds to a lethal ablation zone, but multiple overlapping probes are necessary for successful ablation. Analgesia requirements for cryoablation are typically < that of RFA.

RFA of RCC: Initial CECT Imaging Evaluation

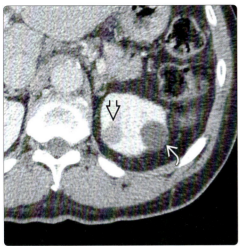

RFA of RCC: Access Site Preparation and Anesthesia

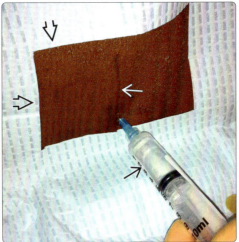

(Left) Axial CECT demonstrates a hypodense renal mass ➨ medially at the same level as a simple cyst ➨. Ultrasound confirmed that the hypodense mass was solid. Review of prior imaging is important in planning access to the lesion. Imaging also shows that hydrodissection is unnecessary, as there are no adjacent structures at risk of nontarget thermal injury. (Right) The skin is marked ➨ after a preliminary CT with a radiopaque grid. After sterile cleansing and draping ➨ the skin, 1% lidocaine local anesthetic ➨ is administered.

RFA of RCC: Cluster Configuration RFA Electrode

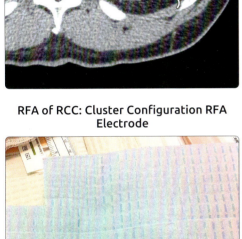

RFA of RCC: Cluster Electrode Placement

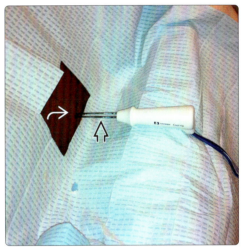

(Left) Photograph shows a cluster RFA probe ➨. The probe consists of 3 prongs attached to a single hub. The design allows a larger area of thermal ablation when compared to a single needle design. Internal cooling of the probes reduces the impedance of the surrounding tissue, enabling a larger ablation. (Right) The probe ➨ is inserted through the skin ➨ to a predetermined depth as measured by CT. The prongs are kept parallel but separate; prongs too close or too far apart may yield a smaller burn.

RFA of RCC: Cluster Electrode Placement

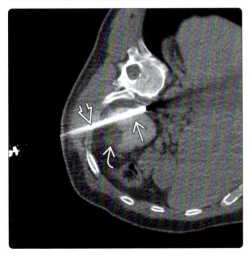

RFA of RCC: Radiofrequency Generator Operation

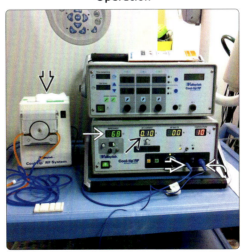

(Left) Axial NECT confirms that there is satisfactory probe ➨ placement through the lesion ➨. Note the simple cyst ➨ at the same level as the mass. (Right) The probe ➨ and grounding pad ➨ cables are attached to the generator. There are displays for impedance ➨ and for current and temperature ➨. During active ablation, the temperature is low as a result of internal cooling. At the end of RFA, the cooling is shut off, and the actual temperature of the ablation is displayed. The electric pump ➨ for providing internal cooling is also seen.

(Left) Two overlapping ablations were performed with adjustment and repeat NECT confirmation of the probe position between each treatment. A postprocedure NECT demonstrates a small posterior collection of perirenal blood ➡ adjacent to the ablation zone ➡, which is a typical finding. (Right) Axial T1WI FS MR performed 1 month post RFA demonstrates T1 hyperintensity ➡ in the ablation zone, which is compatible with coagulation necrosis. Note the T1-hypointense simple renal cyst ➡.

RFA of RCC: Posttreatment NECT Imaging

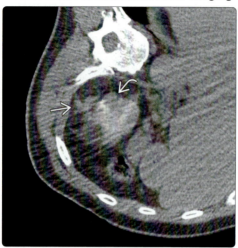

RFA of RCC: Posttreatment MR at 1 Month

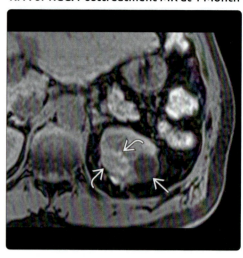

(Left) T2WI FSE 1 month post RFA shows predominantly ↓ T2 signal ➡ in the ablation zone, which is an expected finding. Note the ↑ T2 signal cyst ➡. (Right) Gd-enhanced T1WI FS MR shows no enhancement ➡ in the ablation zone, which is the best imaging correlate of tumor necrosis. Comparison to the pre-RFA CECT shows that the ablation zone encompasses the lesion and a surrounding margin. A thin rim (< 5 mm) of enhancement may occasionally be seen early on, which is a benign ancillary finding.

RFA of RCC: Posttreatment MR at 1 Month

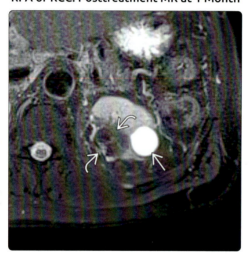

RFA of RCC: Posttreatment MR at 1 Month

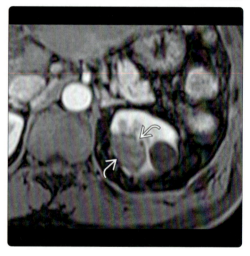

(Left) Coronal CECT shows a large lower pole renal mass ➡. Note that the mass extends centrally, close to the ureter and the renal pelvis ➡. These structures are at risk of nontarget thermal injury during ablation, which could result in a ureteral stricture &/or urinoma. (Right) (A) Scout and (B) axial images from a preliminary NECT for RFA show an externalized ureteral stent ➡ placed immediately prior to RFA. Pyeloperfusion with D5W protects the renal collecting system from thermal injury during ablation.

RFA Planning: Potential Risk of Thermal Injury

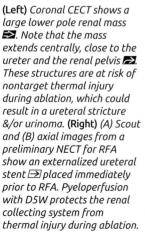
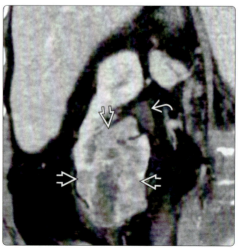

RFA Planning: Need for Pyeloperfusion

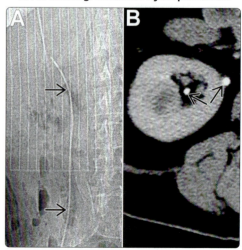

Cryoablation of RCC: Ultrasound Guidance

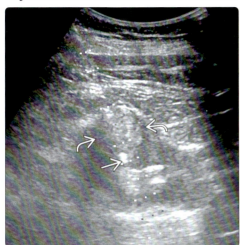

Cryoablation of RCC: NECT "Ice Ball" Monitor

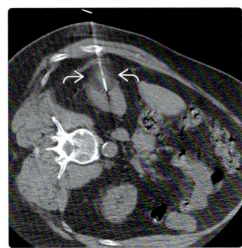

(Left) *Ultrasound guidance may be used for biopsy and initial placement of ablation probes. The distal aspect of 1 of 2 overlapping 17-gauge cryoprobes* ➡ *is shown within the posterior aspect of a biopsy-confirmed (echogenic) clear cell Renal Cell Carcinoma* ➡. (Right) *NECT of the same patient shows a low-attenuation ablation zone* ➡. *Although probes may be placed under ultrasound guidance, "ice ball" shadowing makes it impossible to monitor the ablation.*

Cryoablation of RCC: Baseline CECT

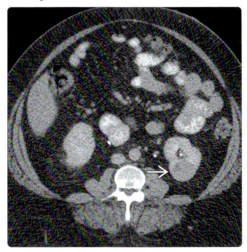

Cryoablation of RCC: Probe Positioning

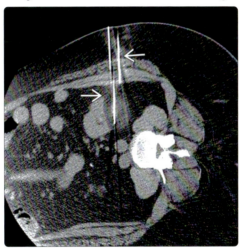

(Left) *Excretory-phase CECT performed on a 57-year-old obese woman with diabetes shows a 2.5-cm nonborder-deforming renal mass* ➡. *A biopsy confirmed clear cell RCC.* (Right) *The patient was referred for percutaneous cryoablation given her significant comorbidities. The lesion was not visualized at either ultrasound or NECT. Overlapping cryoablation probes* ➡ *were positioned after administration of IV contrast.*

Cryoablation of RCC: Early CECT Surveillance

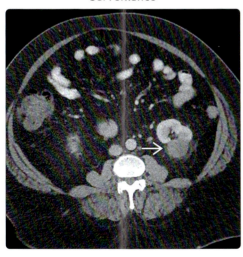

Cryoablation of RCC: Long-Term Surveillance

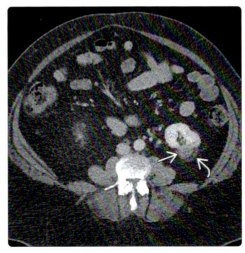

(Left) *Surveillance CECT performed 3 months post treatment on the same patient shows a nonenhancing ablated lesion* ➡ *that is smaller than on previous imaging.* (Right) *Two-year surveillance CT shows a significantly smaller, nonenhancing ablated lesion* ➡ *and a partial peripheral fat halo* ➡. *The renal halo sign is a characteristic feature of renal tumors after RFA, though it may be seen after cryoablation as well.*

Procedures

(Left) *Axial NECT shows a renal mass* ➔ *located posteriorly in the upper pole of the right kidney. The patient was not a surgical candidate due to comorbidities, and the renal mass was an appropriate size for ablation.* (Right) *NECT obtained 10 minutes into the cryoablation freeze cycle shows 1 of the cryoprobes* ➔ *as well as the hypodense "ice ball"* ➔ *encompassing the lesion. The lethal zone is 5 mm internal to the ice ball margin. Typically, a freeze-passive thaw-freeze cycle is performed. Cryoablation may cause less pain than RFA.*

Cryoablation of RCC: Initial NECT Imaging Evaluation

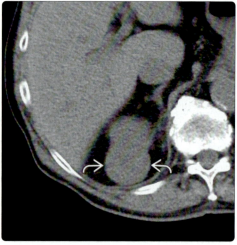

Cryoablation of RCC: Hypodense "Ice Ball" During Freeze Cycle

(Left) *Coronal CECT reconstruction prior to planned RFA demonstrates a solid renal mass* ➔ *in the interpolar region of the left kidney. A pair of renal cysts* ➔ *are also evident. Using a cluster electrode, several overlapping RFA treatments were performed.* (Right) *Axial CECT obtained 3 months after the RFA demonstrates a nonenhancing zone of ablation* ➔, *which appears both to completely encompass the lesion and to extend beyond it with a generous surrounding margin.*

Residual Disease After RFA: CECT Prior to Initial Ablation

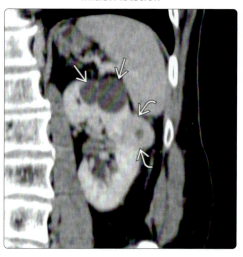

Residual Disease After RFA: CECT After Initial Ablation

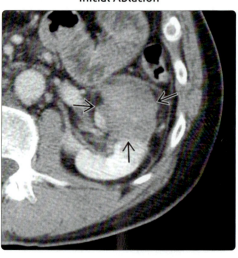

(Left) *Although the axial images showed what appeared to be a satisfactory result, a coronal image from the same CECT shows irregular enhancement* ➔ *along the superior margin of the ablation zone* ➔. *Review of multiplanar reformats may aid assessment of ablation zone margins and is useful in avoiding volume averaging effects.* (Right) *Repeat RFA of the residual disease was performed. CECT 1 month later shows no enhancement in the ablation zone* ➔, *an appearance consistent with tumor necrosis.*

Residual Disease After RFA: Coronal CECT After Ablation

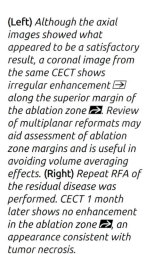
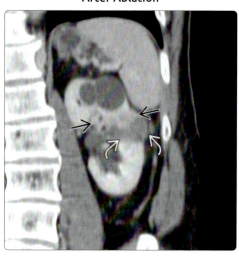

Residual Disease After RFA: Coronal CECT After Retreatment

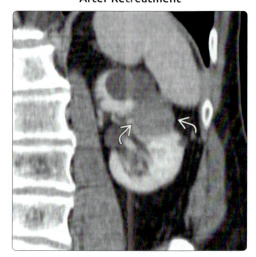

Benign Postablation Ancillary Findings: Initial CECT Evaluation Before RFA

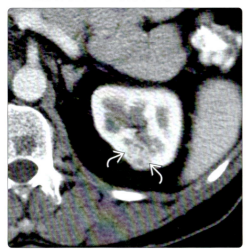

Benign Postablation Ancillary Findings: CECT 1 Month After Treatment

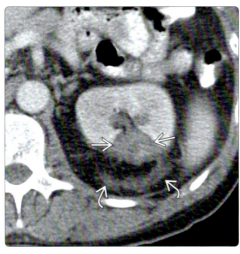

(Left) *Axial CECT obtained prior to a planned RFA demonstrates a small enhancing mass ⮢ in the posterior aspect of the left kidney. The patient subsequently underwent RFA.* (Right) *Axial CECT 1 month post RFA shows a satisfactory lack of enhancement in the ablation zone ➡. However, there is soft tissue stranding ⮢ in the perirenal fat oriented parallel to the renal contour. This is a typical benign finding that occurs after ablation and should not prompt concern for tract seeding.*

Benign Postablation Ancillary Findings: Fat Halo on CECT 9 Months After RFA

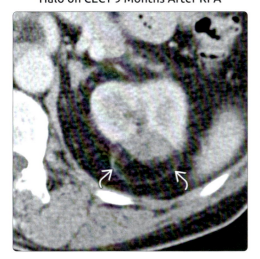

Benign Postablation Ancillary Findings: Extracalyceal Contrast Accumulation

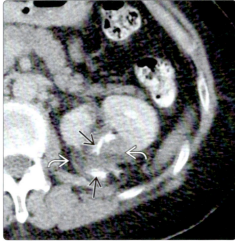

(Left) *Axial CECT obtained 9 months after RFA shows that there has been coalescence of the perirenal stranding into a fat halo ➡. The ablation zone and fat halo may shrink over serial imaging.* (Right) *Axial CECT obtained during the excretory phase demonstrates strands of extracalyceal contrast ➡ in the ablation zone ➡. This may be seen on serial CECT exams but is present only in the excretory phase. In the absence of downstream obstruction in the renal collecting system, this is a benign ancillary finding.*

Benign Postablation Ancillary Findings: Probe Tract Pseudoseeding After RFA

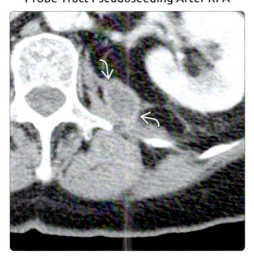

Complication after RFA: Perirenal Hematoma Formation

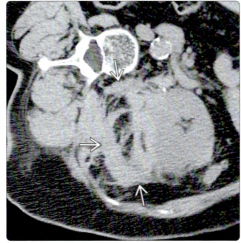

(Left) *CECT obtained 1 month after RFA shows a rim-enhancing density ➡ posterior to the kidney along the RFA probe tract. This abnormality involuted over serial CT studies. While true tumor seeding is exceedingly rare, enlarging or persistent suspicious soft tissue may prompt biopsy.* (Right) *NECT obtained immediately after RFA shows a posterior perirenal hematoma ➡. Mild perirenal hemorrhage can be expected after ablation. Rarely is blood loss significant enough to require or prolong hospital admission.*

AML Embolization: Initial CECT Imaging Evaluation

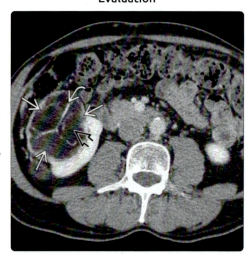

AML Embolization: Initial CECT Imaging Evaluation

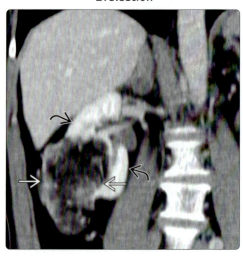

(Left) *Axial CECT shows a large right lower pole angiomyolipoma (AML)* ➡️. *The mass has a large fat component* ➡️ *but also contains numerous enhancing vascular structures* ➡️, *which is typical of AMLs.* (Right) *Coronal CECT shows the large right renal mass* ➡️ *and its relationship to the normal renal parenchyma* ➡️. *Size is a rough measure of the rupture potential of an AML, and tumors > 4 cm are often prophylactically embolized, especially if they are vascular.*

AML Embolization: Initial DSA Imaging Evaluation

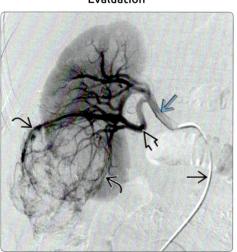

AML Embolization: Superselective DSA via Microcatheter

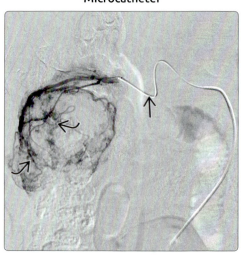

(Left) *Selective DSA via a Cobra catheter* ➡️ *placed in the right renal artery* ➡️ *shows there is a prominent vascular component to the AML and that the tumoral blood supply* ➡️ *arises from an enlarged lower pole arterial branch* ➡️. (Right) *Superselective DSA via a coaxial microcatheter* ➡️ *prior to embolization shows typical intratumoral vascularity* ➡️ *but no arterial aneurysms. The goal of AML embolization is tumor devascularization to limit or prevent growth &/or spontaneous rupture.*

AML Embolization: Renal DSA After Embolization

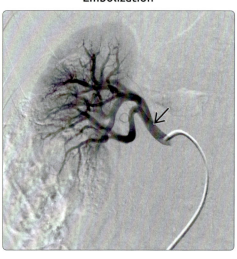

AML Embolization: Renal DSA After Embolization

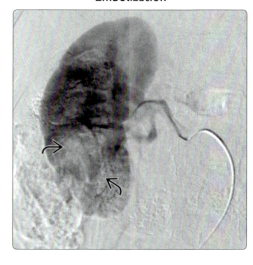

(Left) *After embolization with 300- to 500-μm particles via the microcatheter, a repeat renal* ➡️ *DSA was performed. The arterial phase shows that the AML has been successfully devascularized, as no tumor vascularity is seen. Absolute alcohol mixed with lipiodol has also been utilized for AML embolization.* (Right) *Delayed parenchymal-phase image from the selective renal DSA shows preservation of normal renal tissue with an area of slight hypoperfusion* ➡️ *corresponding to the treated AML.*

Massive AML Embolization: Initial Evaluation With CECT

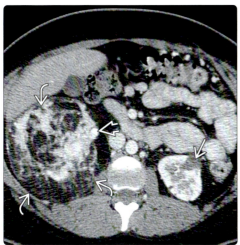

Massive AML Embolization: Initial Evaluation With CECT

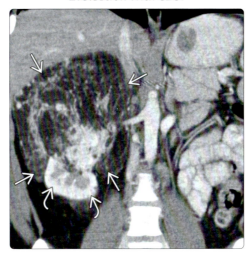

(Left) Axial CECT obtained in a patient with tuberous sclerosis shows an extremely large vascular AML ⇗. A much smaller 2nd AML ➡ is seen in the left kidney. The relationship of the main renal artery ⇒ to the mass is evident. (Right) Coronal CT reconstruction shows the massive size of the AML ➡ and the extent of residual normal renal parenchyma ⇗. It is important to preserve normal renal tissue during embolization, particularly given the number of AMLs.

Massive AML Embolization: Initial DSA Imaging Evaluation

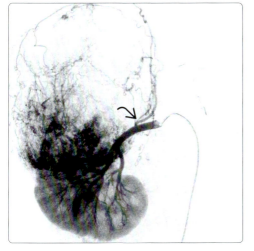

Massive AML Embolization: Initial DSA Imaging Evaluation

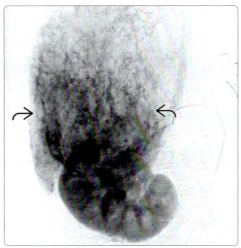

(Left) Arterial-phase renal DSA provides important information regarding the arterial supply and serves as a road map for embolization. The main supply to the AML is through middle and upper pole renal branches, but the AML is also supplied by hypertrophied capsular branches ⇗. (Right) Parenchymal phase from the DSA shows marked vascularity ⇒ of the AML. Although increased size is a predictor of the rupture potential of an AML, tumor composition is important as predominantly fatty tumors are unlikely to bleed.

Massive AML Embolization: Superselective DSA via Microcatheter

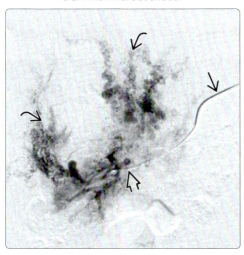

Massive AML Embolization: Renal DSA After Embolization

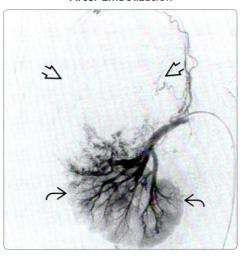

(Left) A microcatheter ⇒ was coaxially introduced through a Cobra catheter ➡ in the main right renal artery and has been positioned more selectively beyond the arterial supply to the residual kidney. DSA shows only tumor vascularity ⇒ at this catheter position. Particle embolization was performed, and additional branches supplying the tumor were also embolized. (Right) Right renal DSA following embolization shows marked tumor devascularization ⇒ and preservation of residual normal renal parenchyma ⇗.

Procedures

TERMINOLOGY

- Transplant renal disease processes
  - Transplant renal artery stenosis (TRAS): Luminal narrowing involving or near anastomosis
  - Inflow aortoiliac disease ("pseudo-TRAS")
  - Renal artery/vein thrombosis
  - Arteriovenous fistula/pseudoaneurysm
  - Graft intolerance syndrome: Flu-like syndrome due to renal transplant rejection
  - Urinary obstruction/leak
  - Perigraft fluid collection (e.g., hematoma, abscess)

PREPROCEDURE

- Review procedure indications; prior imaging
- Review operative history to determine anatomy of arterial/venous/ureteral anastomoses

PROCEDURE

- TRAS: PTA ± stent

- Aortoiliac inflow disease: Stent placement
- Arteriovenous fistula/pseudoaneurysm: Coil embolization
- Graft intolerance syndrome: Ethanol ablation
- Urinary obstruction: Percutaneous nephrostomy/stent; ureteral balloon dilatation
- Perigraft collection: Aspiration/drainage

POST PROCEDURE

- Clinical success
  - TRAS: 82%
  - Arteriovenous fistula/pseudoaneurysm: 57-88%
  - Ureteral balloon dilatation/stenting: 73-100%
  - Lymphocele drainage/sclerosis: 68-100%

(Left) *Graphic shows a renal allograft* ➡ *in the right iliac fossa in a retroperitoneal location with the ureter tunneled into the dome of the bladder. The renal artery* ➡ *and vein* ➡ *are anastomosed to the recipient external iliac vessels.* (Right) *Coronal noncontrast MRA shows normal arterial anatomy of a right renal allograft* ➡. *The donor renal artery* ➡ *is anastomosed to the recipient's right external iliac artery* ➡ *with no evidence of an anastomotic stenosis.*

Renal Transplantation: Normal Anatomy

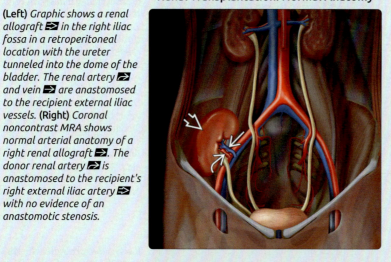

MRA: Normal Transplant Arterial Anatomy

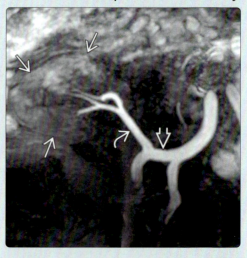

(Left) *Ureteroneocystostomy at the bladder dome* ➡ *is particularly well shown in this patient because of severe reflux. Complications at the ureteroneocystostomy include reflux (despite tunneling techniques), obstruction, and leaks. Assessment of collecting system dilatation after voiding helps to differentiate between reflux and true obstruction.* (Right) *Color Doppler screen shows normal renal vascular anatomy. Note the end-to-side renal artery* ➡ *to external iliac artery* ➡ *and the renal vein* ➡ *to external iliac vein* ➡ *anastomoses.*

Normal Transplant Anatomy: Ureter

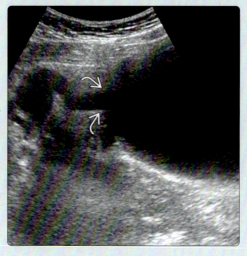

Renal Transplant Anatomy: Color Doppler Map

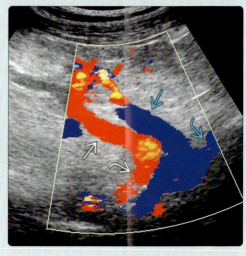

Transplant Kidney RAS: US Evaluation

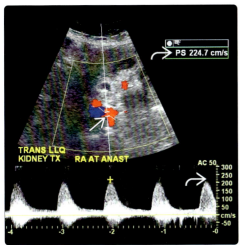

Transplant Kidney RAS: Initial MRA Evaluation

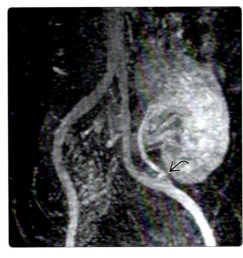

(Left) *Color Doppler US, with the gate* ➡ *at the anastomosis of the donor renal artery to the left external iliac artery, shows markedly elevated peak systolic velocities* ➡, *reflecting a high-grade renal artery stenosis. Common causes of stenoses include anastomotic strictures and vascular clamp injuries.* (Right) *Oblique MIP from an MRA shows an angulation* ➡ *of the donor renal artery near the anastomosis to the external iliac artery, which is the area of the suspected renal artery stenosis.*

Transplant Kidney RAS: Initial MRA Evaluation

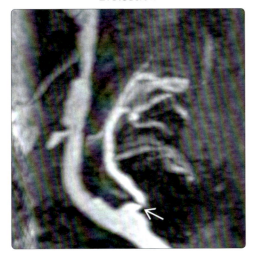

Transplant Kidney RAS: Diagnostic DSA Evaluation

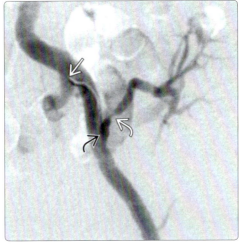

(Left) *Oblique gadolinium-enhanced MRA shows a stenosis* ➡ *of the proximal transplant renal artery in the area of acute angulation near the anastomosis. Based upon the imaging and clinical findings, further evaluation with DSA and potential transcatheter intervention was recommended.* (Right) *A catheter was introduced from a left common femoral approach, and the tip* ➡ *was placed in the external iliac artery proximal to the renal artery anastomosis* ➡. *The DSA confirms a focal severe renal artery stenosis* ➡.

Transplant Kidney RAS: Intravascular Stent Placement

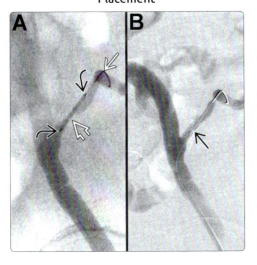

Transplant Kidney RAS: Posttreatment DSA

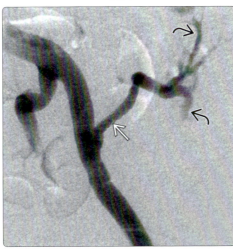

(Left) *Fluoroscopic spot radiographs during stent placement show (A) a balloon-mounted stent* ➡ *advanced over a guidewire* ➡ *that bridges the stenosis* ➡. *(B) After expanding the stent* ➡, *the stenosis has been eliminated.* (Right) *DSA performed after removal of the stent delivery system and guidewire shows an appropriately positioned stent* ➡ *and no residual stenosis. Intrarenal branches* ➡ *fill appropriately, and subsequent images showed no dissection or distal emboli.*

Transplant Recipient Arterial Disease: Evaluation With CT Imaging

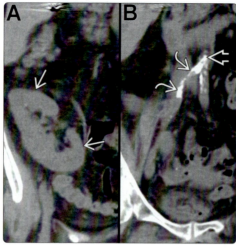

Transplant Recipient Arterial Disease: Evaluation With CO₂ DSA Imaging

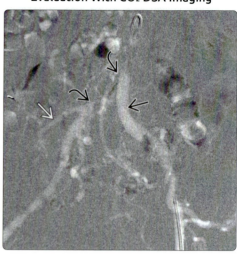

(Left) *Coronal NECT in a failing renal transplant (A) shows a transplant kidney* ➡ *in the right iliac fossa, which was anastomosed end to side to the common iliac artery. (B) Extensive calcified plaque in the right common iliac artery* ➡ *extends into the distal abdominal aorta* ➡. *(Right) DSA from a left femoral access was performed using CO_2 contrast, given the patient's poor renal function. This shows a patent left common iliac artery* ➡ *and an absent (occluded) right common iliac artery* ➡. *The transplant renal artery* ➡ *is patent.*

Transplant Recipient Arterial Disease: Stenting of Iliac Artery Occlusion

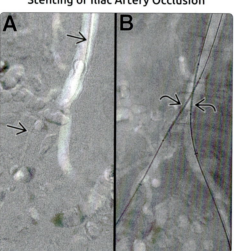

Transplant Recipient Arterial Disease: Postintervention DSA Imaging

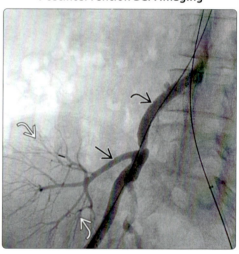

(Left) *(A) The right femoral artery was accessed, and a guidewire and catheter* ➡ *were used to traverse the occluded right common iliac artery. (B) Balloon-mounted stents* ➡ *were introduced bilaterally and were positioned in the common iliac arteries, extending slightly into the distal aorta. They were simultaneously deployed using a "kissing" stent technique.* **(Right)** *DSA after "kissing" stents shows that the right common iliac artery* ➡ *is widely patent. The transplant renal artery* ➡ *and intrarenal branches* ➡ *now fill normally.*

Transcatheter Transplant Ablation: Diagnostic DSA Evaluation

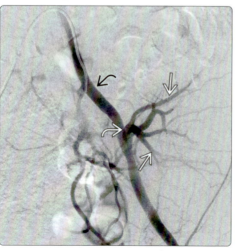

Transcatheter Transplant Ablation: Embolization With Absolute Alcohol

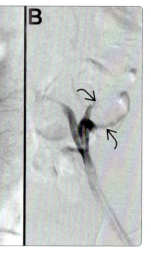

(Left) *DSA in a case of acute transplant rejection and severe hematuria shows a catheter in the left external iliac artery* ➡. *The transplant renal artery* ➡ *and intrarenal branches* ➡ *are patent, and no mass is seen.* **(Right)** *Transcatheter transplant ablation was performed before nephrectomy to control bleeding. (A) After placing a balloon occlusion catheter* ➡ *in the renal artery, contrast was injected, noting the volume used. (B) DSA after injecting a similar volume of alcohol shows nonfilling* ➡ *of branch vessels, ablation.*

Acquired Arteriovenous Fistula: Nonfocal Renal Biopsy

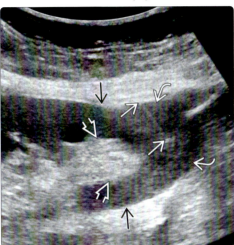

Acquired Arteriovenous Fistula: MRA Evaluation

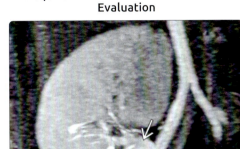

(Left) *Sagittal US obtained during biopsy of a right lower quadrant transplant ⊡ shows the needle of a biopsy device ⊟ within the lower pole renal cortex ⊡. Note the needle trajectory is oriented away from the hilum ⊟ and is parallel to the cortex.* (Right) *Arterial-phase MRA shows premature filling of the renal vein ⊟ due to an arteriovenous fistula. Both pseudoaneurysms and arteriovenous fistulas can occur as a result of a renal biopsy that lacerates branches of the artery and vein within the transplant kidney.*

Perigraft Abscess Drainage: Associated Hydronephrosis on CECT

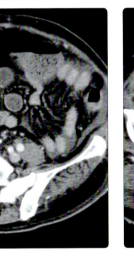

Perigraft Abscess Drainage: Drainage Catheter in Abscess

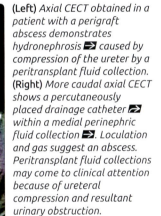

(Left) *Axial CECT obtained in a patient with a perigraft abscess demonstrates hydronephrosis ⊟ caused by compression of the ureter by a peritransplant fluid collection.* (Right) *More caudal axial CECT shows a percutaneously placed drainage catheter ⊟ within a medial perinephric fluid collection ⊡. Loculation and gas suggest an abscess. Peritransplant fluid collections may come to clinical attention because of ureteral compression and resultant urinary obstruction.*

Ureteral Stricture Causing Obstruction: Ureteral Balloon Dilatation

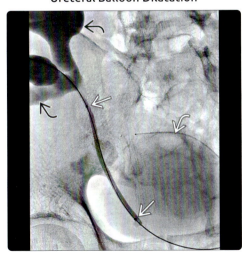

Ureteral Stricture Causing Obstruction: Antegrade Ureteral Stent Placement

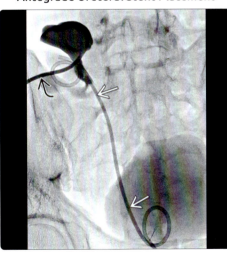

(Left) *Fluoroscopic spot radiograph obtained after percutaneous access to the transplant renal collecting system and contrast injection shows marked hydronephrosis ⊡ due to a long ureteral stricture. A balloon ⊟ was introduced over a guidewire ⊟ and was inflated to dilate the stricture. Ureteral ischemia is the main cause of these strictures.* (Right) *Following balloon dilatation, a double pigtail ureteral stent ⊟ was introduced and was placed across the stricture. Note the safety nephrostomy catheter ⊡.*

(Left) *Axial NECT of the left hemipelvis demonstrates an obstructing calculus ➡ in the proximal ureter of a renal transplant ➡. Dilatation of the renal pelvis ➡ is evident, indicating hydronephrosis. Ureteral stenosis/ischemia is a more common cause of obstruction than calculus.* (Right) *Sagittal US prior to nephrostomy shows marked hydronephrosis ➡ in the transplant kidney. After selecting a lateral calyx for access, local anesthetic is administered using 1% lidocaine, and a dermatotomy is made with a #11 scalpel.*

Renal Transplant Urinary Obstruction: Initial NECT Imaging Evaluation

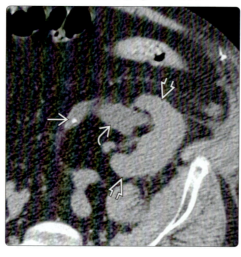

Renal Transplant Urinary Obstruction: Initial US Evaluation

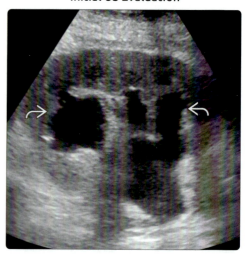

(Left) *US obtained during primary access for percutaneous nephrostomy catheter placement demonstrates a 21-gauge Chiba needle ➡ with the tip ➡ within a lateral calyx ➡ of the transplant kidney.* (Right) *Fluoroscopic spot radiography obtained during nephrostomy after contrast injection through the Chiba needle ➡ confirms that the tip is in a lateral calyx ➡. Nephrostomy catheter placement will now proceed using the 1-stick technique. The injected contrast volume is limited to reduce sepsis risk.*

Renal Transplant Urinary Obstruction: US Guidance During Nephrostomy

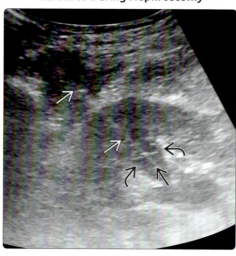

Renal Transplant Urinary Obstruction: Fluoroscopy During Nephrostomy

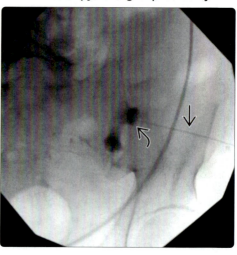

(Left) *A 0.018" guidewire ➡ is advanced through the needle using fluoroscopic guidance. The needle is exchanged for a 6-Fr coaxial dilator-sheath assembly ➡, and the sheath is advanced over the guidewire into the renal pelvis ➡. The dilator is removed, the microwire exchanged for a 0.035" guidewire, and the tract dilated to 8 Fr.* (Right) *Over the 0.035" guidewire, an 8-Fr pigtail nephrostomy catheter ➡ is advanced into the collecting system. Contrast injection confirms the location within the renal pelvis ➡.*

Renal Transplant Urinary Obstruction: 1-Stick Access Technique

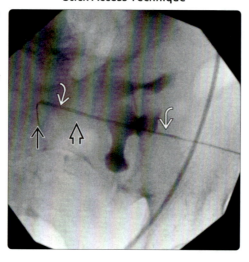

Renal Transplant Urinary Obstruction: Completion Nephrostogram

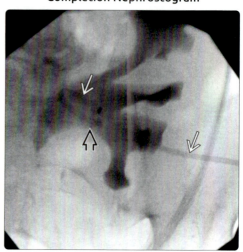

Paratransplant Lymphocele: Initial MR Evaluation

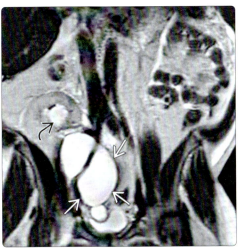

Paratransplant Lymphocele: US-Guided Drainage

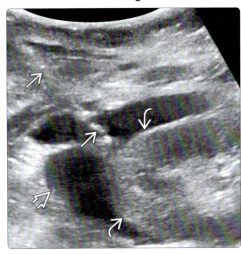

(Left) *Coronal T2WI MR shows transplant hydronephrosis ➔, caused by extrinsic ureteral compression by a surrounding lymphocele ➔. The lymphocele has a typical appearance with multiple septations.* (Right) *US shows an anechoic perinephric collection ➔. An 8-Fr locking pigtail catheter loaded on a trocar ➔ has been advanced into the collection ➔. Once the tip of the assembly is in the collection, the hub is unscrewed, the inner trocar is held still, and the catheter is advanced further into the collection.*

Paratransplant Lymphocele: Persistence After Drainage

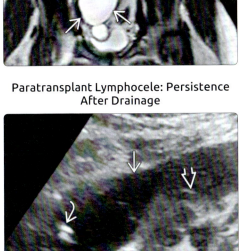

Paratransplant Lymphocele: Postdrainage US

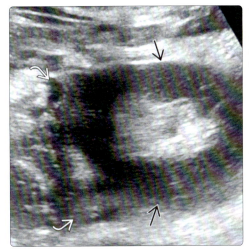

(Left) *Drainage persisted 1 week post catheter placement. US shows the pigtail loop ➔ within the persistent collection ➔ adjacent to the kidney ➔. Lymphoceles are frequently refractory to simple drainage, and sclerotherapy may ultimately be necessary.* (Right) *Postprocedural US shows significant decompression of the collection that previously surrounded the inferior aspect of the kidney ➔. Only a minimal residual collection ➔ remains. A drainage catheter was left indwelling.*

Paratransplant Lymphocele: Lymphocele Sclerotherapy

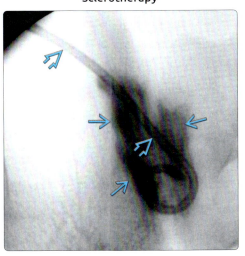

Paratransplant Lymphocele: Lymphocele Sclerotherapy

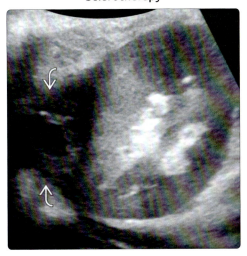

(Left) *In preparation for lymphocele sclerosis, contrast was injected via the drainage catheter ➔ showing a persistent cavity ➔ but no fistula to the collecting system. Sclerotherapy was subsequently performed using a fibrin sealant. 15 mL of sealant were injected into the lymphocele through the catheter.* (Right) *US performed 1 week post sclerotherapy shows interval collapse of the collection ➔. The patient was pain free, there was no reaccumulation of lymphatic fluid, and the hydronephrosis resolved.*

KEY FACTS

PREPROCEDURE

- Indications
  - Adrenal venous sampling
    - Differentiating etiology of primary aldosteronism
    - Used to confirm adrenal gland as source of excess cortisol in patient with Cushing syndrome and adrenal mass on imaging
    - Adrenal venous sampling for pheochromocytomas and paragangliomas
  - Renal vein sampling
    - Determining if renal artery stenosis is etiology of hypertension (renovascular hypertension)
  - Renal venography for diagnosis &/or treatment
    - "Nutcracker" syndrome
      - Pressure gradient > 2 mm Hg between renal vein and inferior vena cava confirms diagnosis
    - Pelvic congestion syndrome
    - Varicocele

PROCEDURE

- Adrenal vein sampling
  - Selective catheterization of each adrenal vein
  - Right adrenal vein more difficult to catheterize than left; should be catheterized/sampled 1st
  - Obtain samples from each adrenal vein before and after adrenocorticotrophic hormone (ACTH) administration
  - High aldosterone:cortisol ratio before and after ACTH, lateralizing to one side is confirmatory of adrenal adenoma
  - Elevated cortisol lateralizing to adrenal vein in presence of adrenal mass on CT/MR is confirmatory of endogenous Cushing syndrome
- Renal venography and renin sampling
  - Discontinue antihypertensive β blockers and ACE inhibitors several days prior to sampling
  - Captopril stimulation (1 mg/kg body weight) 60-90 minutes before sampling increases accuracy

Anatomy of Adrenal Veins

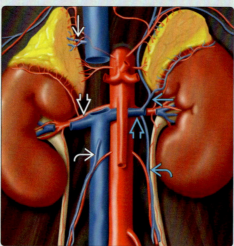

Adrenal Mass

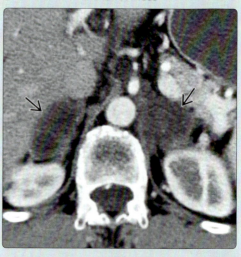

(Left) *Graphic shows that the right adrenal ➡, renal ➡, and gonadal ➡ veins drain directly into the inferior vena cava (IVC); the left adrenal ➡ and gonadal ➡ veins drain into the left renal vein ➡, which courses anterior to the aorta.* (Right) *Axial CECT shows bilateral adrenal masses ➡ in a patient with hypokalemia and diastolic hypertension, suspected of primary aldosteronism. Bilateral adrenal vein sampling was performed for further evaluation.*

Adrenal Vein Sampling

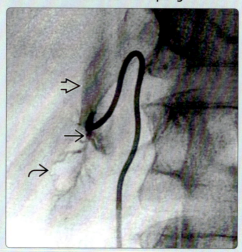

Adrenal Vein Sampling

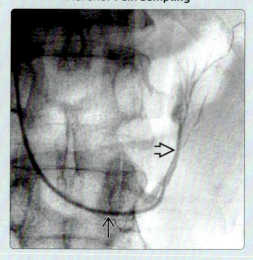

(Left) *Right adrenal venogram shows a short main adrenal vein trunk ➡ draining to the IVC ➡. Note filling of branches within the adrenal gland ➡.* (Right) *Left adrenal venogram shows the catheter ➡ entering the left renal vein, through which a microcatheter ➡ has been coaxially introduced and positioned in the left adrenal vein. After confirming a correct catheter position with gentle contrast injection, venous sampling is performed following cortisol stimulation.*

Adrenal Vein Sampling

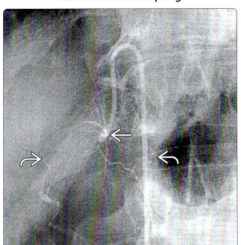

Adrenal Vein Sampling

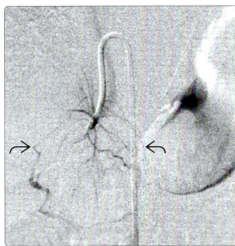

(Left) *Frontal projection from right adrenal venography shows selective injection of the main trunk of the right adrenal vein* ➡ *with a Simmons 1 catheter. The glandular veins* ➡ *are draped around a mass, which was seen on cross-sectional imaging in this patient with Cushing disease. Sampling confirmed this was the source of excess cortisol.* (Right) *Digital subtraction angiography better depicts draping of adrenal veins* ➡ *around the adrenal mass.*

Normal Left Renal Venogram

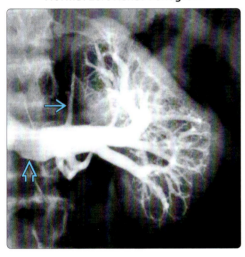

Retroaortic Left Renal Venogram

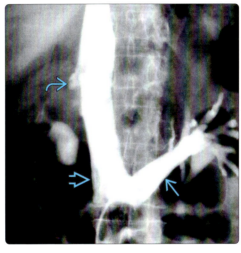

(Left) *Normal left renal venogram shows multiple intrarenal branches draining into the main left renal vein* ➡*. The left adrenal vein* ➡ *drains directly into the left renal vein.* (Right) *Venogram shows a nonconventional course of the left renal vein* ➡ *as it joins the IVC* ➡*. This appearance is typical of a retroaortic left renal vein, which is a well-known anatomic variant. A small portion of the right renal vein* ➡ *is seen entering the IVC at the expected location.*

Circumaortic Left Renal Vein CTV

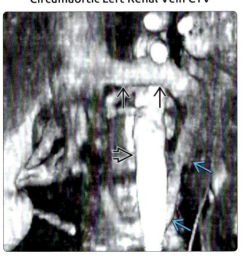

Nutcracker Syndrome

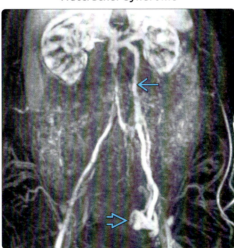

(Left) *3D CTA/CTV of a circumaortic left renal vein shows a normal course of the superior renal vein* ➡ *anterior to the aorta* ➡*, while the inferior vein* ➡ *has a retroaortic course. This anatomy has implications for IVC filter placement.* (Right) *Coronal MRV of suspected "nutcracker" syndrome shows a dilated left gonadal vein* ➡ *and pelvic varicosities* ➡*. Compression of the left renal vein between the aorta and superior mesenteric artery causes renal venous hypertension and gonadal vein reflux.*

Fertility and Sterility Interventions

TERMINOLOGY

- **Hysterosalpingography**: Contrast injection into endometrial cavity with fluoroscopy/imaging
- **Selective salpingography**: Direct selective catheterization of fallopian tubal ostium
  - Contrast injection via catheter during imaging
- **Fallopian tube recanalization**: Guidewire/catheter passage through occluded FT to reestablish patency
- **Fallopian tube occlusion**: Placement of mechanical occluding device into fallopian tubes

PREPROCEDURE

- Selective salpingography indications
  - Differentiate spasm from true obstruction
  - Inadequate fallopian tube opacification by HSG
- Fallopian tube recanalization indications
  - Tubal occlusion despite selective salpingography
- Fallopian tube occlusion indications
  - Prophylaxis against unwanted pregnancy

PROCEDURE

- **Selective salpingography**
  - Advance 4-5-French catheter over 0.035" guidewire; wedge tip in uterine cornual region
  - Gently inject contrast medium; obtain images
- **Fallopian tube recanalization**
  - Advance catheter/guidewire through obstruction
- **Fallopian tube occlusion**
  - Place device in most challenging side 1st
  - Engage 5-French catheter working port in tubal ostium
  - Advance device until 3rd radiopaque marker at tubal ostium; deploy Essure coil

POST PROCEDURE

- Fallopian tube recanalization
  - Procedural success: 71-92%
- Fallopian tube occlusion
  - Efficacy rate of Essure preventing pregnancy: 99.8%

Fallopian Tube Anatomy

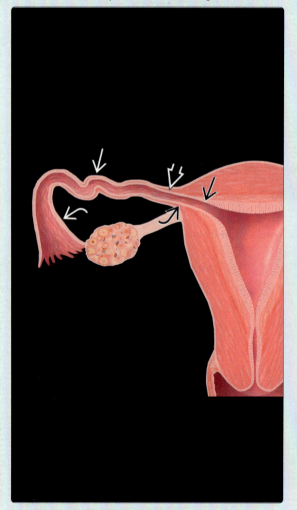

Graphic shows a normal fallopian tube. From the ostium ➡, the interstitial segment ➡ transitions to the isthmic segment at the uterotubal junction ➡. The remaining segments are termed ampullary ➡ and infundibular ➡.

Normal Hysterosalpingogram

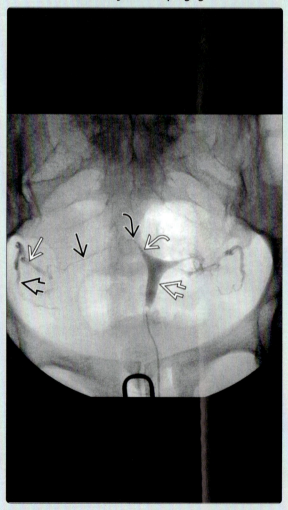

Hysterosalpingogram shows a normal endometrial cavity ➡, the tubal ostium ➡, uterotubal junction ➡, and the isthmic ➡, ampullary ➡, and infundibular ➡ segments. Both fallopian tubes are widely patent.

TERMINOLOGY

Definitions

- **Hysterosalpingography (HSG)**: Contrast injection via cervical canal into endometrial cavity with fluoroscopic monitoring/imaging
  - Normally shows filling of uterine cavity
  - Should also show bilateral fallopian tube (FT) filling
    - Tubal patency confirmed if contrast spills from tubes into abdominal cavity
  - Sensitivity and specificity in detecting pathology
    - Bilateral tubal pathology: 46% and 95%
    - Any fallopian tube pathology: 53% and 87%
- **Selective salpingography**: Direct selective catheterization of fallopian tubal ostium
  - Contrast injection via catheter during imaging
    - Provides direct opacification of fallopian tube
- **Fallopian tubal anatomy**
  - 4 tubal segments
    - Interstitial (intramural)
    - Isthmic
    - Ampullary
    - Infundibular
  - Uterotubal junction located at transition of intramural to isthmic segment of fallopian tube
    - Narrowest portion of fallopian tube
  - Average tubal diameter: 0.8-2.0 mm
    - Increases as fallopian tube courses toward ovaries
  - Average tubal length: 11 cm (range: 7-16 cm)
- **Fallopian tube recanalization (FTR)**: Guidewire &/or catheter passage through occluded fallopian tube to reestablish tubal patency
  - Fallopian tube disease accounts for up to 35% of infertility cases; various causes
    - Infection (chlamydia)
    - Postsurgical
    - Salpingitis isthmica nodosa
      - Inflammation of isthmic segment; characterized by nodular thickening causing obstruction
    - Peritubal adhesions
  - Proximal tubal occlusion often caused by mucus plug/inflammatory debris; also caused by spasm
    - Involves interstitial segment/uterotubal junction
    - Responds fairly well to recanalization
  - Less favorable outcomes with more distal occlusions
    - More often due to scarring/fibrosis
- **Fallopian tube occlusion (FTO)**: Placement of mechanical occluding device into fallopian tubes
  - Type of bilateral tubal sterilization
    - Hysteroscopic transcervical fallopian tube access
    - Placement of Essure device (Conceptus; Mountain View, CA) into fallopian tubes
      - Combined outer nitinol/inner stainless steel coil elicits tissue growth; occludes fallopian tubes
      - During first 3 months device not fully effective
      - Alternate birth control needed during this time

PREPROCEDURE

Indications

- **Selective salpingography**
  - Differentiate spasm from true tubal obstruction
  - Inadequate fallopian tube opacification by HSG
- **Fallopian tube recanalization**
  - Persistent tubal occlusion after selective salpingography
- **Fallopian tube occlusion**
  - Prophylaxis against unwanted pregnancy
  - Medical conditions aggravated by pregnancy

Contraindications

- **Selective salpingography**
  - Active infection
- **Fallopian tube recanalization**
  - Active infection
- **Fallopian tube occlusion**
  - Desire to maintain fertility
  - Pregnancy; recent or current infection
  - Essure device-related contraindications
    - Prior tubal ligation
    - Pregnancy termination/child delivery < 6 weeks before intended placement
    - Immunosuppression
    - Menorrhagia/metrorrhagia of unknown etiology
    - Allergy to nickel

Getting Started

- Things to check
  - Detailed clinical and physical evaluation
  - Allergies
  - Negative qualitative urinary β-hCG (day of procedure)
  - Selective salpingography: Review images/anatomy
  - Fallopian tube recanalization: Document fallopian tubal occlusion
  - Fallopian tube occlusion: Correct procedure timing
    - Perform in follicular phase (day 7-14) of menses
- Medications
  - Preprocedural ketorolac (30 mg)
  - Antibiotic prophylaxis
  - Intraprocedural conscious sedation
  - Paracervical block anesthesia
- Equipment list
  - Speculum
  - Transcervical access catheter/device for hysterosalpingography (various options)
    - Thurmond-Rösch Hysterocath (Cook Medical; Bloomington, IN)
    - 9-French sheath in endometrial cavity
    - 12-French transcervical catheter with balloon
  - Essure device
    - 4.3-French outer diameter delivery system
    - Placed via 5-French catheter working port
  - Catheters for selective FT catheterization
    - 4-French angled-tip catheter
    - 5-French Kumpe catheter
  - Catheter for fallopian tube recanalization
    - Thurmond-Rösch fallopian tube catheterization set (Cook Medical; Bloomington, IN)

PROCEDURE

Patient Position/Location
- Patient in lithotomy position

Equipment Preparation
- Dilute contrast medium to 30%

Procedure Steps
- **Cervical cannulation**
  - Sterilely prepare/drape vulvar and perineal area
  - Introduce speculum; visualize cervix
  - Place 9-12-French occlusive catheter and fix it with tenaculum, external cervical suction, or endocervical/uterine balloon
  - Place 5-French diagnostic catheter: Inject contrast to opacify uterine cavity
- **Selective salpingography**
  - Advance 4-5-French catheter over 0.035" guidewire
  - Gently inject contrast medium
  - Perform contralateral fallopian tube catheterization
- **Fallopian tube recanalization**
  - 3-French tapered catheter preloaded over 0.014-0.018" guidewire
  - Advance catheter/guidewire through obstruction
  - Persistent obstruction
    - Cross with 0.014-0.018" diameter floppy-tip/0.035" hydrophilic guidewire
    - Use firm traction on cervix to straighten uterus
- **Fallopian tube occlusion**
  - Obtain HSG images of both fallopian tubes
  - Place device in most challenging side 1st; should abort procedure if bilateral placement not possible
  - Engage 5 French working port in tubal ostium
  - Advance device through working port into fallopian tube until 3rd radiopaque marker at tubal ostium
  - Deploy Essure coil
  - Perform contralateral device placement

Findings and Reporting
- **Selective salpingography**
  - Selective tubal catheterization: Technically successful in up to 90% of cases
  - Opacification of normal tube in 20-30% of cases with peritoneal passage of contrast
- **Fallopian tube recanalization**
  - Improved tubal diagnosis in 90% of cases
  - Restoration of tubal patency in 40% of cases
- **Fallopian tube occlusion**
  - HSG criteria for grading coil placement and tubal occlusion (3 months follow-up after FTO)
    - Grade I
      - □ Expulsion of coil or > 50% of coil inner length trails into uterine cavity
      - □ Tubal occlusion at cornua
    - Grade II
      - □ < 50% of inner coil length trails into uterine cavity or proximal end of inner coil is < 30 mm into tube from tubal ostium
      - □ Contrast in tube, not past any portion of coil
    - Grade III
      - □ Coil inner length proximal end > 30 mm distal to tubal ostium or coil within peritoneal cavity
      - □ Contrast tracks past coil or into peritoneal cavity
    - Coil placement must be grade II and tubal occlusion must be grade I or II for sterility

POST PROCEDURE

Expected Outcome
- Fallopian tube recanalization
  - Procedural success: 71-92%
  - Pregnancy typically occurs within 6 months of FTR
- Fallopian tube occlusion
  - Efficacy rate of Essure preventing pregnancy: 99.8%
  - Vaginal spotting, pelvic cramping expected afterward

Post Procedure Imaging
- Fallopian tube recanalization
  - Repeat HSG in patients who fail to achieve pregnancy
- Fallopian tube occlusion
  - Follow-up in 3 months with hysterosalpingogram

OUTCOMES

Complications
- Immediate/periprocedural complication(s)
  - Tubal perforation: 2% of cases
    - Often actually submucosal guidewire passage
  - Contrast intravasation
    - Can occur if catheter poorly positioned
  - Infection (extremely rare)
    - Peritonitis: Incidence < 1%
    - Pyosalpinx, endometritis
- Delayed complication(s)
  - Extrauterine (ectopic) pregnancy
    - Tubal pregnancies reported in up to 3% of women after FTR
    - Higher risk after FTR but less than after microsurgical tubal intervention
- Other complications
  - Radiation exposure
    - Ovarian exposure ~ 1 rad (10 mGy)
    - Perform procedures in follicular phase of ovulatory cycle to ensure patient not pregnant

SELECTED REFERENCES

1. Allahbadia GN et al: Fallopian tube recanalization: lessons learnt and future challenges. Womens Health (Lond Engl). 6(4):531-48, quiz 548-9, 2010
2. McSwain H et al: Fallopian tube occlusion, an alternative to tubal ligation. Tech Vasc Interv Radiol. 9(1):24-9, 2006
3. Maubon AJ et al: Interventional radiology in female infertility: technique and role. Eur Radiol. 11(5):771-8, 2001
4. Thurmond AS et al: A review of selective salpingography and fallopian tube catheterization. Radiographics. 20(6):1759-68, 2000
5. Thurmond AS et al: Tubal obstruction after ligation reversal surgery: results of catheter recanalization. Radiology. 210(3):747-50, 1999
6. Lang EK: The efficacy of transcervical recanalization of obstructed postoperative fallopian tubes. Eur Radiol. 8(3):461-5, 1998
7. Lang EK et al: Recanalization of obstructed fallopian tube by selective salpingography and transvaginal bougie dilatation: outcome and cost analysis. Fertil Steril. 66(2):210-5, 1996
8. Thompson KA et al: Transcervical fallopian tube catheterization and recanalization for proximal tubal obstruction. Fertil Steril. 61(2):243-7, 1994
9. Thurmond AS: Selective salpingography and fallopian tube recanalization. AJR Am J Roentgenol. 156(1):33-8, 1991

Fallopian Tube Recanalization (Tubal Occlusion From Salpingitis)

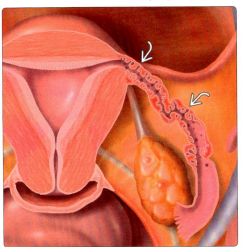

Fallopian Tube Recanalization (Initial Hysterosalpingogram)

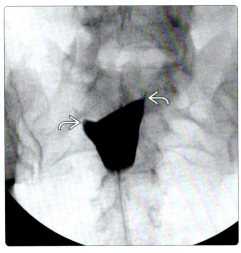

(Left) *Fallopian tube disease accounts for up to 35% of infertility cases with various causes for tubal occlusion. This graphic shows a diseased left fallopian tube* ⇗ *due to salpingitis, which is often due to chlamydia.* (Right) *Initial evaluation is via hysterosalpingography (HSG). After accessing the cervix and endometrial canal, contrast medium is injected and images are obtained. In this case, there is bilateral fallopian tube occlusion at the ostia* ⇗.

Fallopian Tube Recanalization (Selective Right Salpingography)

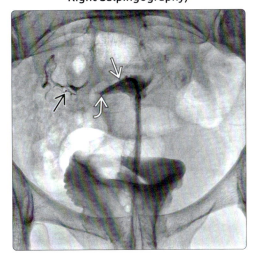

Fallopian Tube Recanalization (Selective Left Salpingography)

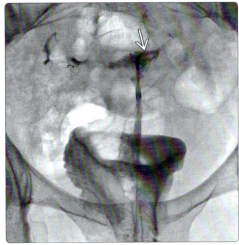

(Left) *The tip* ⇗ *of an angled catheter* ⇥ *has been placed at the right tubal ostium and selective salpingography performed showing a patent fallopian tube* ⇥. *It is not uncommon that proximal occlusion, as seen on a prior HSG, is no longer present (reported in up to 40% of patients).* (Right) *The angled catheter* ⇥ *has been placed in the left cornu where contrast injection fails to fill the fallopian tube, indicating tubal occlusion.*

Fallopian Tube Recanalization (Guidewire Passage on Left)

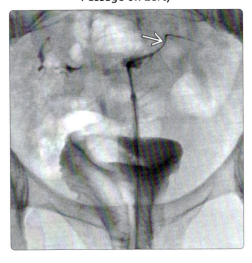

Fallopian Tube Recanalization (Final Hysterosalpingography)

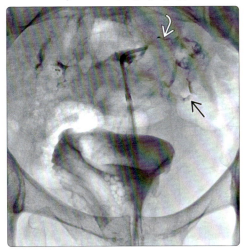

(Left) *After cannulating the fallopian tube orifice, a 0.018" guidewire* ⇥ *has been advanced into the interstitial tubal segment in an attempt to dislodge any occluding debris. More distal occlusions are far less responsive to recanalization.* (Right) *Left salpingogram after guidewire passage shows the fallopian tube* ⇗ *is patent, with free contrast spillage* ⇥ *into the peritoneal cavity. There is a high technical success rate for recanalization, but conception rates are unfortunately much lower and are generally reported at around 30%.*

Fallopian Tube Occlusion (Cannulation of Tubal Ostium)

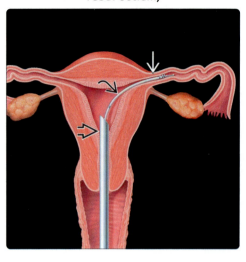

Fallopian Tube Occlusion (Essure Device Placement)

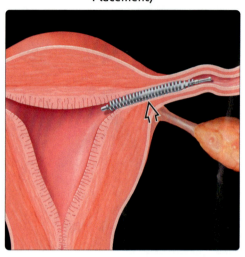

(Left) Graphic shows a transcervical cannula ⊟ in place through which the 4.3-French diameter delivery system ⊟ for the Essure device has been introduced. The left fallopian tube ostium has been selectively cannulated, and the device has been advanced so that it will span the uterotubal junction ⊟ once it is deployed. (Right) Graphic shows the deployed Essure device ⊟ in place. The combined outer nitinol and inner stainless steel coils elicit tissue ingrowth, which will occlude the fallopian tubes over a period of 3 months.

Fallopian Tube Occlusion (Successful Tubal Occlusion)

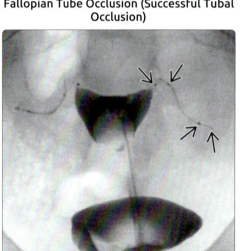

Fallopian Tube Occlusion (Successful Tubal Occlusion)

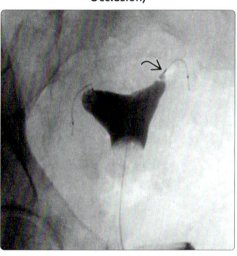

(Left) Partial fill view of the uterine cavity from a hysterosalpingogram obtained 3 months after bilateral Essure placement shows both devices are in satisfactory position. Each device has a series of 4 radiopaque markers ⊟ for determining proper positioning. (Right) Magnified oblique view of the left uterine cornu shows the 3rd radiopaque marker ⊟ of the device at the tubal ostium, the desired position. The device stimulates tissue ingrowth, causing permanent tubal occlusion.

Fallopian Tube Occlusion (Incomplete Tubal Occlusion)

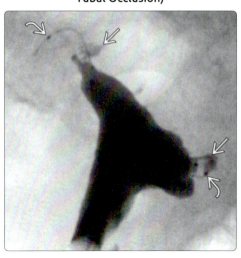

Fallopian Tube Occlusion (Malpositioned Essure Device)

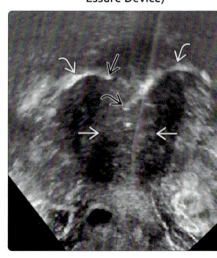

(Left) Hysterosalpingogram 3 months after bilateral Essure placement shows both devices ⊟ in place but contrast ⊟ tracking proximally along each into the tubes. This indicates incomplete tubal occlusion, as contrast should not extend beyond any portion of the coil. (Right) Transvaginal uterine ultrasound shows the endometrial cavity ⊟ and bilateral Essure devices ⊟. The tip ⊟ of the right device is in good position, extending slightly into the cornu. The left device is malpositioned, with the tip ⊟ extending into the uterine cavity.

Fallopian Tube Occlusion (Malpositioned Essure Device)

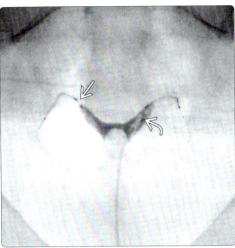

Fallopian Tube Occlusion (Malpositioned Essure Device)

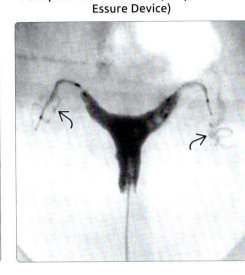

(Left) *Minimal fill view from a hysterosalpingogram 3 months after fallopian tube occlusion procedure shows that the left Essure device tip ➋ extends into the uterine cavity, while the right device is optimally positioned ➡. Less than 50% of the inner coil length should trail into the uterine cavity.* **(Right)** *Total fill view of the uterine cavity in the same patient shows that in addition to a malpositioned left Essure device, contrast fills both fallopian tubes ➘, indicating tubal patency despite the procedure 3 months earlier.*

Fallopian Tube Occlusion (Patent Tubes Despite Essure)

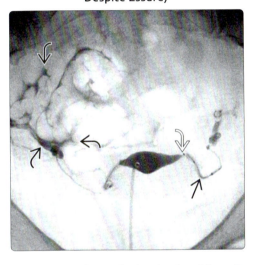

Fallopian Tube Occlusion (Absent Left Essure Device)

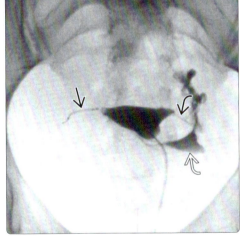

(Left) *Spot radiograph shows a left Essure device ➘ positioned distally in the fallopian tube, with proximal marker ➋ beyond the cornu. Contrast opacifies the fallopian tubes and spills into the peritoneal cavity ➘, indicating tubal patency.* **(Right)** *Spot radiograph shows a right Essure device ➘ in good position, with no fallopian tube filling. There is no device identified on the left, the tube ➘ is patent with free peritoneal spillage ➋. The left device was likely malpositioned and expelled.*

Fallopian Tube Occlusion (Malpositioned Left Essure Device)

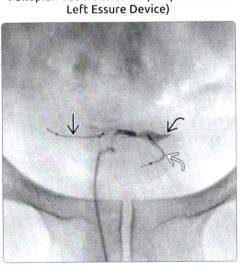

Fallopian Tube Occlusion (Malpositioned Left Essure Device)

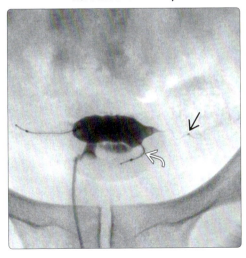

(Left) *Minimal fill view from a hysterosalpingogram 3 months after Essure placement shows the left device ➋ extending through the uterine wall, not into the fallopian tube (contrast opacifies the cornu ➘). The right device ➘ is well positioned.* **(Right)** *Total fill hysterosalpingogram view shows a patent left fallopian tube ➘. During the fallopian tube occlusion procedure, the left Essure device ➋ was advanced into a portion of the endometrial cavity mistaken for the uterine cornu.*

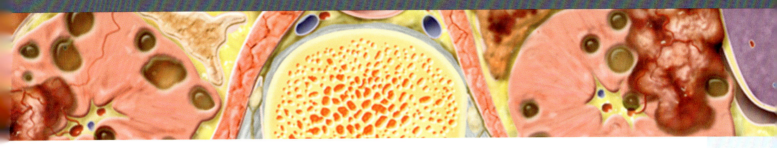

INDEX

INDEX

INDEX

INDEX

INDEX

INDEX

INDEX

INDEX

INDEX

INDEX

INDEX

INDEX

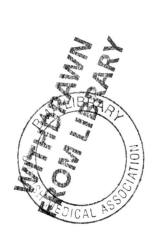